Clinical and Professional Reasoning in Occupational Therapy

Clinical and Professional Reasoning in Occupational Therapy

BARBARA A. BOYT SCHELL, PHD, OTR/L, FAOTA
Professor
Department of Occupational Therapy
Brenau University
Gainesville, Georgia

JOHN W. SCHELL, PHD
Associate Professor
Workforce Education, Leadership, & Social Foundations
University of Georgia
Athens, Georgia

Wolters Kluwer | Lippincott Williams & Wilkins
Health
Philadelphia • Baltimore • New York • London
Buenos Aires • Hong Kong • Sydney • Tokyo

Acquisitions Editor: Emily Lupash
Managing Editor: Andrea M. Klingler
Associate Marketing Manager: Allison Noplock
Production Editor: Beth Martz
Design Coordinator: Stephen Druding
Compositor: International Typesetting and Composition (ITC)

"Introduction", "A Passion for Reasoning", from Decarte's Error by Antonio R. Demasio, MD, copyright 1994 by Antonio R. Demasio, MD. Used by permission of G.P. Putnam's Sons, a division of Penguin Group (USA) Inc.

351 West Camden Street
Baltimore, Maryland 21201-2436 USA

530 Walnut Street
Philadelphia, Pennsylvania 19106-3621 USA

The publisher is not responsible (as a matter of product liability, negligence, or otherwise) for any injury resulting from any material contained herein. This publication contains information relating to general principles of medical care, which should not be construed as specific instructions for individual patients. Manufacturers' product information and package inserts should be reviewed for current information, including contraindications, dosages, and precautions.

Printed in the United States of America

Library of Congress Cataloging-in-Publication Data

Clinical and professional reasoning in occupational therapy / [edited by] Barbara A. Boyt Schell, John Schell.
   p. ; cm.
  Includes bibliographical references and index.
  ISBN-13: 978-0-7817-5914-4
  ISBN-10: 0-7817-5914-5
  1. Occupational therapy—Decision making. 2. Medical logic. I. Schell, Barbara A. Boyt. II. Schell, John W. (John William), 1947-
  [DNLM: 1. Occupational Therapy—methods. 2. Decision Making. WB 555 C6405 2008]
  RM735.C595 2008
  615.8'515—dc22

          2007011691

The publishers have made every effort to trace the copyright holders for borrowed material. If they have inadvertently overlooked any, they will be pleased to make the necessary arrangements at the first opportunity.

To purchase additional copies of this book call our customer service department at (800) 638-3030 or fax orders to (301) 223-2320. International customers should call (301) 223-2300.

Visit Lippincott Williams & Wilkins on the Internet: http://www.lww.com. Lippincott Williams & Wilkins customer service representatives are available from 8:30 am to 6:00 pm, EST, Monday through Friday, for telephone access.

2 3 4 5 6 7 8 9 10

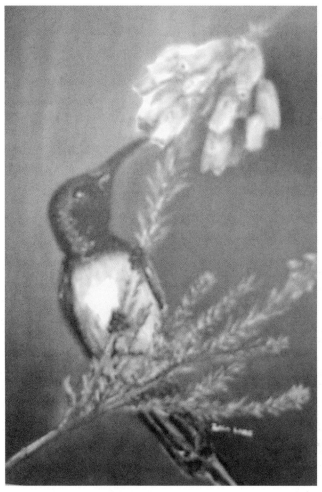

Pastel by Zela Schell

We dedicate this book to the memory of Zela Schell.

She lived a reflective life on earth; found meaning on a higher plane.

It is true that people, not theories, solve problems in professional practice. However, good theories can provide to professionals the lenses for understanding, tools for action, and guides for what to care about in the particular situations they confront. Every so often a field collectively develops a theory that does all three.

Clinical and professional reasoning is such a theory in occupational therapy. This theory has been in the making since the mid-1980s and has had many contributors who have offered various approaches to theory, research, and professional education. Two decades later, it is time for the field to provide a map of the theory's intellectual and practical landscape, summarize its implications for educational preparation, and offer guideposts for research and development. *Clinical and Professional Reasoning in Occupational Therapy* does so remarkably well.

Donald Schön and his books on the Reflective Practitioner are the lynchpin for my connection to clinical and professional reasoning in occupational therapy. When Barbara and John arrived at Georgia in 1990, I had recently published a book on continuing education for the professions. Schön wrote the foreword for that book, and his concept of reflective practice provided its animating spirit. Schön likewise inspired the lineage of clinical reasoning through his work with Cheryl Mattingly and others in the late 1980s. Thus, when Barbara's dissertation research focused on clinical reasoning, we came together with a common intellectual and practical framework for developing the concept of pragmatic reasoning. Those who have labored in the field of clinical and professional reasoning have successfully produced an enduring theory that matters to practice because, like Schön, they understand that the need for rigor and relevance in professional practice are not mutually exclusive. Instead, they have taken theories to the swampy lowland of professional practice and given hope and tools to occupational therapists, their managers, and their educators.

Although there are many reasons why this book will be seen as a signal development for the field of occupational therapy, I will highlight four of them. The first critical contribution is that the book expands the usefulness of the theory by going beyond "clinical reasoning" with its focus on client care. By expanding the focus to include "professional reasoning," the authors move beyond a medical model of treatment by also focusing on the reasoning used by occupational therapists' managers and educators. Second, the book brings to the table the many different approaches (scientific, narrative, pragmatic, ethical, interactive, and conditional) to professional reasoning. By honoring and bringing into dialogue these different traditions, the possibility for future theory development is greatly enhanced. Third, the authors demonstrate practically how and why professional reasoning can and should be used as a basis for educating occupational therapists across the continuum of professional education. Education is demonstratively more effective when it seeks to improve the ways that professionals actually reason and make decisions in their daily practice. Fourth, the last two chapters provide an excellent foundation for future research by offering comprehensive treatments of the methods and substantive results of research on professional reasoning in occupational therapy. The authors provide a number of insights that are likely to lead to continuing developments and breakthroughs in future research.

Occupational therapists need to carry on the field's historical legacy of helping people achieve their full potential and achieve a sense of worth and dignity in their lives. This book offers a wonderful guide to leaders and scholars as they continue experimenting with the design of innovative approaches to practice and education that can improve therapists' professional judgments and the systems in which client care is delivered.

RONALD M. CERVERO
Professor and Head
Department of Lifelong Education, Administration, and Policy
The University of Georgia
Athens, Georgia

ABOUT THE AUTHORS

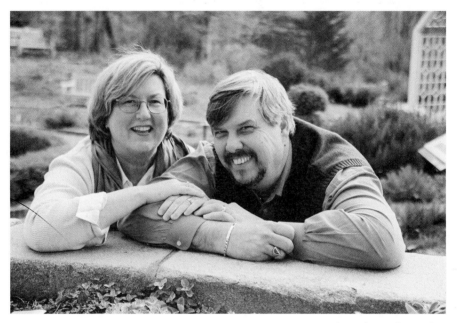

Photo by Helen Kabat

SHAPING PRACTICE: BARBARA'S PURSUIT OF PROMOTING EXCELLENCE IN PRACTICE

Barbara first began to explicitly explore clinical reasoning when she was an occupational manager at Harmarville Rehabilitation Center in Pittsburgh, Pennsylvania. In that capacity, she had oversight of a large department, including over 30 occupational therapy personnel, along with other related professionals and support staff. When she first came to Harmarville, there was a great deal of work aimed at focusing departmental efforts and developing systems to support staff in the delivery of services (Schell & Braveman, 2005). This was during the 1980s, when there was an extreme shortage of personnel and significant turbulence in healthcare as funding mechanisms began to shift from retrospective to prospective systems.

During this same period, Joan Rogers made clinical reasoning the subject of her Eleanor Clark Slagle lecture (1984) and, in the latter part of the decade, the American Occupational Therapy Foundation (AOTF) and the AOTA funded the research project, which came to be known as the *Clinical Reasoning Study* (Mattingly & Fleming, 1994). To progress the department's practices and to support her leadership of this process, Barbara wrote a grant to bring in Wendy Wood (fresh from her master's coursework at the University of Southern California) as a consultant to assist the department to move from what today would be called a medically-based approach to a more occupation-based approach. It was Wendy who first suggested to Barbara that what she was focusing on was clinical reasoning. From this early beginning, Barbara went on to become what she called a "clinical reasoning groupie," closely following the unfolding research of the Clinical Reasoning Study.

After leaving Harmarville, Barbara pursued her doctoral work in Adult Education at the University of Georgia, where she was fortunate to have Dr. Ron Cervero as her advisor. Ron, who is internationally known for his scholarship on continuing professional education, pushed Barbara to articulate her concerns with the limitations of clinical reasoning as it had been described to date. That effort ultimately resulted in her introduction of the concept of pragmatic reasoning to the field (Schell & Cervero, 1993).

Upon completing her doctoral work, Barbara soon became involved in academia, founding the occupational therapy program at Brenau University in Gainesville, GA. This effort required her to move from thinking about how to develop practitioners in the field to how to give them the best possible start. Since that time, Barbara has continued to review and synthesize the literature in numerous publications and to provide continuing education to managers and educators on how to support effective clinical reasoning in practice. Recently, she chose to shift out of administration at Brenau, in order to have more time for research and scholarship on clinical and professional reasoning.

SHAPING PRACTICE: JOHN'S PURSUIT OF LEARNING AND TEACHING

Just as Barbara has a long history of assisting practitioners in occupational therapy management and education, John has an even longer one researching the nature of social learning that can serve as a foundation for effective teaching. After graduating with a degree in Social Studies from Central Missouri State University, John spent many of his early years in Kansas City, Missouri, as a local manager of federally funded employment and training programs. These experiments of the 1960s, 1970s, and 1980s in social engineering aspired to promote a strong American work force among the economically disadvantaged through vocational training and education. Eventually, John's path led through the University of Missouri-Columbia, where he earned his Ph.D. John joined the faculty at the University of Pittsburgh, School of Education before he became a member of the College of Education faculty at the University of Georgia. Currently, John is Program Coordinator for the Educational Leadership Program in the Department of Workforce, Leadership and Social Foundations.

COMBINING FORCES

When Barb and John first met (in their early 30s), they used to humorously tell people that between them they covered health, education, and welfare (after the now-defunct federal agency of the same name). For the first 15 years of their marriage, they both pursued relatively separate career paths, although there was always plenty to talk about between educational and rehabilitation management. However, it became obvious that they were grappling with many of the same concepts and reading some of the same professional literature. Now, for more than a decade, they have enjoyed collaborative projects and consultations.

MORE THAN WORK

In addition to their work together, they enjoy time with their family, which now includes two grown children and their families, including six grandchildren. They also share a love of golf, nature, art, and photography. They share their daily lives with their two dogs, who remind them when it is time to go play. Learn more about Barbara at http://www.brenau.edu/shs/OT/faculty_bio.htm. Learn more about John at http://jschell.myweb.uga.edu and http://jschell.myweb.uga.edu/Discovery.

Thinking About Thinking

This House (This Book)
This [book] is for the ingathering of nature and human nature.
   *It is a [book] of friendships, a haven in trouble, an open room for the encourage-
ment of our struggle.*
It is a [book] of freedom, guarding the dignity and worth of every person.
   *It offers a platform for the free voice, for declaring, both in times of security and
danger, the full and undivided conflict of opinion.*
It is a [book] of truth-seeking, where scientists can encourage devotion to their quest,
where mystics can abide in a community of searchers.
   It is a [book] of art, adorning its celebrations with melodies and handiworks.
It is a [book] of prophecy, outrunning times past and times present in visions of growth
and progress.
   This [book] is a cradle for our dreams, the workshop of our common endeavor.
                                                      —Kenneth L. Patton (1993)

This book is a labor of love. It is the outgrowth of many years of reflection and
scholarship. Daily, we focus on the problem of how to help therapists become
better therapists; help teachers become better teachers; and help students
become better therapists and teachers in their own professional practices. We are
motivated to do this work because we believe that the world will be a better
place if people reach their full potential in the service professions in which they
have chosen to spend their lives.

MINDFULNESS IN PRACTICE

Professionals must have a "mindful" approach to decision making and the
actions taken in practice. This book is based on the idea that strategically
arranged *experiences* yield *articulated* knowledge, which is then metacognitively
examined through *reflection* for meaning. This chain of learning events depends
on an environment that is characterized by openness and honesty. Thomas
Jefferson (1762–1826) stated that "Honesty is the first chapter in the book of
wisdom." Learning to be a professional is an intensely personal experience. It
takes a great deal of courage for teachers and learners to be direct and open to

new or competing ideas. But honesty is necessary; it requires engagement of the brain, the mind, and the heart.

In the quotation above, Kenneth L. Patton (1997) used a powerful vocabulary to describe a community, what today we would call a "community of practice." He uses expressions such as *friendship, encouragement, struggle, freedom, dignity, worth, free-voice, conflict, truth-seeking, quest, art, science, adornment, prophecy,* and *past and present.* All of these expressions are deeply emotional, and all are associated with an ethic of honesty. These words are similes for the act of constructing meaning.

Honesty is required to become reflective practitioners capable of the highest levels of expertise. In the tradition of John Dewey (1910), Jack Mezirow (1978), Donald Schön (1983, 1987), Stephen Brookfield (1995), and many others, we view meaning-making as experience: the articulation of new knowledge, application, and reflection on meaning. This book is about how reasoning, coupled with reflection, can elevate practice.

PURPOSE

Clinical and Professional Reasoning in Occupational Therapy is designed to serve students, supervisors, managers, and educators in academia and occupational therapy practice, as well as scholars interested in clinical and professional reasoning. This comprehensive textbook summarizes current theories and research about clinical and professional reasoning, provides learning activities designed to promote effective reasoning, and recommends strategies for teaching clinical reasoning in academic and practice settings. It can be used by students who want to learn and understand their own reasoning and by those concerned with improving practice through professional development and scholarship.

TERMINOLOGY

The term *professional reasoning* has been added to the more familiar *clinical reasoning* for two reasons. First, colleagues who practice in educational and community settings find the word "clinical" to be one that presumes a medically-based orientation and is therefore inappropriate. Second, there is a significant amount of reasoning related to therapy practice, programming, and so on, which is done by supervisors, managers, and others. It seemed appropriate to acknowledge that this reasoning, though not directed to a specific patient or client, also had aspects similar to clinical reasoning.

ORGANIZATION

The content of *Clinical and Professional Reasoning in Occupational Therapy* consists of summaries of different perspectives about the reasoning that occurs within occupational therapy. Many textbooks provide suggestions about what therapists *should* think about and how they *should* conduct therapy. In contrast, contributors to this text were asked to build their discussions using research, which focused on what therapists actually *did* think about and, subsequently, *do* during therapy. In many cases, research findings from within occupational therapy were combined with salient scholarship from a variety of other disciplines, such as psychology, anthropology, philosophy, nursing, medicine, and physical therapy. Although the units and chapters are related, each can also stand alone, thus allowing the text to be used either in a specific class or used across different courses, depending on the curriculum design. Those outside of the academic sphere can pick and choose materials most relevant to their own needs.

Clinical and Professional Reasoning in Occupational Therapy is organized into four units. Unit I, The Nature of Clinical and Professional Reasoning, focuses on clinical and professional reasoning as they are grounded in human experience. The introductory chapter provides an overview of the definitions of clinical and professional reasoning, as well as a guide to the different facets of the reasoning processes described in Units I and II. After this introduction, Chapter 2 explores how therapist values, culture, and worldview serve as an often unexamined basis on which professional reasoning is situated. Chapter 3 draws from a wide range of cognitive psychology literature to explain how the brain builds experiences into professional knowledge and expertise. Chapter 4 discusses the notion of reasoning as an "embodied" process, or one in which mental work involves not only thought or brain-work but experiences of the whole body. By the end of this unit, readers will appreciate the commonalities of human minds, as well as the individual variances that form the ground upon which each therapist reasons in practice.

Unit II, Aspects of Professional Reasoning, provides in-depth explorations of the different facets of therapists' reasoning. These forms of reasoning may not represent different kinds of reasoning from the perspective of cognitive psychology, but they do highlight how therapists shift their attention to different aspects of the therapy process, and in doing so change the rhetoric and ways of framing problems in practice. Chapter 5 provides an extensive examination of *scientific* reasoning, the kind of thinking that attempts to be objective and that seeks theory, evidence, and the use of logic to understand therapy issues. In contrast, Chapter 6 describes *narrative* reasoning, an aspect of reasoning in which the therapist's attention moves from the objective science to the client's subjective experience. By attending to stories and plot lines, therapists reason about the meaning of health experiences to their clients. Chapter 7 goes beyond the therapist–client relationships to *pragmatic* reasoning, in which therapists attend to the practical issues in delivering care. Both the practice context in which care occurs and the therapist's own skill set are factors that therapists reason about when deciding on what care to actually provide. In Chapter 8, therapists' moral sense and ethical frameworks are examined; these come into play when therapists attempt to choose the right action from among competing options. Chapter 9 emphasizes the communicative nature of the clinical reasoning process as therapists seek to build therapeutic relationship and also summarizes the integrative and conditional nature of the process.

Moving away from understanding the nature and common processes of clinical and professional reasoning, Unit III, Teaching Professional Reasoning, looks at how to teach for effective practice. Chapter 10 tackles the complex topic of *epistemology,* or the study of knowledge and thinking, surveying differing assumptions about knowledge that lead to the discussions in Chapter 11 about how to teach for expert practice. Both sociological and psychological perspectives are examined in these opening chapters, providing groundwork for the examination of teaching practices. Although of obvious use to those in academia, these two chapters also are useful for clinical fieldwork supervisors, managers, and those responsible for continuing competence and professional development. The following two chapters provide case studies on two different curriculums: Chapter 12 demonstrates how to implement a curriculum built around clinical reasoning within a communities of practice model, and Chapter 13 describes curricular approaches to building professional reasoning for evidence-based practice. Chapter 14 moves the reader into professional reasoning about student supervision, describing the co-construction of knowledge that occurs between fieldwork students and their supervisors.

The final unit (Unit IV, Research in Clinical and Professional Reasoning) provides a summary of the scholarship related to clinical and professional reasoning. In Chapter 15, researchers can find a summary of the various approaches to researching reasoning in practice, along with discussions about the relative benefits and liabilities of each approach. Chapter 16 summarizes where the field is in the study of clinical and professional reasoning. What seems to be known, what is not known, and fruitful directions for future scholarship are suggested. The Appendix provides a comprehensive bibliography of research and scholarship on reasoning within occupational therapy, as well as listings of important works from other disciplines.

Features

Many features have been added to enhance the understanding and application of the content. **Learning Objectives** serve to orient the reader as well as assist faculty in focusing learners on core content in the chapter. The **Chapter Outline** at the beginning of each chapter helps readers to quickly find materials, and serves as study resources and summaries of important constructs. **Key Terms** are printed in bold and defined in the chapter. The **Thinking about Thinking** quotations (typically from outside of occupational therapy) have been selected to prompt readers to think about metacognitive issues from different perspectives. The **Learning Activities** at the end of each chapter have been designed to provide students with ways to reflect on their experiences and gain deeper learning. Each activity includes the purpose of the activity, how it connects to major constructs about reasoning, and directions. When appropriate, content for handout materials is provided as well. A **Glossary** of key terms is included as well.

The editors and authors of this book hope to promote professional reasoning. It is our strong belief that effective reasoning, when coupled with systematic reflection, will yield more effective care for those we serve.

CONTRIBUTORS

Martha Carr, PhD
Professor
Educational Psychology & Instructional Technology
College of Education
The University of Georgia
Athens, GA

Wendy J. Coster, PhD, OTR/L, FAOTA
Associate Professor & Chair
Department of Occupational Therapy & Rehabilitation Counseling
Sargent College of Health and Rehabilitation Sciences
Boston University
Boston, MA

Ruth S. Farber, PhD, MSW, OTR/L
Associate Professor
Department of Occupational Therapy
College of Health Professions
Temple University
Philadelphia, PA

Toby Ballou Hamilton, PhD, MPH, OTR/L
Assistant Professor
Department of Rehabilitation Science
College of Allied Health
University of Oklahoma Health Sciences Center
Oklahoma City, OK

Dana Harris, MS, OTR/L
Owner
Tailored for Tots, LLC
Douglasville, GA

Barbara Hooper, PhD, OTR/L
Assistant Professor
Occupational Therapy Graduate Program
University of New Mexico
Albuquerque, NM

Elizabeth M. Kanny, PhD, OTR/L, FAOTA
Associate Professor and Division Head
Division of Occupational Therapy
Department of Rehabilitation Medicine
University of Washington
Seattle, WA

Kristie P. Koenig, PhD, OTR/L
Assistant Professor
Department of Occupational Therapy
College of Health Professions
Temple University
Philadelphia, PA

Barbara A. Boyt Schell, PhD, OTR/L, FAOTA
Professor and Graduate Coordinator
Occupational Therapy Department
School of Health and Science
Brenau University
Gainesville, GA

John W. Schell, PhD
Program Coordinator, Educational Leadership and Associate Professor
Workforce Education, Leadership, & Social Foundations
College of Education
The University of Georgia
Athens, GA

Mary Shotwell, PhD, OTR/L
Associate Professor
Occupational Therapy Department
School of Health and Science
Brenau University
Gainesville, GA

Deborah Yarett Slater, MS, OT/L, FAOTA
Practice Associate
Professional Affairs
American Occupational Therapy Association
Bethesda, MD

George S. Tomlin, PhD, OTR/L
Professor and Director, Occupational Therapy
Schools of Occupational Therapy and Physical Therapy
University of Puget Sound
Tacoma, WA

Carolyn A. Unsworth, BAppSC, PhD, OTR
Associate Professor, Research and Higher Degree Coordinator
School of Occupational Therapy
Faculty of Health Sciences
La Trobe University
Melbourne, Australia

Roxie M. Black, PhD, OTR/L, FAOTA
Associate Professor and Director
Master of Occupational Therapy Program
University of Southern Maine at Lewiston-Auburn
Lewiston, ME

Susan Coppola, MS, OTR/L, BCG
Clinical Associate Professor
Division of Occupational Science
University of North Carolina at Chapel Hill
Chapel Hill, NC

Cathy Dolhi, MS, OTR/L, FAOTA
Associate Professor
Department of Occupational Therapy
Chatham University
Pittsburgh, PA

Ruth S. Farber, PhD, OTR/L
Associate Professor
Department of Occupational Therapy
College of Health Professions
Temple University
Philadelphia, PA

Judith Friedland, PhD, OT Reg (Ont.), OT (C), FCAOT
Professor Emerita
Universtiy of Toronto
Toronto, Canada

Janice Tona, OTR, Ph.D.
Clinical Assistant Professor, Rehabilitation Science
University at Buffalo
Buffalo, NY

ACKNOWLEDGMENTS

Any endeavor such as this builds on many conversations and experiences over time, as well as on the focused efforts of a few close supporters. In that light, Barbara would like to acknowledge all she has learned from her students and colleagues at Brenau University. Dr. Helen Ray, VPAA and Provost at Brenau provided wonderful support for the development of the occupational therapy program and Robin Underwood, in her role as Academic Fieldwork Coordinator, showed how to operationalize a community of practice in support of learning. Barbara also recognizes the contributions of past colleagues from Harmarville Rehabilitation Center and valued colleagues throughout the American Occupational Therapy Association who were instrumental in shaping her understanding of clinical and professional reasoning. Finally, she appreciates Dr. Ron Cervero's role in helping her develop a scholarly approach to this topic.

Likewise, John appreciates the support and stimulation from his colleagues and students at the University of Georgia. His colleagues in the Department of Workforce Education, Leadership and Social Foundations are steadfast in their support of scholarly efforts. It is a culture that actively promotes academic research that influences teaching. John is particularly indebted to those doctoral students he supervised, who have continued to explore the implications of context-based learning and teaching. Dr. Bruce Ott started this research agenda with John in his study of expert-led reflective discussion on academic achievement among respiratory therapist students. Dr. Lora Lindsay was very helpful in examining the community of practice that exists within the Occupational Therapy Program at Brenau University. Dr. Jed Gillespie expanded the idea of communities of practice to the UGA Student Services program while comparing traditional and contextually-based styles of teaching. Dr. Chris Jonick conducted a study of teaching for communities of practice within an electronic learning environment; Dr. Debra Arnold examined the socialization of new teachers, Dr. Rhonda Bevis conducted a study of Clinical Reasoning among Respiratory Therapy practitioners, and Dr. Pete Brannan examined professional development, expertise, and meaning-making among veteran technology education teachers. All of these researchers and their studies have significantly contributed to the development of the Framework for Contextual Learning and Teaching, which is published in Chapter 16 of this book. Currently, there are three new studies that will critically examine aspects of this framework. Specifically, we are interested in instruction that promotes reflectivity and meaning-making among educators in their professional practice. John has a particular debt of gratitude to these fine scholars and their commitment to the profession of teaching.

Both Barbara and John appreciate the great work done by the reviewers, Sue Coppola, Cathy Dolhi, and Roxie Black. In addition to these individuals, Betty Crepeau and Ellen Cohn served as background consultants throughout this project, giving thoughtful opinions and suggestions in response to various editorial quandaries. The advice from all these individuals greatly improved both the quality and comprehensiveness of the book. Likewise, we are indepted to the contributing authors, as well as those who shared their instructional materials.

Last, but certainly not least, we appreciate the patience and steady support of Andrea Klingler, our managing editor at Lippincott Williams & Wilkins. She has kept us anchored throughout the process, and has done so with gentle good humor. Thanks for helping us in this new adventure.

CONTENTS

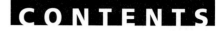

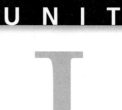

The Nature of Clinical and Professional Reasoning

1

Professional Reasoning as the Basis of Practice

Barbara A. Boyt Schell and John W. Schell

CHAPTER OUTLINE

Definitions of clinical and professional reasoning
    Thinking in context
    Views of clinical and professional reasoning

Putting reasoning in a larger context
Reasoning in a social world
Summary

OBJECTIVES

After reading this chapter, the learner will be able to:

1 Explore the history of research about clinical reasoning in occupational therapy.
2 Define clinical and professional reasoning.
3 Provide an overview of different aspects of clinical and professional reasoning.
4 Appreciate interdisciplinary sources of knowledge related to reasoning in occupational therapy.
5 Understand the importance of content knowledge, experience, and reflection for the development of expertise.

KEY TERMS

Clinical Reasoning
Professional Reasoning

C linical reasoning is a term that first gained prominence in occupational therapy in the 1980s, when Joan Rogers made clinical reasoning the subject of her 1983 AOTA Eleanor Clark Slagle Lecture (Rogers, 1983). Rogers was aware of emerging research in medicine and cognitive psychology, which attempted to explain how clinical decisions were made in medicine. Based on this research, she and her colleague Gladys Masagatani studied a group of 10 occupational therapists doing evaluations to uncover how clinical decisions were made in occupational therapy (Rogers & Masagatani, 1982). They found, among other things, that therapists were often unable to explain why they had done what they had done. In our own experience, this finding is one that is commonly replicated when occupational therapy students ask their clinical supervisors how they "knew" to do a particular therapy action. Rogers stated her concern that if we couldn't describe the reasoning processes underlying our therapy actions, then it would be difficult to systematically improve it and teach it. Rogers' challenge to the profession stimulated a new line of research in occupational therapy aimed at understanding how therapists *actually* thought about what they were doing, not what they were *supposed* to think.

The next chapter in this story came about in the late 1980s as a result of collaboration between the American Occupational Therapy Foundation (AOTF) and the American Occupational Therapy Association (AOTA). A group of theorists and researchers met with Donald Schön to discuss how to "investigate clinical knowledge and expertise within the profession" (Mattingly & Fleming, 1994, ix). Schön was already well known for his book, *The Reflective Practitioner* (1983), in which he described commonalities on how individuals practice in professions as diverse as psychotherapy, architecture, engineering, town planning, and management. His central thesis was that effective professional practice requires a blend of technical know-how, which is combined with reflection during the actual process of practice. Because both AOTF and AOTA were concerned with improving practice and education, the two organizations funded a research project that came to be known as the *Clinical Reasoning Study* (Mattingly & Fleming, 1994). Cheryl Mattingly, Schön's graduate student, teamed up with Maureen Fleming, an experienced occupational therapy faculty member at Tufts University. Their extensive study of therapists at a large medical center in Boston produced findings suggesting not just one clinical reasoning process, but several. This work had tremendous influence on the study of clinical reasoning in occupational therapy. Their subsequent publications in an AJOT (*American Journal of Occupational Therapy*) Special Issue on Clinical Reasoning (Cohn, 1991) and later in their book *Clinical Reasoning: Forms of Inquiry in a Therapeutic Practice* (Mattingly & Fleming, 1994) along with Roger's 1983 Slagle Lecture became and remain core reading for anyone seriously interested in clinical reasoning in occupational therapy.

From that beginning, more than 50 studies have been reported in the occupational therapy literature on clinical reasoning, and many more articles and studies have been published which build on clinical reasoning theory with suggestions on how to improve practice and education. At the very least, this is a wonderful example of how the efforts of a few, supported by member dues and contributions to professional organizations, can benefit many in ways barely anticipated from the beginning. In the appendix of this book is a bibliography of studies and literature about how occupational therapists think in action and how best to educate them to think for more effective action. This list includes several literature reviews that attempt to summarize the work in one fashion or another. The literature on clinical reasoning spans a number of countries. However, in spite of the volume of work, there isn't a book that brings it all together, allowing us to step back and see what we know and what we need to know about this important topic.

The purpose of this book is to provide a current text that summarizes what we know about clinical and professional reasoning in occupational therapy from the work that has been done, as well as to identify where further research is needed. In addition, later units address the implications of this knowledge for education in all its forms, including curriculum planning, classroom education, student fieldwork education, and continuing professional development. The final unit seeks to synthesize the knowledge shared in this book, identify directions for future work, and suggest effective approaches for obtaining that knowledge.

Think About Thinking 1-1

The dilemma of "rigor or relevance" arises more acutely in some areas of practice than in others. In the varied topography of professional practice, there is a *high hard ground* in which practitioners can make effective use of the research-based theory and technique. Moreover, there is the *swampy lowland* in which situations are confusing "messes" incapable of technical solution. The difficulty is that the problems of the high hard ground, however great their technical interest, are often relatively unimportant to clients or to the larger society, whereas in the swamp, the problems of greatest human concern are found (Schön, 1983, p. 42).

DEFINITIONS OF CLINICAL AND PROFESSIONAL REASONING

There are a number of definitions of **clinical reasoning** (Schell & Cervero, 1993; Crabtree, 1998). For purposes of this book, we adopt the definition of clinical reasoning as "the process used by practitioners to plan, direct, perform and reflect on client care" (Schell, 2003, p. 131). Because the term clinical reasoning is associated by some in the profession with a medically based approach, we are also using the term **professional reasoning** in this text. Using the term professional reasoning broadens the discussion to include the reasoning that occurs in non-medical environments, such as schools and community settings, as well as reasoning done by supervisors, fieldwork educators, and occupational therapy managers as they conceptualize occupational therapy practice. For instance, managers make decisions that shape the nature of accepted occupational therapy practices within their settings, and as discussed later in this text, fieldwork supervisors "co-construct" their reasoning with occupational therapy students. Ultimately, the focus of clinical and professional reasoning has to do with framing, implementing, and assessing therapy services, whether the therapist is trying to decide how to evaluate a person who is in an acute care hospital, to coordinate therapy interventions with the teacher for a child with special needs, or to design a wellness program for individuals with persistent mental illness living in the community. This sort of reasoning differs from some other kinds of reasoning, in that professionals must *act* on their thoughts—often without the benefit of prolonged reflection (Schön, 1983).

Thinking in Context

Understanding the thinking that guides practice turns out to be a complicated business, as will be evident to readers. Like any other human endeavor, it is the result of interplay between the person, the context in which the person is acting, and the specific therapy tasks that must be accomplished (for those with an understanding of theories of human occupation, this is going to sound familiar). However, readers should keep in mind that although occupational therapy theories are designed to help us understand our clients, theories about clinical and professional reasoning are focused on the *therapist* and how that therapist goes about doing therapy.

As noted by Schön in the quotation mentioned previously, professional practice requires therapists to traverse a range of problems. Therapists can be guided in their decisions in some cases by fairly straightforward scientific or technical information, but much of actual practice requires a multitude of nuanced decisions and actions, without the straightforward professional guideposts we might wish for. Similarly, research with regard to professional reasoning has attempted to identify the high hard ground of therapist thinking, but also often surfaces on the swampy lowland, where most of us seem to live. Certainly, much of the current research is inadequate to completely comprehend the complexities of reasoning that occur in the real-life context of professional practice. For instance, there is very little research about occupational therapy assistants and how their reasoning may be similar or different from professional level occupational therapists. Likewise, there is little information about how individual differences in therapists affect their reasoning. Because of limitations like these, much of the content of this book represents the best information that we had at the time it was published. Part of our agenda is to raise awareness among the profession of the need for an ambitious program of research using a wide range of hard- and soft-ground methodologies.

Views of Clinical and Professional Reasoning

Because reasoning in practice is a complex process, it is not surprising to find different perspectives on both the nature of the process and the focus or content that therapists reason about. At the risk of oversimplifying, we have chosen in this text to organize chapters by topical areas that represent the terms common to the study of clinical reasoning in occupational therapy. Therefore, those with prior knowledge on this topic will recognize terms that surfaced from prior work by Rogers (1983), Mattingly & Fleming (1994), Schell & Cervero (1993), and Rogers & Holms (1991). These topical areas are summarized in *Table 1-1* for quick reference. The definitions and characteristics of these forms of reasoning are drawn directly from the chapters in this book addressing each topical area.

PUTTING REASONING IN A LARGER CONTEXT

Our present-day awareness of how people use their knowledge in professional practice comes from many disciplines, a number of which are cited in the chapters to come. The next few pages are a very brief overview of the evolution of what we have come to think of today as professional reasoning. We acknowledge that many important contributions and concepts are excluded from our discussion.

TABLE 1-1

Different Aspects of Reasoning in Occupational Therapy

Aspect of Reasoning	Description and Focus	Clues for Recognizing in Therapist Discussions
Scientific reasoning	Reasoning involving the use of applied logical and scientific methods, such as hypothesis testing, pattern recognition, theory-based decision making and statistical evidence	Impersonal, focused on the diagnosis, condition, guiding theory, evidence from research or what "typically" happens with clients like the one being considered
Diagnostic reasoning	Investigative reasoning and analysis of cause or nature of conditions requiring occupational therapy intervention; can be considered one component of scientific reasoning	Uses both personal and impersonal information; therapists attempt to explain why client is experiencing problems using a blend of science-based and client-based information
Procedural reasoning	Reasoning in which therapist considers and uses intervention routines for identified conditions; may be science-based or may reflect the habits and culture of the intervention setting	Characterized by therapist using therapy regimens or routines thought to be effective with problems identified, and which are typically used with clients in that setting; tends to be more impersonal and diagnostically driven
Narrative reasoning	Reasoning process used to make sense of people's particular circumstances, prospectively imagine the effect of illness, disability, or occupational performance problems on their daily lives, and create a collaborative story that is enacted with clients and families through intervention	Personal, focused on the client, including past, present and anticipated future; involves an appreciation of client culture as the basis for understanding client narrative and relates to the "so what" of the condition for the person's life
Pragmatic reasoning	Practical reasoning used to fit therapy possibilities into the current realities of service delivery, such as scheduling options, payment for services, equipment availability, therapists' skills, management directives, and the personal situation of the therapist	Generally not focused on client or client's condition, but rather on all the physical and social "stuff" that surrounds the therapy encounter as well as the therapist's internal sense of what he or she is capable of and has the time and energy to complete
Ethical reasoning	Reasoning directed to analyzing an ethical dilemma, generating alternative solutions, and determining actions to be taken; systematic approach to moral conflict	Tension often evident as therapist attempts to determine what is the "right" thing to do, particularly when faced with dilemmas in therapy, competing principles, and risks and benefits

(continued)

TABLE 1.1

(continued)

Aspect of Reasoning	Description and Focus	Clues for Recognizing in Therapist Discussions
Interactive reasoning	Thinking directed toward building positive interpersonal relationships with clients, permitting collaborative problem identification and problem solving	Therapist concerned with what client likes or doesn't like; use of praise, empathetic comments, and nonverbal behaviors to encourage and support client's cooperation
Conditional reasoning	A blending of all forms of reasoning for the purposes of flexibly responding to changing conditions or predicting possible client futures	Typically found with more experienced therapists who can "see" multiple futures, based on therapists' past experiences and current information

Based on writings by Tomlin, Hamilton, Schell, and Kanny chapters in this text, *Clinical and Professional Reasoning in Occupational Therapy* (2007), and prior work by Rogers and Holm (1991), Mattingly & Fleming (1994).

Our purpose is to *highlight* selected researchers and concepts that have shaped our current thinking on the topic.

Philosophy was the first discipline to deal explicitly with theories of knowledge and the mind. Noticing the practices of ancient craftsmen or artisans, Aristotle came to believe that their work involved thinking and reasoned action (Bernstein, 1983). However, those actions were taken within the artisan's "praxis." Praxis can be defined as reasoned action taken to accomplish a specific task. An expert occupational therapist might approach a client's problem with a goal in mind but careful thinking and reasoning might alter the actions or praxis that he or she might use. As the case continues, the goals may become different as the therapist understands the situation more clearly. Aristotle could be thought of as an early adopter of professional reasoning.

Centuries later, as science emerged, the disciplines of biology and later psychology replaced philosophy as a basis for understanding human reasoning. Theoretical researchers in the late 19th and early 20th centuries drew heavily from Darwin's theory of evolution in which "humans were seen as 'biologically continuous' with the animal kingdom" (Phillips & Soltis, 2004, p.21). As Darwin's theory of evolution became commonly known, researchers of human behavior also incorporated the assumption of progression among humans as a basis for understanding learning and thinking. This form of biology proved to be a strong influence in the development of behaviorism and developmental psychology. Many of the early studies were based on the biological similarities between humans and other forms of animal life. However, it proved to be very difficult to apply scientific principles of deduction to the study of human learning and thinking. Researchers had no reliable way to validate what many viewed as subjective evidence with regard to what was occurring in the human mind. Scientists such as John Watson (1948) contended that it was more appropriate to observe behavior than to ask people what they were thinking. Such perspectives resulted in research shifting from a focus on thinking to a focus on learning as measured by changes in behavior.

Classic theories of behavior emerged as the field of psychology established itself as a separate discipline from biology in the late 19th century. As the field of psychology evolved, Gestalt theories focused on the "tendencies of the mind to pattern and structure experience" became more prevalent (Phillips & Soltis, 2004, p.7). Jerome Brunner (1977) expanded the concept of schemes to illustrate how a given discipline is structured. He argued that learners need a general understanding of the way in which proprietary knowledge is organized. Once a global perspective is gained, learners are then more capable of deciding how problems can be addressed within the context of the field's comprehension of knowledge. These theories eventually led some researchers to compare the human brain with the "revolution in computing and artificial intelligence" (Phillips & Soltis, 2004, p.8).

Jean Piaget, a developmental psychologist who was educated as a biologist, also was concerned with how knowledge was structured and used. He based much of his later work on the assumption that learning and thinking were artifacts of biological functioning (Piaget, 1969). Piaget's research focused on "mental or cognitive structures," which, although unobservable, were the foundation of learning and use of knowledge (Phillips & Soltis, 2004). As a developmental psychologist, Piaget thought of these mental structures as the way in which children organize their minds. This network is developed over three stages (sensorimotor, preoperational, and concrete operation), which are generally associated with the child's age. As the child ages, emerging mental structures assist the child to "interiorize" what Piaget conceptualized as operations (Phillips & Soltis). The impacts of Piaget's scientific work strongly influence our thinking about developmental psychology even today.

Nearly simultaneously, other researchers were examining the relationship of learning and use of knowledge within social contexts. Lev Semyonovich Vygotsky was a Russian child development expert whose work was relatively unknown in the West until the 1960s and 1970s. His contribution was important because it encouraged us to think about human development in light of the interaction of the person within communities. It is evident that his work influenced many Western researchers such as Bruner and even Piaget. Vygotsky's works on zones of proximal development (ZPD) and consciousness were central to understanding how novices thought and how their actions could be facilitated by a teacher with a higher level of skill (The Collected Works of Vygotsky, 1968). Such sociological theories eventually led to the theories of situated cognition (Lave, 1988) and communities of practice (Wenger, 1998). These theories, along with more in-depth discussions of philosophical and psychological perspectives are discussed in more depth in Unit III.

REASONING IN A SOCIAL WORLD

A concurrent movement in Western Europe and the United States during the early 20th century occurred as researchers began to think more seriously about the influence of social relationships on the way humans think and reason. These researchers represented fields that were to become known among academics as the social sciences. Paul Ricœur, a French phenomenologist strongly influenced Martin Heidegger, Hans-Georg Gadamer, Maurice Merleau-Ponty, Jean-Paul Sartre, and Alfred Schütz to examine conscious experience as an existential technique for understanding the meaning of the actions of an individual—or, we could say a person's reflection on his or her experiences that guides and evaluates their professional actions. Alfred Schütz's research extended this work by emphasizing the human ability to capture lived experiences through "flowing consciousness" as they passed from experience into memory (Kauffmann, 1944). Of course, this perspective forms a potent theoretical platform for understanding the reasoning of professionals as they reflect on past, present, or future actions.

Donald Schön (1983) is well known for his work in the area of reflective practice and organizational "systems of learning." Ironically, his own thinking may have been strongly influenced by his avid interest in jazz. Noting his talents as a pianist and clarinet player of some repute, some of his colleagues believe that he was inspired by jazz improvisation leading to his ideas about "thinking in the moment." One could speculate on what impact this had on his work with regard to reflection in action and reflection on action, two core concepts explaining how professionals practice and develop expertise (also addressed later in this text).

Herbert Dreyfus continued the tradition of the existential phenomenology of Heidegger in a book that he co-authored with his brother Stewart titled *Mind over Machine* (Dreyfus & Dreyfus, 1986). This book has subsequently influenced many researchers in numerous professions. It has had a great impact on how many experts think about the processes that shape how novices eventually become experts. Dreyfus and Dreyfus identified five succeeding stages of expertise, beginning with novice and continuing through advanced beginner to competent, proficient, and expert. Novices apply basic rules but do not particularly pay attention to the surroundings. Advanced beginners learn through experience in a variety of situations but still rely on the rules when making decisions. Competent workers may adopt a plan for making a decision based on a limited number of factors to ascertain a conclusion. Proficient workers are more engaged in their task of paying attention to the present situation in light of past encounters with similar circumstances. Experts are more intuitive and take reflexive actions based on past practice and greater understanding of the situation.

In putting reflective thinking in a larger context it becomes clear that the influences of other writers and philosophers such as John Dewey, Kurt Lewin, Carl Rogers, and David Kolb all have contributed to our present-day thinking with regard to reflective practice. We recall this history to reflect on how the "thinking about thinking" has been handed down by several generations of researchers and practitioners. Throughout this text, you will find quotations in Thinking About Thinking boxes, which reflect the thoughts of such scholars.

SUMMARY

This chapter serves as an introduction to the topic of professional reasoning. Our objectives here have been to provide a context that will help you, the reader, to understand the intricacies associated with this highly complex topic. We also want you to appreciate how this topic of reasoning has been derived from many years of research that is arrayed across many professions.

We devoted some space to the history of professional and clinical reasoning within occupational therapy, so that readers can gain a sense of where this work comes from within the profession. Second, we provided operational definitions of clinical and professional reasoning as technical terms that are used in subsequent chapters. It is important to the intention of this book that our approach to reasoning is placed in specific social and physical contexts. With this in mind, we have explored the contexts of thinking in this chapter. In addition, the thinking about reasoning within the profession of occupational therapy has been described.

We also placed reasoning in a larger context, exploring a brief history of the thinking about thinking as a form of reasoning. The larger world of thinking has been described in both psychological and sociological traditions. As Schön (1983) so eloquently noted, practice occurs in both the "high hard ground" and "swampy lowlands," both of which must be addressed if we are to fully understand professional reasoning.

The next chapters in this section of the book begin a more detailed discussion of reasoning and how it has been researched and implemented in occupational therapy practice.

LEARNING ACTIVITY 1-1

Thinking About Thinking

Purpose

The purpose of this activity is for learners to experience the processes underlying everyday practice, using a metacognitive approach.

Connections to Major Clinical Reasoning Constructs

Much of this text is focused on "thinking about thinking" or metacognition. Since readers may not have extensive therapy experience, this activity provides a window to understand how everyday practices are based on tacit knowledge, or things we know but don't put into words. Similarly, the use of reflection and articulation is key to understanding how therapists think in action.

Directions for Learners

1 Think of an everyday activity that you know well, such as taking a shower, riding a bike, or driving a car.
2 Once you identify the activity, think specifically about a recent time that you performed that activity.
3 Using the worksheet provided, answer the questions about the activity itself, your knowledge underlying the activity, and how you gained that knowledge.
4 Discuss within a group what you learned from this reflection, and how it might apply to therapy practice.

1. Identify the activity you are going to reflect on and write it down on top of a grid like the one below.
2. In the left column, put the major steps of your activity in the sequence in which it occurs. Be sure to be as detailed as necessary, so that someone else could follow your steps and do the activity (i.e., for driving a car, the first few steps might be: 1. opened the car door, 2. sat in driver's seat, 3. adjusted the seat, 4. adjusted the rear view mirror, etc.)
3. In the middle column, put down what you "know," which guides you in completing this step.
4. In the last column, under each step of the activity, put down how you learned it.

STEPS OF ACTIVITY	WHAT I KNOW	HOW I LEARNED

REFERENCES

Bernstein, R. J. (1983). *Beyond objectivism and relativism: Science, hermeneutics and praxis.* Oxford: Basil Blackwell.

Bruner, J. (1977). *The process of education.* Cambridge, MA: Harvard University Press.

Cohn, E. S. (Ed.) (1991). Clinical reasoning (Special issue). *American Journal of Occupational Therapy, 45*(11).

Collected Works of L. S. Vygotsky (1968). Volume III, Part 1: Problems of the Theory and Methods of Psychology, Chapter 9: *The Problem of Consciousness,* pp 129–138.

Crabtree, M. (1998). Images of reasoning: A literature review. *Australian Occupational Therapy Journal, 45,* 113–123.

Dreyfus, H. & Dreyfus, S. (1986). *Mind over machine.* New York: Free Press.

Kaufmann, F. (1944). *Methodology of the social science.* New York: Oxford University Press.

Lave, J. (1988). *Cognition in practice: Mind, mathematics and culture in everyday life.* Cambridge: Cambridge University Press.

Mattingly, C. & Fleming, M. H. (1994). *Clinical reasoning-forms of inquiry in a therapeutic practice.* Philadelphia: F. A. Davis.

Phillips, D. C. & Soltis, J. F. (2004). *Perspectives on learning.* New York: Teachers College Press.

Piaget, J. (1969). *Psychology of intelligence.* Patterson, NJ: Littlefield, Adams.

Rogers, J. C. (1983). Clinical reasoning: The ethics, science, and art. *American Journal of Occupational Therapy, 37,* 601–616.

Rogers, J. C. & Holm, M. B. (1991). Occupational therapy diagnostic reasoning: A component of clinical reasoning. *American Journal of Occupational Therapy, 45*(11), 1045–1053.

Rogers, J. C. & Masagatani, G. (1982). Clinical reasoning of occupational therapists during initial assessment of physically disabled patients. *Occupational Therapy Journal of Research, 2,* 195–219.

Schell, B. (2003). *Clinical reasoning: The basis of practice.* In Crepeau, B., Cohn, E. & Schell, B. A B. *Willard and Spackman's occupational therapy.* Philadelphia: Lippincott Williams & Wilkins.

Schell, B. A. & Cervero, R. M. (1993). Clinical reasoning in occupational therapy: An integrative review. *American Journal of Occupational Therapy, 47,* 605–610.

Schnotz, W. (1997). Strategy-specific information in knowledge. In Lauren B. Resnick, Roger Säljö, Clotilde Pontecorvo & Barbara Burge (Eds). *Discourse, tools and reasoning.* NATO ASI series. Series F, computer and systems sciences; vol. 160. Berlin: Springer-Verlag.

Schön, D. A. (1983). *The reflective practitioner: How professionals think in action.* New York: Basic Books.

Watson, J. B. (1948). Psychology as the behaviorist views it. In Wayne, D. (Ed.) *Readings in the history of psychology.* New York: Appleton-Century-Crofts.

Wenger, E. (1998). *Communities of practice.* Cambridge, UK: Cambridge University Press.

Therapists' Assumptions as a Dimension of Professional Reasoning

Barbara Hooper

CHAPTER OUTLINE

OBJECTIVES

After reading this chapter, the learner will be able to:

1 Define and illustrate the concept of assumptions.
2 Summarize the literature related to the connection between professional reasoning and therapists' assumptions about (a) human experience; (b) the human body; (c) how knowledge is obtained and generated; (d) what knowledge is core for occupational therapy; (e) the client's future; (f) the therapist's future; and (g) a future beyond time.
3 Offer an explanation for how assumptions influence professional reasoning.
4 Invite reflection on personal assumptions.

KEY TERMS

Assumption	Perceptual filter
Habits of expectation	Intrinsicality

Professional reasoning involves examining the transactions between how I think and what I do in practice. I examine these transactions through ongoing conversations with myself and others about the many influences that together help me determine the focus of care for a given client or group of clients (Schell, 2003). Therapists' reasoning is influenced by at least four sources: the client, the practice setting, the profession, and the internal values, beliefs, and **assumptions** of the therapist (e.g., Fleming, 1991; Hooper, 1997; Mattingly & Fleming, 1994; Schell & Cervero, 1993; Tornebohm, 1991). Commonly, therapists are cognizant of some influences on their reasoning whereas other influences remain tacit, or outside of awareness. Professional growth takes place as therapists broaden their awareness of the myriad influences and personally held assumptions that shape professional reasoning and guide practice.

Thinking About Thinking 2-1

The range of what we think and do
Is limited by what we fail to notice.
And because we fail to notice
That we fail to notice
There is little we can do
To change
Until we notice
How failing to notice
Shapes our thoughts and deeds.

—From Knots by R. D. Laing

This chapter focuses specifically on how therapists' inner assumptions—specifically assumptions about the human, knowledge, and the future—may influence professional reasoning. This chapter addresses the following questions:

1. What are assumptions?
2. What evidence do we have that assumptions influence professional reasoning?
3. How do assumptions influence professional reasoning?
4. Can assumptions be accessed and changed?

WHAT ARE ASSUMPTIONS?

Assumptions continuously influence all of our actions and emotions in ways big and small. In a social situation, for example, we may assume that the two people with whom we are talking know each other. Consequently, we do not make introductions. As the conversation continues, it becomes apparent they have not met. We reply, "Oh, my apologies. I just assumed you two knew each other," and then offer introductions. In a relationship, we may become irritated with a friend or partner who did not call to say that he or she would be late.

We try to explain our reaction, "I just assumed you'd call. I was worried." These simple examples help illustrate a larger principle: Most decisions, actions, and reactions are guided by a set of assumptions about what is true and desirable.

The Oxford English Dictionary (1984) defines assumptions as that which is taken for granted as the basis for argument or action. In relation to professional reasoning, assumptions can be thought of as an underground component of reasoning that helps to orchestrate actions in practice. Valsiner (1997) defined assumptions as premises or social representations of phenomena, in our case premises or social representations of practice, which are "either explicitly considered to be true or . . . followed implicitly as their truthfulness is felt to be beyond doubt" (p. 23). For example, one therapist may assume that remediating impairments such as range of motion will automatically translate into improved participation in occupation. Another therapist may assume that participation in occupation will improve problems in body function and structures. The course of intervention that each of these therapists configures for clients may vary based on different guiding assumptions. A therapist's assumptions can be clearly recognized and acknowledged or unrecognized and beyond awareness. Either way, assumptions exist anterior to what actually happens in practice and play an influential role in what the therapist perceives is central or peripheral to occupational therapy practice. Assumptions have their roots in the therapist's personal, historical, and cultural context.

Although scholarship related to the influence of a therapist's assumptions on practice is not scarce, piecing together what we know about therapists' assumptions and professional reasoning is challenging. Difficulties arise because relevant work is scattered across a broad range of research topics and sometimes embedded in discussion sections of studies not directly exploring assumptions or professional reasoning. Perhaps most challenging, a broad array of terms are used to describe the intrapersonal dimensions of practice including "values," "beliefs," "expectations," "inner horizon," "worldview," "pretheoretical commitments," "ideological orientation," "personal paradigm" or "personal context," among others. For example, though not studying professional reasoning per se, Peloquin (1993) noted that therapists choose to be with patients in particular ways based on their *beliefs* about caring and competence; in a separate piece (1990) she noted that therapists interact with patients in ways that reflect a *vision* of the therapeutic relationship. Tornbohm (1991) put forward the idea that a therapist's *personal paradigm* regulates intervention and that this paradigm includes "assumptions about persons who are in need of occupational therapy and . . . assumptions about the aspirations of occupational therapy" (p. 452). Schell and Cervero (1993) proposed that a therapist's *personal context* is an important element of pragmatic reasoning. Hasselkus and Dickie (1994) surmised that therapists are satisfied or dissatisfied with their work based on the degree to which personal *themes of meaning* are realized or thwarted. Kielhofner and Barrett (1998) suggested that therapists engage clients in therapeutic activities that support and uphold their own *cultural narrative*. Yet regardless of the terminology and the focus of the scholarship within which assumptions have been discussed, scholars seem to agree that occupational therapists carry a set of personal and professional assumptions and that a good deal of how we view, perceive, understand, and act toward our clients and our work stem from those assumptions.

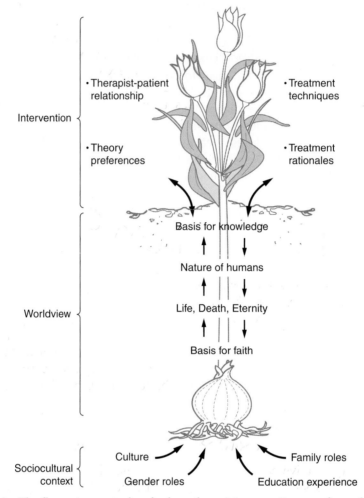

Figure 2-1   The flower is a metaphor for how therapist assumptions are formed, changed, and influence professional practice. The roots represent the sources of our views, whereas the plant above ground continues to form through an interchange of these values with both internal experience and the outside world. (Adapted with permission from *American Journal of Occupational Therapy* 1997, 51 (5), p.331.)

A flower *(Fig. 2-1)* offers a helpful metaphor for conceptualizing how assumptions, though invisible, exert a great deal of influence in action. A therapist's culture, including family, religious, social, and educational experiences, forms the root system from which personal and professional viewpoints arise. Such experiences infuse our lives with various assumptions about reality, human beings, life's purpose, knowledge, higher powers, work, and relationships, to name a few. These assumptions, taken together, establish an internal lens or viewpoint through which we filter, perceive, understand, and interact with events in the external world. This internal viewpoint guides us to particular actions and helps us explain what our actions mean.

Note that although the flower grows from the ground up, it also takes in external events such as sunlight and transports them deep inside, where they are transformative to the life of the plant. Similarly, therapists not only reason from the inside outward to actions, but also take in new experiences or life dilemmas that often alter the makeup of their deeply rooted assumptions. Life dilemmas are often born from conflicts between inner assumptions and outer experiences. Thus, there seems to be a two-way process whereby our assumptions influence how we see and what we do, while at the same time, what we see and what we do affect our assumptions. Professional reasoning, in part, involves engaging in the "conversation" happening between deeply internal and underground assumptions and external daily actions to discover the ways in which they influence each other (see Learning Activities at the end of the chapter).

WHAT EVIDENCE DO WE HAVE THAT THERAPISTS' ASSUMPTIONS ABOUT THE HUMAN INFLUENCE PROFESSIONAL REASONING?

Explicit answers and inner predispositions to the question, "What is the essence of human experience?" can shape how therapists interact with clients and approach clinical problems. Phemister (2001), referring to the reasoning process of rehabilitation counselors, said a counselor's "personal beliefs about human nature will a priori influence any theoretical orientation that is used to address disability" (p. 5). Similarly, occupational therapists' reasoning processes have been linked to their assumptions about an essence of human experience as well as assumptions about the body.

Assumptions About the Essence of Human Experience

In a qualitative case study, an occupational therapist described one essence of human experience as a process of becoming increasingly aware of a divinity within (Hooper, 1997). The therapist believed that humans (a) progressively recognize cosmic universal power as inner personal power and learn to tap that power for peace and resistance to suffering; (b) carry a long evolutionary history of movement within their subconscious, which can be tapped to recover movement patterns now limited by stroke or other trauma; (c) are a single mind-body-soul unity; and (d) are surrounded by protective layers that when diminished make them vulnerable to illness and disease. The therapist explained her practice in accord with these assumptions. For example, she said her intervention approaches increase clients' "awareness of the soul and positive thinking with the mind" (p. 333), which tap their inner power for resisting suffering. Facilitating the client's independence with eating was—for her—a means of reawakening dormant movement patterns within the subconscious of the client. She explained a patient transfer from a wheelchair as a means to calm the mind, "make the soul more aware" (p. 334) so the body will improve. This occupational therapist's assumptions about human experience offered one way she understood and explained her interventions with clients.

Kielhofner and Barrett (1998) conducted a qualitative study of how occupational therapists used goal setting in a work-focused program. Although not looking at professional reasoning specifically, they concluded that occupational therapists' selection of therapeutic activities and processes, what they called occupational forms, is deeply infused with culturally rooted ideas about the nature of human experience. Consistent with particular Western and economic cultural experiences, therapists in this study assumed that human experience is primarily organized around a progressive narrative in which "people progress forward in time, calculate steps of actions, mark passages, and set objectives to get to somewhere in the future" (p. 351). Because of this assumption, the therapists struggled to understand why goal setting and identifying steps to meet goals was not important to some clients. The therapists worked hard to persuade clients of the importance of goal setting, and when one client did not follow through with setting goals for herself, the therapists tended to question the client's motivation. The therapists were unaware of their culturally derived assumptions about human experience as a progressive journey or of how those assumptions influenced the selection of therapeutic approaches, or occupational forms, and the explanations they gave when those approaches were not successful.

The authors concluded, "Therapy is precisely founded on taken-for-granted cultural perspectives. As a consequence, therapists naturally select as therapeutic tools those occupational forms that belong to and reinforce their own conceptions of the world." (p. 351). In other words, the authors argued that therapists select intervention strategies in part from their own "deeply ingrained predisposition" and to sustain their own world view. In this study, the therapists' assumptions about human experience were out of sync with the client's, which had a negative impact on the effectiveness of therapy.

Ward's (2003) phenomenological study sought to understand a therapist's professional reasoning related to therapy with groups of clients in a community-based setting. She interviewed one expert therapist to describe how the therapist was mentally processing her clinical experiences. A good deal of the therapist's professional reasoning was focused on her inner responses to clients, what Ward described as the therapist's inner horizons. "Inner horizons are those ideas and fantasies that form the sense of self" (p. 630). While not stated specifically in these terms, I can imagine the therapist in this study reflecting on her inner responses to clients, and in those responses discovering her assumptions about what clients' needed and what they would likely achieve through occupational therapy.

Seeking to understand connections between therapists' assumptions about human nature and professional reasoning, Mekkes (2003) interviewed three occupational therapists who worked together on the same team of a rehabilitation hospital and who were identified by their colleagues as "expert." The three therapists described how they viewed the connections between their assumptions and their practice as occupational therapists. Their descriptions are summarized below. The therapists held unique assumptions about the nature of human experience and gave unique reasons for why they did what they did with clients, even as they used similar interventions. The therapists' assumptions about human experience seemed to give rise to the way in which they understood the intervention approaches they selected. Sometimes assumptions about human experience may have held more weight than the scope, domain, theoretical foundations, and research base of the profession; thus in relaying the practices of these therapists, I am not endorsing the techniques they used.

CASE STUDY 2-1

Jane

An occupational therapist for 19 years, Jane believes people are essentially good, even though that good does not always show. At their core, people share common needs to "love and be loved," to "learn," to "strive to be better," and to "care." It is important for Jane not to judge her patients if their values are in conflict with hers; her job is to "help heal them." She explained her practice as "really honing in on caring for patients and helping people to deal with tragedy. Their lives have been interrupted and they need help working through it." Jane described her work as creating an "environment that provides the opportunity for clients to heal as best as they can." She attributed many of her beliefs to her religious and cultural experiences.

Jane saw the techniques she used as helping to create a healing environment. Her primary intervention approaches included "a lot of the basic techniques taught in school" as well as "some techniques learned through continuing education." She relied heavily on neurodevelopmental treatment (NDT) approaches, "handling techniques," and other motor control strategies. She also incorporated alternative techniques such as brain gym exercises, craniosacral techniques, myofascial techniques, acupressure, and myofascial release, believing that these gave the same sensorimotor input as NDT. Jane also relied on a "strong gut level" feeling in her interactions with clients, their families, and even students. Her instincts enabled her to "walk in and really have a pretty good idea" of the recovery a patient would make. Life experiences and professional experiences, as well as verbal and nonverbal cues from the patient, informed her "gut level" impressions.

In summation, Jane viewed human experience as essentially good yet interrupted by tragedy and in need of restoration. Consequently, she interpreted her work as an occupational therapist as providing restoration through her skills in neuromotor interventions. For Jane, interventions focused at the impairment level were assumed to be doorways into a more global healing experience for the client.

John

An occupational therapist for 12 years, John saw his role as "providing an opportunity for patients to find ways that they can heal themselves or ways to compensate or accommodate to their change." John attempted to create an environment that "allows patients to find a path or way through their dysfunction toward function." He stated, "We don't fix people. Doctors and mechanics fix things." Instead, humans have "innate drives to be normal and balanced, to have power over their environment, and to find purpose in life by what they are doing." By tapping these drives, occupational therapists provide opportunities for clients to find meaning in their lives again. Thus, for John, the meaning that an activity holds for an individual was primary in his reasoning, whereas the physical performance was secondary. He emphasized the importance of his interactions with clients, believing the unique contribution of occupational therapists is the ability to immerse with the patients and connect with "the true essence of the human being." This immersion allows therapists to "find out what the true essence of the human is and connect with it and to find out what that person is feeling." The essence of the person is revealed through verbal interactions or by clients "trusting me and allowing me to be with them."

John believed he connected with the essence of his clients as he engaged them in basic and instrumental activities of daily living (ADL) such as cooking. By watching a specific patient perform an ADL, "I figured out something about him and his personality. I immersed into therapy with him. That's what OT is about." For John, an essence of human experience involves expressing innate drives toward agency, normalcy and meaning. Consequently, John believed his therapeutic interventions offered opportunities for clients to tap and express these essential drives. Interventions that targeted impairment level problems were assumed to better position clients to express innate needs for agency and purpose.

Sally

An occupational therapist for 20 years, Sally described her work as helping clients "listen to their inner guidance." In her view, illness is a physical manifestation of an internal dysfunction, and the true source of a patient's problem is a failure to see and hear the answers they have inside. Her work was rooted in a desire to "heal" others through her interactions and enable clients to see and hear those answers by helping them listen to their inner god. The therapeutic interaction in her view involved two equal persons who interact comfortably, which allows "both of us [therapist and client] to be happy and feel loved . . . and have this exchange of peace." "We can sit together and kind of gel and to know things about each other." Sally felt so strongly about the importance of basing her practice on these core assumptions that "if the only things I could use were the things I had learned when I was in school . . . then I would say I will leave the field and find something else to do."

In practice, Sally used a variety of methods she described as "holistic" and were, in her view, well suited to occupational therapy, which she saw as holistic in the same vein. Some of the interventions she used included Feldenkrais exercises, craniosacral techniques, acupressure, vision circles, energy work, and esoteric healing. She began treatment by "actively listening to what the [client's] body needs." She would "try something and see if it feels right, then trust that inner feeling." Adaptive equipment or adaptive strategies were used as "last resorts."

In the above examples, therapists' assumptions about an essence within human nature and experience, or who clients were, generally helped explain why they did what they did with clients. Consistent with the foundational beliefs of occupational therapy, these therapists had very optimistic views of human potential and they described their practice as means for tapping that potential. Each held strong assumptions about the power of the therapist-client interaction as vital to healing and reinstating meaning and purpose. Consequently, each emphasized interactions with clients as one of their most important clinical actions, even if aimed at varied ends.

The degree to which Jane, John, and Sally accepted and held on to their assumptions as "the way things are" was not clear. But these vignettes help illustrate how some practices that are adopted by therapists may actually fall outside theoretically based and evidenced-supported occupational therapy. That is, if one's assumptions are accepted uncritically and in isolation from the larger conversations of the profession, then the practices that ensue from these assumptions may be adopted uncritically as well and gradually become solidified as "the way things are," or what is most central to occupational therapy.

Assumptions About the Body

In addition to assumptions about an essence of human experience, Mattingly (1994a; 1994b) identified two sets of assumptions therapists hold about the human body that also inform occupational therapy practice. She suggested that occupational therapists, because of their relationship with biomedicine, view the body "as machine," but because of their professional roots in phenomenology also view the body as "the lived body." In her study, assumptions about the body as machine often lead therapists to focus on identifying dysfunction and designing diagnosis-specific interventions. Assumptions about the body as lived experience sometimes lead therapists to view engagement in daily living tasks as experiences whereby patients learn to reconstruct the self and re-embody the world.

There may be other body metaphors within practice that we have yet to explore. For example, the therapist I interviewed in the case study mentioned above (Hooper, 1997) at first glance seemed to focus on biomechanical dysfunction, or the body as machine. But her reasoning was rooted in her belief that the body improved only after the mind and spirit were calm. This assumption led her to use biomechanical interventions as means to address a client's agitation, depression, and distraction, which she saw as barriers to biomechanical improvements. The therapist also believed that biomechanical interventions could elicit movement patterns stored in the subconscious from all of evolutionary history. Thus, her view of the body seemed rooted in a third metaphor, Body as Means. Body as Means was also apparent in the above case of Sally (Mekkes, 2003), who believed the body is a litmus test to the degree one is listening to an inner god and that disease is an outward manifestation that one has stopped listening. Therefore, occupational therapy for her was not so much about the body, even though from an outside observers' perspective, the body was a large focus, but about reconnecting to one's inner truth through body-focused interventions.

In summation, preliminary evidence suggests that assumptions about the nature of human experience or the physical body influence how therapists think about and enact occupational therapy practice. Although largely unrecognized, the connection between assumptions about the human and practice seems powerful, perhaps in some cases even more powerful than current theory or evidence as an influence on professional reasoning (see Learning Activities 2-3 and 2-4 at the end of this chapter).

WHAT EVIDENCE DO WE HAVE THAT ASSUMPTIONS ABOUT KNOWLEDGE INFLUENCE PROFESSIONAL REASONING?

Explicit answers and inner predispositions to the questions: "How is knowledge obtained and generated" and "What is considered 'core' knowledge for occupational therapy" can shape how therapists interact with clients and approach clinical problems.

Assumptions About How Knowledge Is Obtained and Generated

To further understand assumptions about how knowledge is obtained and generated, it is helpful to turn to scholars outside of occupational therapy. Researchers in education, for example, suggest that adults progress through stages or sets of assumptions about how knowledge is acquired (Baxter Magolda, 1999; Belenky, Clenchy, Goldberger & Tarule, 1996; Kegan, 2000; King & Kitchener, 1994). The stage, and associated assumptions, a student has acquired will guide the actions a student takes in the learning process. For example, a student who assumes that knowledge about occupational therapy exists "out there" somewhere, packaged, complete, and crated like a container in a warehouse may expect instructors or the authors of books and journal articles to have access to that knowledge. The student may assume that as the primary keepers of and authorities over the knowledge, instructors and authors in occupational therapy are responsible to deliver it thoroughly and clearly. Working from this assumption, the student may select actions in the learning process focused on receiving knowledge from others. The student may be frustrated by assignments that do not lead directly to the knowledge, but rather require him or her to evaluate articles for what the author overlooks and what is yet to be known about a topic, or to create a personal practice model that synthesizes present models in the profession, or to generate a new program in a community agency that does not have occupational therapy or an insurance reimbursement system.

Generally, educational research suggests that we begin with a view of knowledge, like the example above, as certain, outside the present learning or clinical situation, and generated by and obtained from experts. From there, we move through various stages toward a view of knowledge as uncertain, existing both outside and inside the present situation, and generated and obtained through a continuous remodeling or construction process within a social group such as the profession of occupational therapy. In this stage, knowledge is not like a container housed in a warehouse somewhere; it is more like an improvisational comedy troupe. The troupe develops repeating themes out of its shared experience but builds a new "show" from those themes in response to each unique audience and venue. Similarly, practitioners in occupational therapy bring their shared understandings developed through immersion in the field's literature and build a mostly new "show" out of those themes in response to each unique client and practice venue. This view of knowledge is called "contextual knowing" (Baxter Magolda, 1999) and "constructed knowing" (King & Kitchener, 1994), but the important point is that in education one's assumptions about knowledge influence actions taken in the practice of learning.

The links established by educators between assumptions about how knowledge and actions taken in the learning process may have parallels in occupational therapy, although they are not as clearly established at this time. In the following vignettes, collected by Pace, Vernon, and Yenny (2000), therapists' assumptions about knowledge seem to play a role in how they understand and enact occupational therapy.

CASE STUDY 2-2

Jackie and Pamela's Prescriptive Views of Knowledge

Both Jackie and Pamela had approximately 10 years of experience in occupational therapy, and both women's' careers have been lived out in primarily medical model settings such as acute care and rehabilitation. In telling their career and clinical stories, Jackie and Pamela seemed to prefer highly prescriptive forms of knowing as the basis for their clinical actions and favored generalized checklists as guides for intervention. For example, Jackie stated "if it's a hip patient, they have to have a reacher, they have to have certain things in order to comply with their hip precautions. Those [specific pieces of adaptive equipment] are considered pretty essential now to go home with." Similarly, in the following scenario, Pamela follows what appears to be a prescriptive discharge plan regardless of the unique situation of the client:

> *Pamela:* We have assessed your shower and gotten you equipment you need. I will recommend that you need a shower chair and grab bars as we discussed.
> *Client:* I don't need grab bars. There's nowhere to put them up. I live in a mobile home, the walls are too thin. I'll get along fine without them; I always have.
> *Pamela:* I understand, but I still need to recommend the grab bar.

The therapist's assumptions that clients with particular diagnoses receive particular assistive devices prevented her from hearing the needs and desires of the client and exploring with the client alternatives for addressing safety. Most of the clinical stories Jackie and Pamela told seemed rooted in biomedical knowledge and implied that what counts as core knowledge for occupational therapy remains fairly static and exists outside of the therapist–client interaction and as such transcends the need for continual critical inquiry. "Some things have worked well in the past and they are still working. It's kind of hard. It's like why change it if it's not broken? I think that's the reason why I kind of resist a few things." Similarly, Jackie expressed that for several years she felt that what she had learned in school was "how I have to do it" and that there are still areas of knowledge that she "probably won't change, that I am stubborn about."

These therapists' view of knowledge as prescriptive seemed to set them up to consistently engage clients using approaches that were therapist-centered and favored procedural reasoning. Knowledge organized prescriptively and used as a checklist seemed to preclude allowing clients to discover adaptations and solutions that worked within their unique circumstances.

Pat's Hierarchical View of Knowledge

Pat has been practicing occupational therapy for approximately 20 years, a career that has ranged widely in terms of both settings and client populations. Her current practice is primarily in home care. Pat's career and clinical stories reflected much more flexibility and attention to the client's current and future situation than did Jackie and Pamela's. But while always considering the client's interests and life stories, she continually organized and used knowledge in a hierarchical structure. That is, Pat believed the "basics" or "core" of occupational therapy knowledge resided in knowing body structures as a *prerequisite* to occupational performance, stating "if I did not have the knowledge base that I have in terms of systems of the body, there's no way I could do what I am doing." Consequently, while considering the whole-life context of her clients, Pat still believed that therapy *begins* with remediating performance components. In fact, if a client is referred to an occupational therapist who doesn't understand "the balance system and how hip flexors work and how to push up with triceps in the transfer, they are going to be out of luck." The following scenarios suggest how hierarchical ways of knowing helped direct Pat's practice in particular ways:

> With the stroke patient I just saw, I'm not just going to look at him as being some-one who's got a hemi and just deal with that. I'm gonna look at his posture. I'm gonna look at how he's shifting his weight in his transfers. I'm gonna look at his balance when he's standing and then sitting down . . . . So, I'm looking at him developmentally. . . .

Similarly,

> It's not me just going in and moving a shoulder. It's me going in and moving a shoul-der and feeling a joint that's tight and teaching a patient how to relax that shoul-der. [Or teaching them] what muscles are now working that weren't working before, or how to visualize decreasing that pain because they just had a joint replacement. Or teaching them that, 'OK, you don't have full range now. But you've got enough range that if you want to make the sign of the cross when you're saying your prayers you can do it.'

From Pat's assumptions that knowledge is hierarchical, her intervention often started with remediating components and moved to functional tasks. She tended to combine procedural and narrative reasoning, and her clinical actions tended to reflect both client-centered and therapist-centered practices.

Brenda's Situated View of Knowing

Like Pat, Brenda has practiced occupational therapy for more than 10 years, and like Pamela and Jackie, many of those years were in settings dominated by the medical model. At the time of the observation, she had been a therapist in home care for approximately 9 years. From Brenda's career and clinical stories, it became apparent that she viewed knowledge as something that the client and the thera-pist constructed together out of the particularities of each client's situation. What "counted" as occupational therapy knowledge for Brenda was rooted in the needs and wants of each individual in a particular context. "The reality is . . . . where is the aggravation, or the indignation [for this particular person]?" Consequently, Brenda's practice was not prescriptive nor did her interventions draw upon a body of authoritative, hierarchical knowledge, beginning at a common point with most clients. Instead, what constituted occupational therapy for Brenda was open and tentative and was formed within the parameters of each case.

> But I mean, his very first goal was – 'What do I need to do so that my mother doesn't have to be here?' She can go back to work if you can toilet yourself and get to the kitchen to get yourself something to eat, even if somebody's already made it'. It was such a big deal to him when his mom didn't have to be there.
> I also knew there wasn't a real good connection between doing upper extremity exercises and getting back to what he wanted to do. . . the fact was he was still having to have his sister shave him. And so I remember that person, saying 'let's see

if we can figure out a way for you to sit up and prop up your arms' because he hated having somebody else shave him.

By holding her understanding of core occupational therapy knowledge tentatively, and by creating knowledge within the therapist–client context, Brenda was able to allow clients to express their inherent agency and re-create lives that made sense to them. Consequently, her professional reasoning was dominated by narrative and conditional thinking as she worked to understand the occupational stories of the client within the social and physical contexts in which the person lived, and the meanings of the illness for both the client and the family.

> They are very often at the point where they've just gone through an entirely dis-orienting experience, they're back home, and the environment where they may have had more control before is now an environment where they need assistance. The bowling trophy up on the mantel is just a reminder that you can't get out of the chair by yourself, let alone fling a bowling ball. And so, those rhythms are disrupted.

Although Brenda realized that an understanding of the underlying physical aliments is an important aspect of clinical treatment, she tended to engage in less procedural reasoning than the other three therapists. She focused almost entirely on the life story and histories of her clients.

> [Your] life may not look like it used to but we'll get it back to something that looks like a life that you'll like. [If] I come in and [say] 'you've had a stroke. Well, let's just measure your arms and let's do this and let's do that.' I can come up with a ton of goals from that, but it's not necessarily going to mean anything [to you].

In the above vignettes, the specific combination of professional reasoning modes addressed in subsequent chapters of this book (procedural, interactive, narrative, and conditional reasoning) may have been influenced in part by each therapist's assumptions about how knowledge is obtained, generated, and utilized, whether prescriptive, hierarchical, or contextual/constructed. The development of more complex forms of professional reasoning, then, may involve among other things transforming one's assumptions about knowledge. Simultaneously, the practice of more complex professional reasoning may itself be a process that presses the therapist toward new assumptions that knowledge is contextual and constructed. That is, expert professional reasoning makes demands on therapists to assemble knowledge about a client, a diagnosis, occupational needs, a practice model or models, available and absent evidence, a practice setting, and their own experience and viewpoints into a particular construction of what intervention will be *in this case*. The nature of knowledge about interventions and diagnoses and client needs is not fixed, prescriptive, or authoritative, but uncertain and assembled in context. Thus, a therapist's assumptions about how knowledge is obtained, generated, and utilized in practice will influence professional reasoning, but simultaneously the practice of more complex professional reasoning rests on and calls for the development of particular assumptions about knowledge.

Assumptions About What Knowledge Is Core to Occupational Therapy Practice

It is difficult to find research in occupational therapy specifically framed to study the connection between therapists' assumptions about what constitutes core knowledge in the field and their clinical practice. But there are studies that seem to address this link indirectly. For example, Burke (2001) studied the "theoretical perspectives used by occupational therapists during pediatric evaluation situations and the variation of perspectives among therapists" (pp. 49-50). I see the therapists' fundamental assumptions about *what* knowledge, or theoretical perspective, is most central to practice as another important aspect of her work. In order to understand "how the therapists' perceptions of their work are informed by the occupational therapy conceptual models they use" (p. 49), Burke observed four occupational therapists during a pediatric evaluation, each using the same evaluation tool. Findings suggested that therapists enacted and made sense of the evaluation based on two divergent views of practice: a medical/scientific view and an occupational view. A medical/scientific view led therapists to concentrate on physical signs of the client's problem and target issues related to the symptom or problem in the evaluation process. An occupational science perspective led therapists to emphasize the human as an occupational being in need of meaningful engagement and to focus on breakdowns in occupations within particular social and temporal contexts, as well as the individual's important activities across multiple roles. Burke also found that therapists working from an occupational perspective addressed medical issues once and occupation issues 14 times in the first 10 minutes of the evaluation, whereas therapists working from a medical/scientific perspective addressed medical issues seven times in the first 10 minutes of assessment and did not address occupation issues at all.

In this study, what Burke (2001) called theoretical "perspective" led to different kinds of information being solicited even when therapists used the same evaluation tool. Burke saw the clinical actions associated with an occupational perspective as more likely to represent the unique and vital contribution of occupational therapy, not duplicating the language and practices of other disciplines serving pediatric clients. "Of greater issue is that these differences represent contrasting definitions of the intent of occupational therapy" (p 59). Burke's study helps illustrate that what therapists adopt as core knowledge influences clinical actions. However, there is a possibility that different models of practice rest upon and demand different assumptions about how knowledge is obtained and generated and that the alignment to a therapist's personal knowledge beliefs may make one model more attractive than the other (see Learning Activity 2-5).

WHAT EVIDENCE DO WE HAVE THAT ASSUMPTIONS ABOUT THE FUTURE INFLUENCE PROFESSIONAL REASONING?

Hasselkus and Dickie (1994) suggested that "our therapy exists in the shadow (or the light) of the end; that is, in our hopes and images of the future and what we will be able to bring about for our patients and for ourselves" (p. 153).

Assumptions about the future seem to fall within at least three categories in the occupational therapy literature: the future of the client, the future of the therapist, and the ultimate future beyond time.

The Future of the Client

Hasselkus and Dickie (1994) studied the satisfying and dissatisfying experiences of occupational therapists working with adults who had experienced a cerebral vascular accident (CVA). Therapists' assumptions about the future of the client were expressed as "expectations" about what would occur in the near future as a result of rehabilitation. Therapists expected clients to make improvements related to their "arm and hand." That is, they expected the client's immediate and short-term future to entail neuromotor change in the upper extremity and return of function. As a result of this expectation, therapists selected treatment approaches and techniques they believed were associated with neuromotor recovery and often persisted with those approaches even after a client's recovery seemed to plateau. Some therapists viewed their role as facilitators of the neuromotor changes that did occur, even though they recognized that a large part of recovery after CVA is spontaneous. Therapists also expected that clients' would regain enjoyment in occupations that had been meaningful before their stroke and would be able to return home. These assumptions about the course of clients' near futures served not only to guide therapeutic approaches but also as criteria by which the therapists judged the success of their therapy. When the therapists' expectations for a client's future were thwarted, they felt dissatisfied with the therapy experience. Hasselkus and Dickie concluded that "occupational therapy in stroke practice was driven by expectations" (p. 636).

Similarly, in an ethnographic study of therapists' professional reasoning, Mattingly (1991, 1994) found that occupational therapists infused a story of the future onto clients with whom they worked and that these future-stories guided actions in treatment. Therapists imagine a certain future and then imagine how they might guide the patient toward achieving that future. Therapists reasoned about "how to guide their therapy with a particular patient by using images of where this patient is at now and where this patient might be at some future time when the patient will be discharged" (p. 240). How therapists *imagined* the future of a patient gave them "a basis for organizing [intervention] tasks." Although therapists in the study continually revised their stories about clients' futures, these stories consistently served as one means to structure therapy.

The Future of the Therapist

In addition to assumptions about clients' futures, Hasselkus and Dickie (1994) found that occupational therapy practice was intimately tied to the therapist's vision of his or her own future, or personal process of becoming. Satisfying therapy experiences were those that supported the therapists' image of his or her own future and image of the possible good, times when "the essence of our being-in-the-world as occupational therapists is made manifest" (p. 153). This is consistent with Mekkes (2003) study, in which all three participating therapists described their work as contributing to their desire to be positive role models to others and bring good things into their lives. Peloquin (1997) suggested that therapists, like patients, are in the process of "making worlds and making lives. "From behind the label 'therapist' emerges a person who hopes to make a difference and a connection . . . we can see acts of making within the roles of patient and therapist" (p. 168).

The Ultimate Future Beyond Time

The specific difference each therapist believes he or she is making may be rooted in assumptions about the ultimate good to which therapists see their work contributing in a future beyond time. In the case study I conducted (Hooper, 1997), the therapist reported that her work helped individuals to fight suffering and overcome difficulty. Fighting suffering was related to how one reaches a better status in the afterlife. For her, occupational therapy was not just about helping her clients achieve better function now; it was also part of helping them accomplish improved status, more peace, and less strife in an afterlife. In the case examples used earlier in this chapter from Mekkes' (2003) study, Sally described her work as helping clients reconnect with the god or light within. She, too, held a view that her work connected to a future beyond this place. Thus sometimes therapists see their work as serving an ultimate good. These assumptions may not directly influence the treatment approaches therapists select but rather offer a way of explaining why they do what they do. In other words, assumptions about the ultimate future to which occupational therapy contributes may not lead to specific clinical actions, but to an explanation of what lies at the heart of a therapist's practice.

HOW DO ASSUMPTIONS SHAPE PROFESSIONAL REASONING?

Assumptions shape what therapists see, affect the interpretation they make, and guide what course of action they select. Specifically, *how* assumptions guide perception and action may be understood in light of the evolution of assumptions into **"habits of expectation"** (Mezirow, 1991). That is, through the reinforcement of culture, experience, and language, one's assumptions about humans, knowledge and future, among others, may be said to "gel" into habits of expectation. In turn, habits of expectation act to selectively determine the scope of our attention by filtering information and guiding perceptions toward what to notice, what to ignore, what is relevant, and what is irrelevant. Thus, habits of expectation provide a basis for judging and selecting and interpreting what an experience means. It is as if this internal perceptual screen sets us up to see, act, and interpret in habitual ways. Therefore, assumptions play an influential role in action by (a) filtering and directing attention, (b) guiding and constricting choices, and (c) interpreting the meaning of an act or experience (Mezirow, 2000). In occupational therapy practice, this means that assumptions can serve as one means by which therapists filter their attention, prioritize and select actions, and construe meaning about what clients need. Tornbohm (1991) argued that, depending on the level of understanding therapists have about their own assumptions or paradigms, their assumptions or paradigms could support, limit, or contradict clinical actions.

The concept "habits of expectation" helps explain the role of assumptions when they seem consistent with action, but it doesn't explain instances when assumptions appear to limit or contradict clinical action. Barris (1987) identified such a limitation when therapists believed or assumed that mutual rapport with clients was necessary to the therapeutic process yet, at the same time, interviewed clients using unbalanced interactions between themselves and patients and unconsciously maintained control by asking questions, disregarding patient's comments and dominating conversations. Borell, Gustavson, Sandman, and Kielhofner (1994) found that the staff at a day hospital program for clients with dementia held certain assumptions about what clients needed and how they should be treated, but did not always choose actions consistent with those assumptions. The staff assumed that stimulating activities should be provided and that some measure of control must always be enforced. To maintain control, the staff did not allow patients to clear their own plates after meals, believing that too many people moving around the dining room could contribute to anxiety or chaos. Although barring table clearing allowed the staff some control, it had the additional effect of limiting or reducing the patient's activity level, despite a commitment to providing stimulating routines.

How assumptions both guide actions and, at times, conflict with actions may be understood in light of Grene's (1971) concept of belief clusters. Studying the role that teachers' beliefs played in practice, Grene suggested that practitioners hold beliefs or assumptions in clusters. Some belief clusters may be closely aligned to one another, whereas other belief clusters remain very separate and "as long as the incompatible beliefs are never set side by side and examined for inconsistency, the incompatibility may remain" (Richardson, 1994, p. 91). Tornbohm (1991) related contradictions between assumptions and actions to the therapist not having a paradigm broad or deep enough for satisfactory and consistent intervention.

In summation, as **perceptual filters**, assumptions form the screen through which therapists view and understand therapeutic experiences. A therapist's assumptions become a habituated way of seeing clinical events and focus attention on specific cues within the therapy environment. From behind that screen, certain professional actions emerge on a "horizon of possibility . . . that represents values regarding ends, norms and criteria for judgment" (Mezirow, 1991, p. 62), whereas other equally valid, if not better, actions do not. Therapists' assumptions can be more or less coherent and integrated with action.

What If Our Assumptions Are Limiting to How We Practice?

According to Mezirow (1991), "there is much evidence to support the assertion that we tend to accept and integrate experiences that comfortably fit our frame of reference and discount those that do not" (p. 35). Therefore, the structure of assumptions through which we "come to perceive and understand ourselves and the world we inhabit" can also "limit and distort what we are able to perceive and understand" (Dirkx, 1998, p. 4). Overcoming limited perspectives involves "reflection on assumptions that formerly have been accepted uncritically . . ." (Mezirow, 1991, p. 5).

But if assumptions are largely tacit, how do we access, reflect on, and modify them? Two processes have been described in the education literature that may help. One process is more cognitive or rational and one takes a more imaginative approach to reflection. The cognitive-rational approach asks us to reflect on the content of our actions along with the process and premises within our action (Mezirow, 1991). Reflection on content involves thinking about what happened. Reflection on process involves thinking about how we were perceiving, thinking, judging, feeling, and acting within what happened. Reflection on premises involves thinking about *why* we perceive, think, feel, or act as we do in situations like the one that happened. Premise reflection can lead us to discover influential taken for granted or tacit assumptions. Premise reflection is the dynamic by which our assumptions "become transformed" (Mezirow, 1991, p. 111).

The more imaginative approach to reflection draws attention to the images that emerge in the mind's eye, or the metaphors that come to mind, as we work with clients and think about our practice (Dirkx, 1998; Dirkx, 2000). In adult learning, these images and metaphors are believed to be a window into assumptions, beliefs, needs, and desires that are tacit. This approach invites adults to enter into an internal, exploratory dialogue with such images to gain deeper awareness of themselves in relation to their practice and the world (Dirkx, 1998). For occupational therapists, this approach would involve shifting reflection from what happened in practice and why to reflecting on the images and words that suddenly come to mind or play consistently like a movie in the back of our minds as we work with a given family, client, group or population of clients, or a particular setting. In the case examples in this chapter, one therapist used the metaphor of "healer" to describe her practice, one described herself as "enabler," one said she "merges" with the client, one said, "we don't fix things, mechanics fix things." These are all images that upon reflection, upon entering a dialogue with, can open a door into tacitly held assumptions that may be influencing practice.

PROFESSIONAL REASONING: THINKING IN AN INWARD DIRECTION

Chapter 1 defines and subsequent chapters discuss several types of reasoning used by occupational therapists, including scientific, procedural, interactive, ethical, narrative, pragmatic and conditional reasoning. Professional reasoning is often discussed in terms of how the therapist is thinking about and assembling external phenomena, such as the client's diagnosis and symptoms, the occupations a client wants and needs to perform, the expectations and engagement of the family, the constraints of the practice setting, and the possible futures a client may inhabit. For example, when a therapist uses procedural reasoning, he or she is usually "thinking about the patient's physical performance problems" (Burke, 2001, p. 50). When a therapist uses interactive reasoning "the therapist works to understand the patient as a person" (p. 51). When a therapist uses conditional reasoning, "the therapist thinks more deeply about the whole condition involving the person, the illness, the family, the physical environment, and society" (p. 51). Each of these forms of reasoning involves consideration of *outward* phenomena, thinking outward toward the client. But this chapter has highlighted consideration of inner phenomena, or thinking in an *inward* direction to the self.

SUMMARY

Reflection on one's assumptions about human beings, knowledge, the profession and the future, and on how those intrapersonal truths link to practice is as important as processing external cues related to the client's condition and context. Thus, one aspect of professional reasoning involves asking how is what I'm doing "out there" reflective of who I am and the assumptions I hold "in here" [inside myself]? How do my explanations of what I do "out there" reveal the assumptions I hold "in here?" What do I tell myself about the ultimate worth of my work and how is that being played out in what I do with clients? How is what I do with clients revealing what I assume to be true about humans, knowledge, and the future? The answers to these questions constitute the stories we tell ourselves about work as an occupational therapist, and those stories in turn influence what we do and why we do it.

Some may think such esoteric questions are more spiritual in nature than clinical. And perhaps the literature on spirituality in occupational therapy helps further clarify the intrapersonal dimension of professional reasoning with which this chapter has dealt. In describing how occupational therapists address spirituality with clients, Hammel (2001) proposed substituting the term "spirituality" with the term **"intrinsicality."** Intrinsicality is "a personal philosophy of meaning with which we interpret our lives. . . .that informs life choices and life satisfaction" (pp. 186, 190). Although therapists consider the intrinsicality of each client, I have suggested in this chapter that we also consider our own intrinsicality, our individualized sets of assumptions about humans, knowledge, and the future through which we interpret and enact our work. These assumptions may mediate our actions with clients and our interpretations of what constitutes occupational therapy by influencing how we configure the other aspects of clinical reasoning discussed in this book. For example, the therapist who assumes that scientific, objective knowledge supported with hard evidence constitutes "real" knowledge may give more weight to the procedural aspects of reasoning and less weight to information obtained through the client's narrative, and may not recognize the embodiment of practice as a legitimate form of knowing. Alternatively, the therapist who assumes that "real" knowledge is located in the particular experiences of the individual client within a social context may rely heavily on interactive, conditional, and narrative types of reasoning. Assuming that client interaction is the core of practice, a therapist may not stand back to recognize the larger system-wide assumptions that exist in the practice setting (part of pragmatic reasoning). In addition, the ethical issues that "grab" each therapist may vary based on how the therapist believes human beings are related to each other, to higher powers, to activity, to the medical system, and to society. Of course, as the stories in this chapter indicate, the relationship between assumptions and practice is much more messy and obscure than these simple examples illustrate. More commonly, assumptions seem to remain partially veiled, and the links with action are often contradictory or even untraceable. The obscure nature of assumptions and the shadowy ways they influence practice emphasize the importance of teaching students to tune into and discern assumptions the best they can.

LEARNING ACTIVITY 2-1

Cultivating Links Between Assumptions and Action

Purpose

To trace assumptions into particular actions

Connections to Major Professional Reasoning Constructs

- Assumptions
- Perception or ways of seeing
- Actions based on assumptions or perceptions

Directions for Learners

We've all had experiences sometimes called "aha" experiences. "Aha" experiences can happen when we are unaware of a set of assumptions we hold; then something happens and those assumptions are brought into new light.

Can you think of an experience like that? It may have been assumptions you held about gender, about learning, about a group of people, about a "truth" you held dear, about money or about occupational therapy. Try to recapture the details of that experience by doing the following:

1 Draw two plants like the one in Figure 2-1. One plant represents your experience before that "aha." The second plant represents your experience after the "aha." On the stem of plant one, draw the beliefs and assumptions that came into light. On the petals, draw the actions that were related to those assumptions; and
2 On the stem of plant two, sketch your new or newly developing assumptions. Trace the assumptions outward to the actions they support. Compare the two for the influence of assumptions on action.

LEARNING ACTIVITY 2-2

Explaining Professional Reasoning

Purpose

To define and explain in your own words how assumptions are related to other elements of professional reasoning

Connections to Major Professional Reasoning Constructs

- Elements of professional reasoning
- Importance of assumptions to professional reasoning

Directions for Learners

Imagine yourself working as an occupational therapist. A student has come to your setting for his Field Work Level I experience. In your own words:

1 Explain to the student professional reasoning and the sources of information therapists need to consider; and
2 Include an example of why therapists' own assumptions are important to consider in professional reasoning.

LEARNING ACTIVITY 2-3

Cultivating Links Between Views of the Human and Practice

Purpose

To illustrate the influence of assumptions on actions taken in practice

Connections to Major Professional Reasoning Constructs

- Assumptions about human experience/body

Directions for Learners

1 Pick any three assumptions about the human mentioned either in the literature reviewed or the stories provided in this chapter;
2 Draw three more tulips; and
3 Illustrate the underground assumption in relation to its outer actions.

LEARNING ACTIVITY 2-4

Cultivating Personal Assumptions

Purpose

To "dig up" tacitly held assumptions about the essence of human experience.

Connections to Major Professional Reasoning Constructs

- Assumptions about human experience/body

Directions for Learners

1 Drawing upon your personal, spiritual, professional experiences, complete the following sentences as spontaneously as you can.
   - Human beings at their core are . . . OR human experience is essentially about. . . .
   - By that, I mean. . . .
   - An individual is valuable because. . . .
   - By that, I mean. . . .
   - As a therapist, these beliefs influence my practice by. . . .
2 Think of a person you greatly admire and hold in highest esteem, a person you would love to model your life after.
   - Describe the qualities of that person.
3 What do those qualities teach you about what you value about human experience?

LEARNING ACTIVITY 2-5

Cultivating Links Between Practice and Assumptions About Knowledge

Purpose

To "dig up" and reflect on tacitly held assumptions about knowledge

Connections to Major Professional Reasoning Constructs

- Assumptions about knowledge known to be true.

Directions for Learners

The first three exercises focus on personal experiences not specific to occupational therapy. The assumptions we hold about knowledge in the rest of life can become a window helping us look at our assumptions in professional experiences.

1 Think of a time in your life when you believed something to be absolutely "true," then discovered what you believed was largely a product of where you grew up or how you were raised or when you grew up. [*Note:* This doesn't mean the belief was not valid, but simply that it was more culturally shaped than you had realized.]
   - What was the belief(s) you held?
   - What happened to cause you to see the belief in a whole new light?
   - What features of the belief that had previously been invisible came into view?
2 Try to map your experience using the tulip diagram.
3 What did that experience teach you about what we know and how we know it?
4 Can you apply what you learned from your personal experience to how you view knowledge in occupational therapy?
   - For example, what knowledge do you believe is "true" for the profession?
   - What cultural influences have shaped your assumption?
5 What can be said about knowledge based on your personal and professional experiences?

REFERENCES

Barris, R. (1987). Professional reasoning in psychosocial occupational therapy: The evaluation process. *Occupational Therapy Journal of Research, 7,* 147–162.

Baxter Magolda, M. (1999). *Creating contexts for learning and self-authorship: Constructive-developmental pedagogy.* Nashville, TN: Vanderbilt University Press.

Belenky, M. F., Clenchy, B. M., Goldberger, N. R. & Tarule, J. M. (1996). *Women's ways of knowing* (2nd ed.). New York: Basic Books.

Borell, L., Gustavsson, A., Sandman, P. & Kielhofner, G. (1994). Occupational programming in a day hospital for patients with dementia. *Occupational Therapy Journal of Research, 14*(4), 219–238.

Burke, J. P. (2001). How therapists' conceptual perspectives influence early intervention evaluations. *Scandinavian Journal of Occupational Therapy*, 8, 49–61.

Dirkx, J. M. (1998). Transformative Learning Theory in the Practice of Adult Education: An Overview. *PAACE Journal of Lifelong Learning*, 7, 1–14.

Dirkx, J. M. (2000). *Transformative learning and the journey of individuation*. ERIC Clearinghouse on Adult Career and Vocational Education, [microform: 1 v]. Columbus, OH: ERIC Clearinghouse on Adult Career and Vocational Education Center on Education and Training for Employment College of Education the Ohio State University.

Fleming, M., H. (1991). The therapist with the three-track mind. *American Journal of Occupational Therapy*, 45(11), 1007–1014.

Hammell, K. W. (2001). Intrinsicality: Reconsidering spirituality, meaning(s), and mandates. *Canadian Journal of Occupational Therapy*, 68(3), 186–194.

Hasselkus, B. R. & Dickie, V. A. (1994). Doing occupational therapy: Dimensions of satisfaction and dissatisfaction. *American Journal of Occupational Therapy*, 48(2), 145–154.

Hooper, B. (1997). The relationship between pretheoretical assumptions and professional reasoning. *American Journal of Occupational Therapy*, 51(5), 328–338.

Kegan, R. (2000). What "form" transforms? A constructive-developmental approach to transformative learning. In J. Mezirow (Ed.). *Learning as transformation: Critical perspectives on a theory in progress* (pp. 35–70). San Francisco: Jossey-Bass, Inc.

Kielhofner, G. & Barrett, L. (1998). Meaning and misunderstanding in occupational forms: A study of therapeutic goal setting. *American Journal of Occupational Therapy*, 52(5), 345–353.

King, K. P. & Kitchener, K. S. (1994). *Developing reflective judgment: Understanding and promoting intellectual growth and critical thinking in adolescents and adults*. San Francisco: Jossey-Bass.

Mattingly, C. (1991). The narrative nature of professional reasoning. *American Journal of Occupational Therapy*, 45(11), 998–1005.

Mattingly, C. (1994a). Occupational therapy as a two-body practice: The body as machine. In C. Mattingly & M. Fleming, H. (Eds.). *Professional reasoning: Forms of inquiry in a therapeutic practice* (pp. 37–63). Philadelphia: F.A. Davis.

Mattingly, C. (1994b). Occupational therapy as a two-body practice: The lived body. In C. Mattingly & M. Fleming, M. H. (Eds.). *Professional reasoning: Forms of inquiry in a therapeutic practice* (pp. 64–93). Philadelphia: F.A. Davis.

Mekkes, M. (2003). *The influence of occupational therapist's worldview on professional reasoning: A Qualitative study*. Unpublished, Grand Valley State University, Grand Rapids, MI.

Mezirow, J. (1991). *Transformative dimensions of adult learning*. San Francisco: Jossey-Bass.

Mezirow, J. (2000). *Learning as transformation: critical perspectives on a theory in progress*. San Francisco: Jossey-Bass.

Pace, J., Vernon, D. & Yenny, C. (2000). *Understanding professional reasoning and clinical actions through the exploration of therapists' assumptions*. Unpublished master's thesis, University of North Carolina, Chapel Hill.

Peloquin, S. (1990). The patient-therapist relationship in occupational therapy: understanding visions and images. *American Journal of Occupational Therapy*, 44(1), 13–21.

Peloquin, S. (1993). The patient-therapist relationship: beliefs that shape care. *American Journal of Occupational Therapy*, 47(10), 935–942.

Peloquin, S. (1997). Nationally speaking. The spiritual depth of occupation: making worlds and making lives. *American Journal of Occupational Therapy*, 51(3), 167–168.

Schell, B. (2003). Professional reasoning: The basis for practice. In E. B. Crepeau, E. S. Cohn & B. A. B. Schell (Eds.). *Willard & Spackman's occupational therapy* (10th ed., pp. 131–140). Philadelphia: Lippincott Williams & Wilkins.

Schell, B. & Cervero, R. (1993). Professional reasoning in occupational therapy: An integrative review. *American Journal of Occupational Therapy*, 47(7), 605–610.

Törnbohm, H. (1991). What is worth knowing in occupational therapy? *American Journal of Occupational Therapy*, 45(5), 451–454.

Valsiner, J. (1997). Basic assumptions underlying psychological research. In J. Valsiner (Ed.). *Culture and the development of children's action: A theory of human development* (pp. 23–66). New York: John Wiley & Sons.

Ward, J. D. (2003). The nature of professional reasoning with groups: A phenomenological study of an occupational therapist in community mental health. *American Journal of Occupational Therapy*, 57(6), 625–634.

3

Information Processing Theory and Professional Reasoning

Martha Carr and Mary Shotwell

CHAPTER OUTLINE

The role of information processing
Information processing as a model
  Working memory
  Long-term memory
Metacognition and self-regulation
Automaticity

Expertise theory and information processing
Integrated knowledge base
Differences in strategy use
Automaticity through experience
Regulation of problem solving
Summary

OBJECTIVES

After reading this chapter, the learner will be able to:

1 Understand the role of information processing as a part of professional reasoning.
2 Describe theories explaining cognitive aspects of reasoning including frame, ACT*, and Dual Code theories.
3 Describe the impact of metacognition upon professional reasoning.
4 Articulate how the novice to expert continuum applies to cognitive components of professional reasoning.
5 Be able to apply what we know about information processing to a specific case.

KEY TERMS

Information processing

Working memory (or short-term memory)

Long-term memory

Cues

Metacognition

Automaticity

Expertise

I n this chapter, we explore the mental processes that are fundamental to reasoning. A major portion of this discussion comes from information processing literature in psychology. The first part of the chapter is devoted to helping you understand how our brains organize and process information that is used in professional reasoning. Such concepts as long-term and working memory are argued. The next section of the chapter describes several theories that may explain cognitive aspects of reasoning. Such theories as Frame, ACT*, and Dual Code are used as a foundation. In the middle of the chapter, we discuss "thinking about our own thinking" or metacognition. Next, the novice to expert continuum is compared with some of the components of professional reasoning. The last portion of the chapter is devoted to application of these aspects of information processing in the form of a case study depiction of professional reasoning.

Thinking About Thinking 3-1

We know most at this point about what knowledge acquisition is not—namely, the incremental accumulation of facts or associations.

—Deanna Kuhn (2002)

THE ROLE OF INFORMATION PROCESSING

Information processing refers to the organization of our memories and the processes used to learn and use information in those memories. To frame this chapter, we are using a case to help illustrate how information processing is involved in clinical reasoning. As seen later on in this chapter, we store many significant memories for later use. These memories are organized into frames or scripts. Many professionals have "frames" or "scripts" of experiences that include "what works" and "what doesn't work." We also store memories related to our senses including memories of smells, sounds, and images. We use these memories to interpret and understand what we experience. The Case Study below describes a case in which Mary (the second author of this chapter) discovered a client whose situation challenged her clinical reasoning processes.

CASE STUDY 3-1

Mary and Leslie

Mary's Reflection

The case of Leslie challenged me clinically and made me question my clinical reasoning. Having been an occupational therapist for some 22 years, I was confident in my clinical skills. While completing my doctorate, I decided to take on some clinical work. I had just started working in a private practice pediatric setting and assumed the caseload of a therapist who recently relocated to another state. Having worked in many settings with many types of children, I did not expect to encounter any surprises in this setting even though I had not treated pediatric clients for about 3 years. The case of Leslie is memorable because I can recall feeling "blown away" after the first therapy session.

When I was given my new caseload, I contacted each family and asked questions about the child's interests to help guide me in planning occupation-based sessions, as was my usual practice. When I contacted Leslie's mother to set up an appointment, I asked her about Leslie's interests, functional abilities, and her mother's goals for Leslie. Mom informed me that Leslie liked to read and play in her room, but she was "not into age-appropriate things like Barbie's, baby dolls, or playing school." Since the time of year was around Halloween, I asked if she was going to dress up for Halloween. Leslie's mother reported that Leslie was not interested in dressing up and that it was enough work getting her into regular clothes, let alone a Halloween costume. She then informed me that Leslie was a "PT/OT co-treat, so the PT would fill me in on the specifics about Leslie."

Background on Leslie

Leslie was a 9-year-old girl with a diagnosis of autism, who was being seen in an outpatient clinic for occupational, physical, and speech therapy. She had received occupational therapy since she was 2 years old. Leslie's occupational therapy goals were to improve her performance in activities of daily living, to improve her ability to tolerate textures and sensations such as movement, and to maximize her ability to attend and participate in daily life tasks. Notes written by the prior therapist indicated that most of the treatment sessions were focused on getting Leslie engaged in any purposeful activities.

"Once You Pop, You Can't Stop"

Ellen, the physical therapist, was out sick for my first visit with Leslie. Leslie came into the setting "on fire" as Mom explained, stating: "She (Leslie) had a rough day at school. . .I have my younger son in the car sleeping. . .I'll be back in an hour" (what felt to be one of the longest hours of my life). I knew from the clinic director that this child had "sensory integrative issues" so I chose a therapy area that had suspended equipment. Leslie was nonverbal, so I tried to connect with her by showing her toys and equipment that she might be interested in. She immediately ran for the toy closet and pulled out the "popper," which is a toy probably familiar to most of us (Fig. 3-1).

Many children use this "popper" toy in an imaginative or imitative way to pretend they are vacuuming or mowing the lawn. Leslie took the toy and "plopped" down on the floor and just started looking at the balls. Leslie made eye contact with me and smiled, then went back to looking at the colored balls inside the popper. The next week I found out that other therapists hide this toy and the Barney toy when Leslie comes in, to prevent her from playing with these objects in a nonpurposeful manner at the expense of engaging in any other activity.

Finding the Problem Space

My typical flow of a therapy session with children who have sensory integrative deficits is to incorporate vestibular, tactile, or proprioceptive activities into

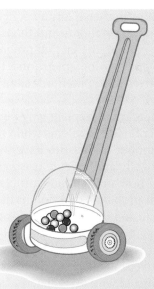

Figure 3-1   Popper toy.

activities. Usually, I have information about the child to make the sessions more geared toward the interests of the child or the family, but in this case, Leslie was nonverbal and her Mom had also not offered much information, so I believe that I began focusing on deficits rather than strengths. Leslie just sat on the floor and I made several attempts to lure her over to any suspended equipment to get her moving. When I touched the "popper" in an attempt to shift attention to more purposeful activity, Leslie held on tightly as if to let me know she wasn't going to let go of the toy.

I know that I "froze" several times during the session. I was also new to this practice, and I didn't want the other therapists to think that I was inept. After several attempts to lure Leslie toward equipment that might help her, I finally decided not to fight her and I began using the popper to lure her to change her activity pattern. We began to play a tug-of-war game with the popper, which I could justify as giving her proprioceptive input. I followed this by pulling the popper toward the ball pit, where I lured Leslie into for more proprioceptive input. After this activity, I was able to use the popper to briefly lure her onto a suspended swing all the while using the popper to pull her back and forth on the swing.

When doing therapy with children who experience sensory integrative dysfunction, I usually start with more gross and sensory motor activities leading up to more functional activities appropriate for each child. With Leslie, I never made it beyond the suspended equipment during a 50-minute session. I was relieved to at least have gotten Leslie to move off the floor, but felt that the session was somewhat wasted by my "trying to figure out what to do."

At the end of the first session, Mom cheerfully picked up Leslie stating "I have to get my son to an appointment, so I'll see you next week." Driving home, I kept racking my brain for what I could have done differently. I hoped that next week, the physical therapist who had worked with this child for the past 2 years might give me some insight into Leslie's behavior as well as fill me in on "what worked" with this child.

Mary, the therapist in this case example, activated a script or frame that had previously worked with other clients and then based Leslie's therapy session on that frame. As she reflected on the lack of progress during the session, Mary realized that she was not going to be able to use the usual default techniques. She thought about alternatives to the methods she typically used and was able create an alternative approach.

Cognitive researchers try to explain why people like Mary are able to quickly assemble solutions to complex problems while remaining able to flexibly respond to new situations. A number of theories have been proposed to explain both our tendencies to automatically and quickly use well-learned approaches to problem solving and to explain how more expert problem solvers can be thoughtful and flexible in dealing with problems that do not fit the mold. As you read this chapter, you will learn about the different theories that explain problem solving and how these theories may be applied to occupational therapy.

Our ability to process information, to draw conclusions based on that information, and to make decisions depends to a large extent on what we know, how our knowledge is organized, and our capacity for simultaneously considering different types of information from different sources. To make an appropriate decision about treatment, health practitioners must coordinate information from a number of sources, including data from assessments, client history, and what the clinician sees, hears, or feels with what is known about a client's diagnosis. As practitioners gain experience and knowledge, they are better able to coordinate the many sources of information with their knowledge. As a result, experienced practitioners can make fast and accurate diagnoses of situations and make an appropriate intervention plan. Less experienced practitioners, in contrast, may not be able to attend to all relevant information, may not be able to distinguish between what is important and what is not important, and will be less able to coordinate what they are experiencing with what they know. In addition, more novice practitioners may be slower and less accurate in evaluation and intervention planning (Robertson, 1996b). Here, we deal with what we know about the development of expertise from the perspective of cognitive psychology and information processing theory. First, we discuss some of the basic mechanisms and structures that make up our cognitive systems. Much of the research and theory described is the seminal work in the area. We then discuss the development of skill in the form of higher-order metacognitive reasoning and automated processing. Finally, the development of expertise and how it might be applied to occupational therapy is presented.

INFORMATION PROCESSING AS A MODEL

Information processing is a model of cognition that uses metaphors from computer programming as a way of understanding the mind. Atkinson and Shiffrin (1968) proposed that information processing involves two systems, working memory and long-term memory, which work together to allow us to learn, comprehend, and respond to our experiences.* The first type of memory, **working memory**, also

---

*A third memory system called sensory memory or sensory register also exists but is not discussed here because it is not involved in processing or long-term storage of information.

called **short-term memory,** mediates our perceptions of the world with our memory or knowledge of the world. The primary purpose of working memory is to process, but not store, information. It is considered a memory because information is stored longer than it is perceptually experienced. This enables us to make sense of the incoming information and to reflect on what we experience.

The second system involved in information processing is the **long-term memory,** which is considered a storage system for both declarative knowledge and procedural knowledge (Anderson, 1983). Declarative knowledge is what we know. For example, much of the scientific information we use in clinical reasoning, such as our knowledge of diagnostic sequelae, which helps us understand a client's medical prognosis, would be considered declarative knowledge. Procedural knowledge is the ability to do something such as perform various intervention or assessment techniques. Fieldwork experiences require students to use declarative knowledge to define problems, whereas students must use procedural knowledge when implementing assessments and interventions. Both procedural and declarative knowledge are stored in the long-term memory. There is also some evidence that we store sensory experiences in long-term memory such as memories of odors or sounds.

Our ability to learn and to respond to our experiences is determined to a large degree by the way the two systems work together to coordinate what we are experiencing with what we know. As shown in *Figure 3-2*, new information comes into working memory, and we interpret our experiences by activating information in long-term memory that seems to be related to what we are experiencing. When we walk into a new situation, we interpret what we are experiencing using information pulled from long-term memory (long-term storage system) into working memory (processing system). Decisions about what has happened and needs to be happening occur in working memory as we reflect on what we know and what we are experiencing. Our responses to our experiences are constructed in working memory and, frequently, acted on. For example, in the case described, Mary had prior knowledge about children with autism, as well as knowledge about using activity as therapy. She pulled this information from her declarative memory, along with her knowledge of what toys and equipment would appeal to a child of this age.

We also retrieve procedural knowledge stored in long-term memory that tells us how to carry out the procedures. For instance, Mary remembered to sequence therapy so as to move from more gross motor to more fine motor activities, and to weave in vestibular, tactile, and proprioceptive activities. We compare in working memory what we are seeing, feeling, and hearing with retrieved memories (in this case, what children with autism look and act like in therapy). We then respond by carrying out the necessary procedures based on our assessment. Part of what made this case challenging for Mary was the disconnection between what she had experienced with other children and the behaviors of *this* child.

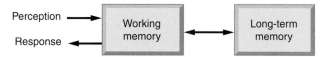

Figure 3-2   Working memory processes information, whereas long-term memory stores information.

Working Memory

Working memory is best described as the system in which the work of thinking is done. It is the system in which we comprehend what we experience, connect what we are seeing or hearing with what we know, reflect on what can or cannot be done, and plan for the future. It is the system that allows us to regulate our behavior and thoughts. For example, processing in working memory may allow us to realize midway through an intervention that the intervention is not working and to shift to a different intervention.

Working memory is surprisingly limited in its capacity. The capacity of working memory was initially thought to be limited to seven plus or minus two items (Miller, 1956). This means that if you were to read a list of numbers, letters, or words, you would be able to remember between five and nine of them. Miller was working for Bell labs when he did this research, and it is one of the reasons why telephone numbers contain seven digits. Miller may have been overoptimistic in his conclusions. More recent research suggests that we can hold only about four items in working memory and can really only actively attend to a single item at any given time (Verhaeghen, Cerella & Basak, 2004). That is a pretty limited capacity, given the importance of working memory for thinking, learning, and problem solving. Practitioners must attend to many factors during the course of one treatment session including performance skills, client factors, activity demands, and environmental demands related to occupational performance. It can be overwhelming, particularly for the novice practitioner, who may have difficulty determining the salient aspects of performance on which to focus with the client (Robertson, 1996b).

We get around limitations in working memory by relying on long-term memory as a storage system for information that is not being immediately used in working memory. This allows working memory to be allocated to comprehension, problem solving, and reflection, as opposed to storage. Individuals with considerable discipline-specific knowledge can rely on long-term memory when solving problems within that discipline because they have a considerable amount of information stored in long-term memory compared with novices (e.g., Lesgold, Rubinson, Feltovich, Glaser, Kopfer & Wang, 1988). This decreases cognitive overload problems common in people just entering a field.

We process information in working memory in a number of ways. We can process and represent sensory-based information including images, sound, smell, taste, and touch (Conrad, 1964; Shepard & Metzler, 1971). We also use a purely semantic means of representing information in working memory (Wickens, Born & Allen, 1963). Semantic representation is not linked to senses but is linked to the way in which we organize and use information. For example, an apple, a banana, and a kiwi are all considered members of the fruit category even though they are visually different from each other, do not taste the same, do not all have the same textures, and do not have similar-sounding names. They are categorized together semantically because our culture has decided that they are all forms of fruit.

Working memory is a temporary memory. Unless information in working memory is attended to, it will be forgotten. Once we shift our attention, decay of the information in working memory begins to occur. It is stopped only if we refocus our attention on that information and reactivate it in working memory. We also forget information through interference when new information replaces old information in working memory (Waugh & Norman, 1965). For example, a therapist who has just seen patient "x" is on her way to report on patient "x" in a team conference. If nothing distracts the therapist, the new information will remain in her working memory when she enters the conference. She may lose the new information in working memory, however, when she meets a colleague, who brings up patient "y." The information about patient "x" is replaced in working memory with information about patient "y" through interference.

Most adults are aware of the limits of working memory and the tendency for attention to be distracted. As a result, we use mnemonic devices or memory strategies to help us remember. For example, most people write notes or create lists with the understanding that they are unlikely to remember the information otherwise. Many of us in today's current practice would be lost without "sticky notes" or our personal data assistants (PDA). In the example above, the therapist may have thought that she was safe in not making a note of the new information on patient "x" because she was just about to go to a conference on that patient. Unfortunately, even a short conversation can produce interference (forgetting) of information in working memory.

So far, working memory appears to be very fragile and limited. How can such a system enable us to comprehend what we read and hear, do complex problem solving, reflect on our problem solving, and plan for the future? The answer is that long-term memory is used extensively by working memory to store knowledge, and that knowledge is accessed as needed by working memory. People who are more expert in their professions do not have larger working memory capacity. Rather, they possess a rich store of knowledge in long-term memory. This means that the working memory is less efficient for young children, whose brains have not yet fully matured, who have less working memory capacity than adults, and who have less information stored in long-term memory. Working memory is also less efficient for people just beginning to learn a discipline, because they have less knowledge stored in long-term memory and that knowledge is not as easily accessible as that of experts within that discipline.

Working memory is least efficient when something completely new is being learned. For instance, if a student who knows nothing about neurodevelopmental intervention techniques is learning how to provide intervention, the information about the intervention (e.g., reducing tone) is represented entirely in working memory or externally in a textbook or notes. Students in such situations are slow in progressing through the procedures and frequently must refer to some external aid, such as notes or a textbook, to refresh their memory of what needs to be done. The slowness is due to the many demands being placed on working memory in the form of the need to hold relevant information in memory and the need to coordinate what needs to be done with that information as the student shifts attention from information about what needs to be done to actually carrying out the procedure. As students gain experience with the task, knowledge about the task is shifted to long-term memory. Repeated practice reinforces connections in memory making task completion more fluent and less dependent on working memory (LeFevre, Bisanz & Mrkonjic, 1988; Zbrodoff & Logan, 1986).

In professional reasoning, information in long-term memory is cued by information in working memory. In the case of Leslie, a typical script or frame for therapy was activated in long-term memory and brought into working memory. The thought processes that occurred when it was apparent that this "typical" approach was not working took place in working memory. As a part of the therapist's reflections on the problem, alternative approaches stored with the activated frame or script were brought into working memory and implemented. In the following text, we talk about three theories that describe the organization and storage of information in long-term memory.

Long-term Memory

Research on long-term memory focuses on issues other than research on working memory. Capacity, for instance, is not an issue. The brain is estimated to have more storage capacity than a large university library. Instead, theory and research on long-term memory focus on how information is organized in long-term memory and how we use that information to interpret and respond to the world. The focus is also on how organization can help or hinder encoding (moving) information into long-term memory and retrieval of information from long-term memory.

The following discussion of three theories of how information is organized in long-term memory constitute only a few of the theories dealing with the organization of long-term memory. These three theories have been selected to present different aspects of long-term memory. Information about these theories is from the original work on the theory. Barsalou's (1992) frame theory assumes a purely semantic representational code and focuses on how we organize and connect related knowledge when multiple possibilities exist for relationships among items of knowledge. Frame theory might explain how we select from a number of options to create a particular therapy for a patient with unique needs. Anderson's propositional network and ACT* model focus on how declarative and procedural knowledge develop in relation to each other. Anderson's theory explains, for instance, the knowledge of the therapist and the skill of the therapist. Dual Code theory focuses on the existence of sensory coding in long-term memory and its implications for memory. Dual Code theory explains how therapists use their senses to collect and interpret information about a particular patient.

Frame Theory

According to Barsalou (1992), our long-term memory comprises frames that include semantic concepts, their attribute-values, structural invariants, and constraints. These frames are similar to the scripts described by Schell (2003), which are used to guide clinical reasoning, except that frames are more structured and complex than scripts. Frames make it easier to describe the rich, complex knowledge involved in therapy and the many options occupational therapists have for therapy. There may be several types of interventions, for example, to improve the cognitive processing of individuals with autism. From the perspective of frame theory, each intervention includes a number of attribute-values, constraints, and structural invariants. For example, the intervention *sensory integration therapy* would include a number of attributes-values including vestibular, proprioceptive, and tactile interventions. The attributes are basically characteristics or components of the therapy. Each attribute includes values that would be different ways in which the component could be carried out or modified. There may be a certain order (structural invariant) for attribute-values so that some components always follow or precede others. Some attributes of intervention(s) may have to occur together (constraints), whereas other attributes may be optional or not linked to other attributes. For example, in providing "brushing" as an intervention in a sensory integration frame of reference, the therapist typically links this input with joint compressions. In contrast, vestibular activities are often "stand alone" interventions.

Frames are theoretically similar to schemes (Bartlett, 1932) and scripts (Schank & Abelson, 1977) except that frame theory better specifies how knowledge is organized in memory and is more flexible in that it describes the organization of knowledge about a topic as well as a sequence of events. Frames can describe, for example, the organization of all the knowledge that a therapist has in regard to working with individuals with autism. This frame would also have information about the diagnosis as well as about different interventions used during therapy. In this way, frames are good at organizing complex, related information. Frames describe possible ways in which a particular goal can be reached and also describe the constraints of ways to meet a goal.

As we learn, we construct frames that become increasingly complex as we include more concepts, attribute-values, structural invariants, and constraints. Part of the development of expertise involves the refinement of knowledge through the acquisition of attribute-values, structural invariants, and constraints. Expertise is more than knowing facts. It also involves knowing how these facts are related to each other, when things tend to occur consistently together, and when and why they do not. A frame that includes sufficient attribute-values, structural invariants, and constraints allows an individual to make accurate judgments about situations and to make inferences about what is happening based on the organization of the information in the frame. If we apply this theory to the case of Leslie (Box 3-1), the therapist (Mary) activated a frame that included attribute-values related to sensory integration strategies for intervention with each strategy being a separate attribute and being accompanied by the different ways that the strategy could be carried out (value). She was also attending to the structural components of intervention in terms of the typical order and timing of how therapy sessions "should" progress (structural invariants). Mary activated frames related to developmental theory as well as frames for sensory integration theory to guide the therapy session. These frames are linked in Mary's memory because sensory integration theory is based in neuroscientific as well as developmental theory. Although past experience suggests that the intervention Mary created should work, it became clear that the activities used "as is" were not working. At this point, reflection on the problem and comprehension of the situation and the problem took place in working memory. Once Mary realized that holding on to the "popper" was not a constraint on the intervention, she modified her frame regarding this type of therapy to include attributes-values that involve making a game out of using a favorite toy. As Mary altered her frame about therapy and began to act on that revised frame, Leslie began to participate in the therapy session. Mary was able to obtain her goal of having Leslie reduce her gravitational insecurity, as evidenced by Leslie's ability to tolerate suspended equipment and later in her therapy to ascend and descend stairs without assistance. Mary also enriched her frame about this form of therapy to include activities that allow the patient to guide the therapeutic session.

The ACT* Model

Anderson (1983) proposed that long-term memory comprises two separate systems of declarative and procedural knowledge. This theory is unique in that it describes how we store semantic, conceptual knowledge as well as how we store information necessary for carrying out actions. Declarative knowledge is what we know or can declare, whereas procedural knowledge is knowledge about how to do something (actions). For example, the therapist may be able to describe how to position a patient to carry out a particular therapeutic activity (declarative knowledge) in addition to having the ability to do so (procedural knowledge). Although both declarative and procedural knowledge tend to co-exist, this is not always the case. When just learning a particular therapy, a novice therapist may be able to describe what needs to be done in detail but not be able to do it. Expert therapists are able to describe a procedure for an intervention by calling on information stored in declarative memory *and* to carry out the procedure by accessing procedural knowledge.

Information from procedural and declarative knowledge interacts, and can be acted on, only when it is activated and brought into working memory. Procedural knowledge and declarative knowledge work together in working memory to allow us to understand and respond to our experiences. As can be seen in *Figure 3-3*, all reflection, thought, and problem solving occurs in working memory. For example, when a child with sensory integrative dysfunction begins to escalate his or her arousal level to the point of having difficulty focusing, the therapist activates and retrieves information in declarative memory about how to modulate the child's activities to help the child "re-group" and be able to focus more effectively. This information is brought into working memory, where the therapist can reflect on how it can be applied in this specific instance. Likewise, the actual activity of modulating activities requires information in procedural knowledge being activated and retrieved into working memory, where it can be acted on.

Reflecting on Mary and Leslie, we can see that Mary has information about sensory integration principles and behavioral theory stored in declarative memory. Likewise, her intervention goals are stored in long-term declarative memory. In terms of her procedural memory, Mary has practiced her pediatric treatment sessions so that her ability to carry out procedures is relatively automatic. Based on information stored in declarative memory about clients like Leslie, she typically

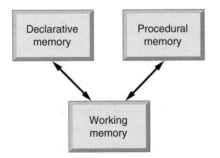

Figure 3-3   Working memory interacts with both declarative memory, which stores the "know what," and procedural memory, which stores the "know how."

tries to encourage sensory and gross motor activities first in a session (to prime the neurological structures) and then helps the child proceed to occupation-based fine and perceptual motor tasks as the child's sensory system becomes more organized. This knowledge and the knowledge used to create the activities were stored in declarative memory, but the actions Mary took to set up the activities and her actions and statements to Leslie were the result of procedural knowledge. Of particular note were the uses of both procedural and declarative memory to help this child be able to transition from one activity to the next without a "meltdown" or extreme emotional response.

Much of skill development occurs as we refine our declarative and procedural knowledge while it is activated in working memory. Many therapists can remember taking lab experiences in school or having to demonstrate a skill to a clinical instructor, where we "verbally talked ourselves" through the process using declarative memory. As our declarative and procedural knowledge become refined with experience, we rely increasingly on retrieving well-learned knowledge and skill from long-term memory. This lessens the demands on working memory. A novice practitioner will have substantial demands placed on his or her working memory because knowledge in long-term memory is not optimally organized and cannot be fluently accessed and used by working memory. This may be why the student fieldwork experience or the first year of employment can be exhausting for many practitioners. With experience and the development of skill, this process becomes automated, allowing the practitioner to more deeply reflect on details that a novice may not recognize. Robertson (1996b) recommends that opportunities should be provided for students to analyze problem solving during fieldwork to allow for the development of schemata "based on a sound understanding of the context" (p. 215). Such reflections allow for the development of a richer declarative knowledge.

Dual Code Theory

Paivio's Dual Code theory (1971) is a departure from frame and propositional ACT* theory in that it assumes that knowledge is represented in memory using sensory-based codes of sight, hearing, smell, touch, and taste rather than semantic representation. Most theories including frame theory and Anderson's ACT* model assume that all knowledge in long-memory is semantically represented or coded. Specifically, Dual Code theory assumes that we possess two systems for representing information in long-term memory. In the verbal system, language-based information is stored as verbal codes similar to the semantic representations of frame theory and the ACT* theory. According to Clark and Paivio (1991), in this system we use visual (print), auditory, and articulatory (speech) to represent language in long-term memory. The nonverbal system includes sensory-based representations of shape, sound, actions, and emotions. The two systems are not separate, but interact with each other to allow us to understand and respond to the world. So when you hear the word *tone* (as in muscle tone), information from both verbal and nonverbal systems is activated. The verbal (language-based) representation of the word *tone* is elicited from your verbal system, and sensory information about *tone* (e.g., visual image, kinesthetic senses, and emotions) is elicited from the nonverbal system. In this way, you retrieve both knowledge about dealing with tone and related sensory and affective information about tone from long-term memory. If you really like dealing with tone, you will have a positive emotional reaction to the word *tone* as well as knowing what tone is. You might picture a prototypical case including sensory information about good and poor tone.

Paivio argued that theories that assume only a semantic representation of information need to explain how emotion is semantically coded and how emotion is reconstructed from this coding. Similarly, these theories must explain how sights, sounds, touch, taste, and smell might be semantically coded similar to language-based knowledge, semantic knowledge. Dual code theory addresses the question of how semantic knowledge, sensory knowledge and emotions are represented and integrated in response to our experiences. When we are faced with a situation we activate not only what we know about the situation and topic but memories of sights, smells, proprioceptive sensations, and emotions related to that situation. In the case of Leslie, Mary had sensory-based visual, auditory and tactile memories stored in long-term memory that allowed her to select the most appropriate toys to use in therapy from an array of stimuli. She selected specific items based on their color, the noise they would make and their feel based on these non-verbal, sensory-based long-term memories. She also had verbal knowledge about why items with these characteristics would be most helpful in therapy for specific children.

Summary of Long-Term Memory Theories

Frame theory, ACT* theory, and dual code theory are informative because they describe how we organize information in long-term memory. They also present different views of how this information is coded in long-term memory. Frame theory provides an explanation of how complex phenomenon can be represented in memory. ACT* theory explains how procedures (actions) might be represented in long-term memory and how these procedures interact with declarative knowledge. Dual code theory provides an explanation of how we might code emotions, images, taste and other sensory experiences into long-term memory. The three theories are not in agreement with each other in that frame theory and ACT* theory assumes a strictly semantic representation with even actions being semantically represented in long-term memory. Dual code theory assumes that sensory and emotional experiences can be represented in long-term memory. We do not know yet which, if any, of these theories best explains the organization and coding in long-term memory. At this point we will consider what each theory says about our ability to recognize patterns, how these patterns might cue different diagnoses and recommended interventions (*Table 3-1*).

All three theories assume that it is the organization of our knowledge that affects how we recognize patterns. Knowledge, whether it is semantic or sensory, is organized as a function of repeated experience and it is the match between this organization and what we are perceiving that allows us to see patterns. Expert clinicians have more patterns stored in memory, which may allow them to predict outcomes of interventions with far more accuracy than would a novice clinician (Robertson, 1996). Further, an expert clinician typically has knowledge organized in such a way that she can discriminate indicators of a particular problem, can articulate which occupational performance factors tend to co-occur together, what client factors tend to occur for a particular diagnosis, and how a disease or condition might affect occupational performance. The cognitive structures of the expert clinician are organized in such a way that this information is tightly linked in memory after repeated experiences with patients.

TABLE 3-1

Cognitive Functions and Memory

	Long-Term Memory	Working Memory
Semantic Coding	Yes, see Anderson's ACT* theory Frame theory	Yes, much of the coding is semantic because that is how it is stored in long term memory.
Perceptual Coding	Yes, see Paivio's Dual Code theory	Yes, visual, verbal and other sensory codes likely in working memory.
Capacity	Unlimited	About 4 items can be held in working memory but only one can be attended to at any given time.
Forgetting	Probably occurs as we blend new information with old making it difficult to remember the "original" information	Information decays if we don't periodically attend to it to keep it active. Interference can also be a problem if new information overwrites old information or causes us not to attend to old information.
Organization	Semantically organized based on our level of expertise and other experiences	We organize information based on how information is organized in long-term memory.

Practice settings provide a considerable amount of information that might or might not be useful for correct assessment and intervention. If a novice and expert clinician walk into the same situation they often will come to very different conclusions about the situation because they will see different cues as important. **Cues** can be anything in the environment that prompt the therapist to consider a specific diagnosis. A cue can be a smell, information from the client, something the therapist sees or a combination of these. Both the novice and expert clinician will listen to client complaints or descriptions of limitation. They will get sensory information about client through sight, sound, smell or touch. They will draw different conclusions about what is important to consider based on differences in the richness of their frames and sensory-based memories. Specifically, the ability to determine what is important as a cue is a function of the knowledge organized in frames and sensory-based representational networks, not what is available in the environment. Experts have more and richer knowledge stored in frames and as declarative and sensory-based memory. It is the organization of this knowledge that allows them to recognize patterns in cues. Expert practitioners will quickly assess the situation and focus the important cues using what they know about the situation. Novices may not even be aware of important cues because their long-term memory is not organized in such a way that they can recognize the relationship between cues and a particular diagnosis.

In the case of Leslie, Mary was not a novice but was reentering practice on a part time basis while earning her doctorate. Mary had not been in pediatric practice on a regular basis in three years. She found herself struggling to "find information in her brain's file cabinets" to solve the "popper dilemma" with Leslie. Much of the rich information that was stored in long-term memory was inaccessible because it had not been recently activated and brought into working memory. In addition to not practicing recently in pediatrics, Mary was also new to this outpatient clinic and may have had many distracters, such as understanding the schema of practice in this context not to mention treating clients in an open and distracting setting. As a result, she was not able to work at the expert level that she had achieved when she had worked full time in a familiar setting.

METACOGNITION AND SELF-REGULATION

Although much of the pattern recognition that occurs as a function of expert organization in long-term memory is automatic, experts also differ from novices in their ability to metacognitively reflect and to regulate problem solving. **Metacognition** is essentially cognition about cognition (Flavell, 1979) and is a contributor to expert problem solving. According to Flavell (1979), metacognition allows us to reflect on our knowledge and actions in two ways. First, we possess metacognitive knowledge about our own knowledge and its limitations. For example, by early elementary school children know that they are capable of forgetting, that distractions will cause them to forget something that they have just learned, and that there are strategies for improving memory. Second, we possess the ability to monitor and reflect on our problem solving to determine whether a solution is likely to be successful or whether we have succeeded or failed at all. For example, successful mathematics students are more likely to stop periodically during problem solving to assess the effectiveness of their solution (Schoenfeld & Herrmann, 1982). Less successful students do little planning at the beginning and rarely stop to check whether the solution is working.

Metacognition is apparent in the problem solving of adults in the workplace. Adults, for example, take notes because they are aware of the limitations of working memory and because they know that they are unlikely to remember detailed information about particular clients. They also are aware of clients' working memory limitations so they provide written directions for the clients to follow. The ability to monitor or reflect on an ongoing intervention is critical because unanticipated events may alter the effectiveness of an intervention. In addition, individual differences in the way a client responds to an approach may cause a practitioner to alter the intervention to make it more effective. If the practitioner is not monitoring the effectiveness of the intervention, he or she will not be aware of the need to make changes.

Metacognitive knowledge about cognitive limitations and the ability to monitor the effectiveness of an intervention emerge with experience within a particular domain (Bransford, Sherwood, Vye & Rieser, 1986). When we first learn a new topic, much of our learning is not metacognitive in that we are learning basic knowledge and skills and solving basic problems. We are focusing on the declarative and procedural knowledge of what we need to know and do and are less fluent in these areas. That leaves little room in working memory to consider whether it is working well. Our lack of experience also makes it difficult to reflect on the effectiveness of a treatment because we have not had sufficient experience to know when it is and is not effective. As our knowledge and skills become more complex and as we take on more difficult problems we become increasingly able to make decisions about the best approach to problem solving (Demetriou, Christou, Spanoudis & Platsidou, 2002).

The more experienced we become at a task or more knowledgeable in a domain, the less we rely on working memory to hold the information that we are actively processing. Rather, the information is stored in long-term declarative and procedural knowledge. One outcome of this is that working memory is freed for other tasks, including monitoring and evaluation of outcomes. No longer are we focusing on exactly what needs to be done but focusing instead on evaluating the effectiveness of what has been done. We notice things that we might not have been able to notice before because our attention had been focused on basic activities.

As we develop frames that contain complex information about a domain of knowledge, we are better able to use that knowledge to assess situations and to determine whether our choice of interventions is being effective. This occurs, in part, because metacognitive knowledge about our own and our clients' limitations is stored as a part of the frame. We are able to take that information into consideration when deciding on a course of action. Similarly, as our procedural knowledge becomes more compiled, it becomes more fluent and requires less thought. At this point, we can shift our attention to determining whether the outcome of our actions is effective. Finally, as clinicians make connections among different sounds, sights, smells, and other sensory information, they become better able to see and respond to patterns. When interventions are not effective, the experienced clinician may see a model that suggests the reason for that failure and a new course of action. What we know and the complexity and organization of that information influence our ability to monitor our activities and to assess the effectiveness of problem solving.

The emergence of metacognition allows us to self-regulate because we can now consider information about the effectiveness of our actions and take that information into consideration when altering an intervention. The process of self-regulation itself improves our knowledge and skills in that we can alter what we know as a result of our experiences. Frames change as a function of our experiences. Experience and feedback from that experience likewise informs our declarative and procedural knowledge. As metacognitive knowledge and monitoring emerge with experience and as fluency in retrieval from memory emerges the ability to learn from experience is thought to improve (Crowley, Shrager & Siegler, 1997).

AUTOMATICITY

Metacognition helps us to learn more efficiently by allowing us to intentionally alter what we know and do as a function of experience (e.g., Kuhn & Pearsall, 1998). The emergence of **automaticity** through repeated practice is another part of the learning process. Automaticity occurs as we solidify our knowledge and skills so they become both fast and efficient at problem solving. With practice we become more fluent in our ability to retrieve information from declarative memory and to compile procedures (Anderson, 1983). We more swiftly process what we experience and more quickly match what we experience to what we know. From the perspective of frame theory, certain attribute-values in frames become more likely to be activated and brought into working memory. This results in faster performance and further frees working memory space. When this happens, an individual can focus on learning a more complex, intellectually demanding task or can deal more efficiently with such a task.

Metacognition and automaticity can work together in that as we self-regulate and correct our knowledge and actions through repeated experiences we are also practicing retrieving that knowledge and making the actions. Metacognition can also improve the outcome of practice by allowing the individual to be aware of necessary changes that will result in more accurate performance in addition to faster performance.

Expertise Theory and Information Processing

So far, the focus of this chapter has been on the knowledge and skills that make up the information processing system. We now shift to discussing how changes in knowledge and skills over a period of years results in the emergence of expertise. **Expertise** is defined as the experience and knowledge to work at a high level in a given domain. A novice, in contrast, is just beginning to learn a new domain and may be slow and inefficient in problem solving. This occurs because when a new discipline is first being learned, the learner has little understanding of the overarching principles that guide problem solving within that domain. The declarative and procedural knowledge of a novice includes basic ideas about the domain and individual actions, but the declarative knowledge has not been integrated into complex frames and the procedures have not been compiled into larger, complex procedures. Over a period of time, typically at least 10 years, the knowledge of the novice increases and reorganizes to better represent the knowledge of an expert. According to Benner (1984), as professionals gain experience, they become increasingly able to rely on knowledge that is a result of years of experience, to use their expert knowledge to select important cues from the setting and be more reflective in interacting with clients.

Part of this developmental process occurs as a function of practice and the emergence of automaticity. Another part of the developmental process occurs as the individual reflects on and responds to inconsistencies between what he or she knows and new information he or she is learning. As expertise emerges qualitative changes occur in the way practitioners in a discipline organize their knowledge, respond to problems, and repair problem solving. In summation, expertise depends on the emergence of a number of skills and knowledge states that are interdependent in their development. Expertise includes a rich, integrated knowledge base, qualitatively different strategies, automaticity in problem solving, and the ability to reflect on problem solving when necessary.

Integrated Knowledge Base

As we learn, we not only increase the amount of knowledge in memory but qualitatively change the way that knowledge is organized. For instance, young children's knowledge tends to be organized on a single level with little understanding of how ideas, such as horse or dog, might be hierarchically organized into an animal category (Ornstein & Naus, 1985). Over time, children begin to develop an understanding of the features that connect knowledge and create frames for organizing this knowledge. The changes in knowledge that novices undergo as they participate in a new discipline are similar to those of children. Unlike preschool-aged children, however, individuals learning a new discipline are provided by that discipline with a structure to organize their newly acquired knowledge. The discipline also provides the learner with experiences designed to teach the discipline's organization to the learner. The role of the learner is to construct and reconstruct his or her own knowledge so that it increasingly resembles that of the discipline. For example, when you began learning about occupational therapy, the books you read included basic information and provided an organizational frame for that information. When you began to learn intervention techniques, a rationale was provided for the actions that made up the intervention. As new knowledge and skill were acquired, you used information from occupational therapy teachers and textbooks to organize that knowledge. An expert occupational therapist has well-developed frames, including an array of attribute-values, structural invariants, and constraints that provide the structure for that knowledge. In addition, he or she likely possesses significant sensory-based knowledge related to the profession. The richness of the frames in declarative knowledge and the sensory memories derived from much experience result in what Benner (1984) called practice based on experience.

Research based on the development of expertise in medical doctors may be helpful in explaining the development of expertise in occupational therapists. A theory by Schmidt and Boshuizen (1993) takes Anderson's ACT* theory and applies it to the emergence of expertise in medical doctors. Knowledge begins as causal networks of propositions that are compiled or chunked into larger units over time and experience. Over time, the acts of compilation and chunking result in increased speed and automaticity. It is further assumed that "illness scripts" similar to the frames described above emerge out of the compiled and chunked networks.

Specifically, low-level detailed concepts are clustered together to create higher-level concepts. From the perspective of frame theory, lower-level concepts take on the role of values to higher-level attributes. More expert physicians match these illness scripts or frames to the symptoms presented by a new patient, whereas novices might search among related propositions for information that will help them diagnose a medical problem. This can be seen when comparing the diagnostic skills of medical school students and practicing family physicians. In diagnosing, the students actually reported more ideas than the practicing family physicians (Boshuizen, 1989). This suggests that the practicing family physicians have reorganized their knowledge to focus on diagnoses that best matched the symptoms and that were most likely to be seen in practice. Instead of activating any frame that might be applicable to the situation, they activated frames that most closely resembled similar situations encountered in the past.

Expert knowledge improves experts' ability to encode and maintain information in working memory. This occurs because the expert can see patterns in information that a novice would not see. This ability allows the expert to organize complex information into manageable and understandable forms. Chess masters, for instance, can identify and remember complex chess patterns when the chess pieces are organized in a way that is usually seen in chess play (Chi, 1987). The chess experts' advantage is not in their better memory, but in their ability to chunk what appears to the novice to be unrelated information into patterns. In a clinical setting, the elaborate frames of an expert clinician provide the means of interpreting what may seem to be unrelated information as meaningful and interconnected. Expert knowledge in the same way enables us to better and more easily comprehend texts dealing with the domain of expertise so that experts get more from domain-specific texts than novices (Schneider & Bjorklund, 1992). In this way, an expert clinician not only picks up the right cues but organizes that information in working memory according to what he or she knows about the domain.

Research on the organization of expertise knowledge indicates that experts use this organization to help them understand and respond to their experiences at a much higher level than novices. The expert can also use their knowledge to fill in information that was not presented to them. They can infer from what they know about the topic information that may not be evident from actual observation. Experts can see patterns and can use those patterns to activate underlying principles. In summation, what experts see and hear is very different from what a novice sees and hears. Experts see patterns and cues not evident to novices and have a deep understanding of what these patterns mean and the course of actions that are possible.

An expert occupational therapist differs from a student in occupational therapy or a beginning therapist in that his or her knowledge is organized so that the expert can easily interpret a situation. For example, if an occupational therapy instructor and student walk into a patient's room and see that the patient is lethargic, cannot move one side of their body, and appears to be having swallowing difficulties, the student may know that what they are seeing and hearing is important but will not know how all this information interacts to result in a particular diagnosis and intervention plan. Furthermore, the student will have difficulty prioritizing which actions should be taken first; whereas the experienced clinician has procedural memory to call on for acting quickly in this situation. For the novice therapist, the information will be in memory, but the experience required to elaborate on the information and make connections has not occurred and, as a result, the student will not know what is important and how the different pieces of information fit together and lead to intervention X. For the student to decide that intervention X is necessary, he or she has to fit all the bits of the puzzle together until the big picture and intervention are evident.

As novices move toward expertise, what would be considered individual pieces of information are combined as a result of experience. For example, as occupational therapists gain more experience, they notice that lethargy, swallowing difficulties, and hemiplegia often co-occur in patients who have had stroke. Experienced therapists notice how these symptoms affect or are likely to affect an individual's ability to engage in daily activities and routines that are important to that person. Eventually, large amounts of information are combined into single frames to which the expert can quickly and accurately respond to provide very customized intervention that may seem effortless when viewed by the novice practitioner.

Differences in Strategy Use

Emerging expertise is characterized by changes in strategies for problem solving. Toglia (1998) defines strategies as "organized approaches, routines, or tactics that operate to select and guide the processing of information" (p. 8). The strategies that novices and experts develop are a function of improvements in the quality and quantity of their knowledge on a subject. A novice's strategic approach to problem solving is more exploratory, whereas the problem solving of an expert tends to focus on proving or disproving a single hypothesis that is created based on years of experience diagnosing problems (Hunt, 1989). When confronted with a wide variety of information about a client, therapists must select appropriate strategies for intervention (Toglia, 1998). The types of strategies used depend on the level of expertise of the therapist.

Research in medicine suggests that novices tend to use *backwards reasoning* from the information given in the problem with the goal of finding some end product. The novice is not sure as to the correct path to take to reach this end product and may try a number of different avenues before a solution is reached (e.g., Hunt, 1989). This approach is data driven in that the novice does not have a conceptual framework to guide problem solving. This method is useful when an individual does not have well-developed frames or networks that can be used to guide problem solving (Patel & Groen, 1991). It is, however, time consuming, since a novice physician or therapist will consider a large number of hypotheses about possible diagnoses. Each hypothesis must be tested, with some hypotheses taking more time than others to discredit. Novices, through the backward reasoning strategy, follow a number of dead end paths to a diagnosis before they find the correct diagnosis. From the perspective of frame theory, their frames comprise a number of attribute-values representing the potential diagnoses, but there is little structural invariance or constraints on this knowledge that would streamline the process of diagnosing the problem.

In the case of the expert, the *forward reasoning* strategy is used. This strategy can be used when someone has enough knowledge to create a mental flowchart showing the possible paths and subgoals needed to solve a problem. Another requirement of this strategy is sufficient experience to know which paths on the flowchart are most likely to result in the correct diagnosis. This knowledge is most likely to emerge through repeated experience with a problem and its potential solutions. Through repeated experiences, structural invariants and constraints are placed on the process of diagnosing a problem. The expert possesses a substantial body of information about a topic and has had considerable experience working with that topic knowledge. This allows the expert to take a very different, less time-consuming approach to problem solving, which involves making and testing a "best guess" hypothesis rather than exploring multiple hypotheses. From the perspective of occupational therapy, an expert therapist has a frame that might include a number of interventions to improve an individual's performance but uses interventions that they know are more likely to work together to achieve a goal.

Research in the area of medical expertise shows that experts use rich and integrated knowledge to frame their problem-solving approach. For example, Joseph and Patel (1990) found that physicians with different levels of expertise differed in the timing of the development of hypotheses about an endocrinology problem and their ability to test the hypotheses. Domain experts were able to develop diagnostic hypotheses with much less information about the problem than physicians without domain specific expertise in endocrinology. Experts use their rich knowledge to generate good hypotheses about a diagnosis and then focus on proving or disproving a specific diagnosis. Such a tactic would be much less useful for novices who might not have sufficient experience and knowledge of the field to generate good hypotheses.

For the beginning occupational therapist, there may be many interventions that will work for a given occupational performance problem. Each client, however, may have unique issues that determine which intervention is the most effective. The beginning occupational therapist will consider a number of interventions and evaluate the effectiveness of each intervention before making a final decision. In contrast, an expert occupational therapist initially recommends an intervention based on the prior performance of this intervention in similar cases and evaluates the effectiveness of that intervention to determine whether it will or will not be the best method for this particular patient. As a novice occupational therapy practitioner, Mary initially worked in psychiatry. She reflects:

> I was working in a day treatment program that closed and in an effort to keep my job, I accepted a position in the same organization as a "neuro" therapist treating patients who had experienced strokes. I can recall the awkward feeling of "not knowing anything" when thrust upon this new intervention context. With only 2 years of experience, I began treating every client who had a stroke the same way. The only technique that I could recall was to place the recovering extremity in a gravity eliminated plane, so I used skateboard exercises with every client for about the first week of being in this new setting. Soon, I realized that what worked for one individual did not always work for others. I quickly went back to intervention textbooks, watched other clinicians and sought expert advice and opinions about individual cases to enhance the intervention I provided.

Automaticity Through Experience

One characteristic that distinguishes experts from novices is the speed with which they are able to process information and make sound decisions based on that speeded processing (Chi, Glaser & Farr, 1988). There are several reasons for this advantage by experts. As noted above, experts have highly integrated knowledge of a topic. We know that highly integrated knowledge of this sort allows experts to quickly access domain-specific knowledge. This occurs because it has been frequently accessed in the past (Anderson, 1982). A reason for this increased speed and the close-knit nature of the expert's knowledge is that experts have had years of experience and practice. This experience and practice reinforce connections and make accessing related information fluent and automated.

Experts also have an advantage in their ability to create retrieval cues while organizing information that is being encoded into working memory. This makes it easier for them to hold substantially more information than novices in working memory because they use the retrieval cues to organize during encoding and retrieval. For example, Chase and Ericsson (1981) found that over a period of months a study subject was able to remember over 100 digits read to him over a short period of time. He did this by organizing these digits into three- and four-digit race times, a topic in which he had some expertise. During retrieval, the subject would use his knowledge of race times to retrieve the digits. In an occupational therapy setting, this might mean that an expert occupational therapist might quickly and efficiently encode information about a new patient by organizing that information using a frame for initial diagnoses of occupational performance problems. For instance, knowing a client has a history of depression in addition to the presenting hand injury would prompt the experienced therapist to watch for problems the client might have in initiating and sustaining routine tasks (common occupational performance problems associated with depression)- all of which could have a negative impact on the person beginning to use his injured hand, and thus affect the overall outcome. The speed and superior memory performance of experts, therefore, are a result of processing automaticity developed through practice and training rather than innate memory ability.

Another benefit of automaticity is that it frees working memory space to allow experts to consider information that a novice would not be able to consider. In some cases, freed working memory space is used to plan ahead and prepare for the next challenge. For example, one reason why expert typists are so fast is that they are not looking at the words they are typing. Rather, they are looking several words ahead (Norman & Rumelhart, 1983). This gives experts an advantage in that they can prepare in advance. From a broader perspective, the forward reasoning strategy allows experts to act in the same way in that they are aware of the steps of problem solving from start to finish. The ability to set up problems shortens solution time because experts do not have to stop and think about the next step during problem solving. Expert therapists will be more efficient and effective in dealing with patients as a result of their ability to quickly encode information about the patient and to select the most likely intervention to succeed.

Citing the work in cognitive psychology, Unsworth (1999) notes that expert learners are able to analyze information more deeply in constructing memories; they can adapt learning strategies and set goals for expanding their knowledge; and they demonstrate superior short-term semantic and general memory. Furthermore, Unsworth asserts that experts are able to use more inferences, more abstract principles, and self-regulation strategies to monitor their learning and reasoning processes.

Regulation of Problem Solving

So far, expertise seems to be something that develops automatically, without much reflection or thought. All you need is practice. Ericsson (2001) points out that this is true for people who want to achieve an everyday level of expertise. That is, being good at something but not achieving at the highest levels of a domain. In fact, most people do just that and are quite competent in their work. True expertise in which the person is among the best in a field is depends on more than practice.

According to Ericsson (2001), expertise is characterized by the ability to control performance and to alter outcomes. The ability to fine tune performance to fit different situations emerges out of *deliberate practice*. Deliberate practice includes three components: a desired performance goal, a representation of how to achieve the goal, and a representation of the outcome of performance (Ericsson, 1998). An expert knows what he or she wants to achieve, creates a plan to achieve this outcome, and then reflects on whether the desired outcome has been achieved. Through reflection, improvements can be made during the next attempt to solve the problem. Through repeated goal setting, practice, and reflection, the emerging expert hones his or her skills to achieve a desired outcome. For frames to improve and become more efficient, therapists need to attend to the outcomes of their intervention choices. For procedural knowledge to become more fine tuned, the therapist must reflect on whether his or her actions need to be changed to better meet a goal. As therapists reflect on and distinguish between similar, but different smells, touches, sounds and sights in working memory, their ability to quickly and accurately assess variables affecting performance improves.

With experience, most occupational therapists are good at what they do. Some occupational therapists achieve excellence in their practice that far exceeds the skill level and performance of most occupational therapists. They differ from the average occupational therapist in that they are interested in constantly improving their skill level and performance. They constantly reflect on their choices and how to improve on the decision-making process and outcomes. It is through this reflection that small, cumulative changes occur in performance. Occupational therapy educators sometimes voice their worry about students or novice therapists who think "they get it," stating that they would hire a practitioner who is able to question their practice in lieu of a "dangerously overconfident" practitioner. As we saw in the case of Mary with 20+ years of experience, she continued to challenge her assumptions and knowledge to learn from the case of Leslie (*Table 3-2*).

TABLE 3-2

Differences in Novice and Expert Cognition

	Novice	**Expert**
Knowledge organization	Poorly integrated; frames simple and less well organized	Highly integrated; frames complex and well organized
Strategy use	Working backward from the problem presented with no specific plan for problem solving	Working forward based on a plan for solving the problem from start to finish
Ability to see patterns	Does not see patterns in information because the patterns do not exist in long-term memory	Can quickly recognize patterns in information because the patterns match or cue patterns stored in long-term memory
Automaticity	Low automaticity with novice having to think through each step with each step being separate from the others	High automaticity with expert quickly and efficiently because the steps have been combined into larger steps
Ability to use cues	Poor in determining cues and their importance	Knows what cues to look for and why they are important
Ability to learn new information	Slower at learning new information related to the topic because novice lacks the integrated knowledge in which to insert the new information	Fast learning of topic-related information because a highly integrated frame system exists; expert plugs the new information into appropriate spot

SUMMARY

Although there are individual differences in the amount of information that we can hold in working memory and in the speed with which we process information, much of learning and thought is dependent on factors that can be controlled and that change with experience. Working memory has a very limited capacity, but this capacity can be greatly expanded using memory strategies and using well-organized knowledge stored in long-term memory. The organization of long-term memory becomes more compact and streamlined with experience and makes retrieval of information into working memory easier and faster. As learners gain more knowledge and skill within a domain, they can reflect on what they know, what they need to know, and the means of achieving learning goals. At this point, learning is increasingly regulated by the learner.

The most important thought that you should take away from reading this chapter is that the learning and development of expertise, whether it be average expertise or elite expertise, is dependent on a number of systems working together. Not one single system is responsible for learning and expertise. Expertise is not a result of memorizing facts, nor can expert strategies be taught and used independently of expert knowledge. Instead, working memory, knowledge organization in long-term memory, strategies, and self-regulatory skills all work together to allow expertise to emerge. Since knowledge is better organized in long-term memory, it allows for more complex strategy use. This, in turn, frees working memory to focus on other aspects of a problem. Self-regulation of cognition and reflection on the problem-solving situation result in changes in procedural and declarative knowledge in long-term memory, which, in turn, alter future performance.

CASE STUDY 3-2

Mary and Leslie: Post-Script

Mary's Reflection

Although the first session was not a roaring success in my eyes, I later came to learn a lot more about sensory integration theory as well as client-centered care. In a more detailed review of her medical record, I noticed that Leslie had also been given the diagnosis of atypical autism. While she was socially interactive, she had many "obsessive" behavioral traits limiting her performance.

As I got to know Leslie's mother, she taught me many strategies (which she learned through "trial and error") that seemed to work with Leslie. Mom informed me that Leslie loved swimming. Although swimming would not only be a client-centered intervention, it was also more practical because it would keep Leslie contained for the therapy session rather than always running off to a toy closet to look for the "popper" or the Barney toy. The first time I took Leslie to the pool, it took me 30 minutes to get her dressed until mother informed me that the only place she would dress was while sitting on the commode.

I came to realize that as Leslie moved, she had severe gravitational insecurity, which is why she avoided using suspended equipment. Slowly, I focused on providing more proprioceptive input to help Leslie learn more about her body in space. The aquatic therapy provided resistive exercise as well as reducing the effects of gravity on Leslie's body. Although Leslie still has developmental delays, her gravitational insecurity has improved, allowing her to move more comfortably within her environments and has helped Leslie to explore and learn more effectively.

LEARNING ACTIVITY 3-1

The Blooming Onion

Mary Shotwell

Purpose

This activity is based on a paper done by Nkanginieme* (1997) who applied the six levels of Bloom's Taxonomy to teaching medical students to "make conscious" when they make clinical diagnoses.

In this activity, the learner enhances their case analysis skills through "peeling back the layers of the onion" and getting at deeper levels of information processing. At the more superficial levels, declarative knowledge is required. At deeper levels, learners use associative knowledge and then integrate information.

Furthermore, deeper levels of knowledge should challenge the student to integrate information from pathophysiology, occupational therapy theory, and intervention. They must also consider contextual factors such as family, culture, and system issues that affect intervention.

Connections to Major Clinical Reasoning Constructs

This activity helps the student to make transparent their "information processing" and to apply declarative, procedural, and associative learning as they analyze a specific clinical case. Bloom's six levels are as follows:

1 *Knowledge*—to recall, identify, or recognize facts that pertain to this case
2 *Comprehension*—to translate or extrapolate information
3 *Application*—to be able to relate, transfer, or associate information to a case or other cases
4 *Analysis*—to discriminate or distinguish the important points about this particular case
5 *Synthesis*—to combine, formulate, specify, or constitute factual and analytical information with features pertinent to this case
6 *Evaluation*—to be able to validate, argue, reconsider, and/or appraise one's decisions and interventions

Directions for Learners

1 Students are presented with a case giving as much information as is known.

2 Students start by recording their declarative knowledge of medical conditions, system issues, OT theory and interventions.

3 Students then translate this factual knowledge into possible reasons for symptoms, signs, client concerns (e.g., a client with a C-5 quadriplegia would have concerns about performing self-care because of being unable to use the hands).

4 Students take results of an evaluation or self-report and apply this information to their client in terms of explanations for reasons or performance.

5 Students then summarize all pertinent information, plausible explanations for strengths and deficits in occupational performance, and contextual factors that might make an impact on intervention;

6 Students generate an intervention plan with appropriate justification for each of the goals;

7 Students evaluate these goals and intervention plans by arguing opposing views, possible outcomes of various interventions, and generating alternative intervention approaches;

8 Finally, students evaluate the intervention in terms of its effectiveness.

*Nkanginieme, K. E. O. (1997). Clinical diagnosis as a dynamic cognitive process: Application of Bloom's Taxonomy for educational objectives in the cognitive domain. *Med Educ Online* Available from: URL. http:// www.med-ed-online.org/issue2. htm#v2, 2(1).

LEARNING ACTIVITY 3-2

Finding the Problem Space
Mary Shotwell

Purpose

This activity is based on Robertson's* (1996) theories of "what constitutes a problem" and definition of the **problem space.**

This activity helps learners develop a quality rationale for specific problems in occupational performance and how they might be addressed.

Connections to Major Clinical Reasoning Constructs

Uses Robertson's model of finding four aspects of a problem:

1 *Initial situation*—Learner interprets current information and recalls information from long-term memory

2 *Goal*—determine the outcome the problem solver seeks
3 *Actions or operators*
4 *Restrictions*

Directions for Learners

1 Given a specific case, the learners identify important points about the case or determine the goal of solving this problem.
2 Using current knowledge, learners document what they know about this case and the situation in general (e.g. diagnosis, past experiences, etc).
3 Learners then consider missing information and steps with regard to acquiring such information (e.g., there may be a critical pathway, research evidence, rather than trial and error problem solving).
4 To determine the most appropriate course of action, learners should aggregate data from their knowledge of the specific case, additional resources required, and anticipated results.
5 Finally, learners ascertain what strengths and barriers exist for the client and the therapist (e.g., therapist's lack of expertise).

Worksheet: Finding the Problem Space

Important points. The goal of solving this problem is to understand:

_____

_____

Things I know from clients I have worked with in the past that are similar in this case:

_____

_____

Resources I can go for more information about this problem:

_____

_____

Possible paths to this solution and likely outcomes:

_____

_____

What operators and restrictors can influence my interventions?

_____

_____

*Robertson, L. J. (1996). Clinical reasoning, Part 2: Novice/Expert differences. *British Journal of Occupational Therapy*, 59, 212–216.

LEARNING ACTIVITY 3 - 3

Rogers and Holm Diagnostic Reasoning Question Matrix
Mary Shotwell, based on Rogers & Holm*

Purpose

This activity provides support to learners as they develop their skills in framing problems requiring occupational therapy intervention.

Connections to Major Clinical Reasoning Constructs

Provides scaffolding needed to help students find the "problem space." Over time these become more automated strategies, requiring less conscious attention.

Directions

1 Identify a client in your fieldwork setting or work from a case provided by your instructor.
2 Reflect on each of the questions and note your comments.
3 After completing the activity, consider how you might address a similar situation the future.

Problem Sensing Phase

Comments

1 *Domain of occupational therapy*
- Does this problem concern problems with occupational roles?
- If so, what are the role performance problems?
- What is the occupational status of the client?

2 *Practice considerations*
- Does the setting limit the scope of OT practice?
- Is there a specific FOR/theoretical base that drives practice in this setting?
- Does the setting regulate the types of diagnoses seen?
- Are there physical resources that might enhance or restrict the assessment/intervention process?
- Are there fiscal/policy issues that have potential to influence assessment/intervention?
- Are there specific "turf" or issues in a multidisciplinary setting that hinder or enhance assessment/intervention?

3 *Therapist factors*
- What is the therapist's level of experience/expertise with this type of client?
- What is the therapist's frame of reference for working with this type of client?

4 *Patient factors*
- Is the client pathology consistent with expected occupational performance deficits?
- Where is the client in terms of the "course" of their condition (acute, recurrent, exacerbation, chronic, etc?
- Are there developmental or age-associated changes that would influence our assessment/intervention?
- Is/are there specific reasons listed in the referral for OT?

Problem Definition Phase

Cue acquisition
Have I searched the data field accordingly? Are there other areas I need to screen/assess?
- Subjective data such as patient concerns?
- Objective data such as performance components/skills?
- What cues in the case/my environment led me to attend to a specific stimulus?
- Is there an appropriate critical pathway, cue sheet, clinical protocol, or practice guideline for this type of client?

Hypothesis generation
- Are there specific cues that I can cluster to explain the client's occupational performance?
- Which data were most important in my initial hypothesis? Are there data I might have missed?
- Are there any cues to know that my initial hypothesis is on target?
- Is there any protocol/pathway available that can help me question my hypothesis?

Cue interpretation
- Have I taken time to interpret cues I have before going and gathering more data?
- Can I group cues that might be indicative of function or dysfunction?

Comments

Hypothesis evaluation
- Have I weighed the evidence supporting each hypothesis against the hypothesis rejecting a particular course of action?
- Are the cues I am finding (reliable) consistent?
- Do the cues I find represent the phenomena I think I am evaluating?

Problem Representation

- *Data known*—What information do I have about this case?
- *Knowledge*—What information can I recall about this diagnosis? Context? or population?
- *Environment/context*—What factors outside the diagnosis or the individual might influence assessment/intervention?

Limiting the Problem Space

- Which factors are most important to attend to at this time?
- What are the possible paths I might choose to solve this problem?
- Which path(s) are the most feasible in this situation?
- *Pattern matching*—What prior knowledge do I have that can be applied to this situation? Are there any patterns seen in previous clients that might be used in this case?
- *Trial and error*—PS vs. means-end/ planning methods. Do I try one thing at a time to see whether or not it works? Or, do I start with the goal and then go backward to see how I can get to the goal?

Memory Strategies

Accumulation vs. transformation of data
- Do I merely keep locating new facts about the case? Or, do I continually use resources and questioning to ascertain what data are pertinent to this case?

Chunking
- Am I able to take associations made and store them as chunks in my memory?

Comments

Schema

■ Can I take information about this case, recall old chunks of information in relation to this case, and create a new schema for storage the next time a similar case arrives?

*Developed from Roger, J. C. & Holm, M. B. (1991). Occupational therapy diagnostic reasoning: A component of clinical reasoning. *American Journal of Occupational Therapy*, 45, 1045–1053.

LEARNING ACTIVITY 3-4

Mind Mapping
Mary Shotwell

Purpose

The purpose of this activity is to provide a visual representation of one's clinical reasoning process.

Students can choose to use standard visuals such as a flow chart, a fishbone diagram, a "story web", or any other visual that shows linkages and association between various pieces of information in relation to a case.

The goal of this activity is to help learners reconsider any associations, or to change the "map" slightly to gain new perspectives about the case.

Connections to Major Clinical Reasoning Constructs

This activity focuses on having a student illuminate her metacognitive processes. It also helps demonstrate the power of associating information to formulate our plan of action with a client. By reflecting on the representation the learner may find other associations that enhance their information processing.

Directions for Learners

1 Learners are presented with a specific case (student or teacher generated);
2 Instructors can have students each do their own "mind map" or just focus on one learner's mind map (which might take the whole seminar session).;
3 The mind map should be a 2- or 3-dimensional model of how a case is understood. Suggestion: use a diagram of the brain while making comments with regard to how lobes of the brain and other structures might process information;
4 Students then share their diagrams and discuss differences in processing. Learners encourage learners to challenge assumptions of their classmates;
5 As time permits revise the mind map to facilitate a new way of thinking about the case.

REFERENCES

Anderson, J. R. (1982). Acquisition of cognitive skill. *Psychological Review, 89,* 369–406.

Anderson, J. R. (1983). A spreading activation theory of memory. *Journal of Verbal Learning and Verbal Behavior, 22,* 261–295.

Atkinson, R. C. & Shiffrin, R. M. (1968). Human memory: A proposed system and its control processes. In W. K. Spence & J. T. Spence (Eds.). *The psychology of learning and motivation: Advances in research and theory* (vol. 2, pp. 89–195). New York: Academic Press.

Barsalou, L. W. (1992). Frames, concepts, and conceptual fields. In A. Lehrer & E. F. Kittay (Eds.), *Frames, fields, and contrasts: New essays in semantic and lexical organization* (pp. 21–74). Hillsdale, NJ: Erlbaum.

Bartlett, F. C. (1932). *Remembering: A study in experimental and social psychology.* New York: Cambridge University Press.

Benner, P. (1984). *From novice to expert: Excellence and power in clinical nursing practice.* Menlo Park, CA: Addison-Wesley Publishing Company.

Boshuizen, H. P. A. (1989). *On the development of medical expertise: A cognitive psychological approach.* Doctoral dissertation, University of Limburg, Thesis Publishers, Haarlem, The Netherlands.

Bransford, J., Sherwood, R., Vye, N. & Rieser, J. (1986). Teaching thinking and problem solving. *American Psychologist, 41,* 1078–1089.

Chase, W. G. & Ericsson, K. A. (1981). Skilled memory. In J. R. Anderson (Eds.), *Cognitive skills and their acquisition* (pp. 141–189). Hillsdale, NJ: Erlbaum.

Chi, M. T. H. (1987). Representing knowledge and metaknowledge: Implications for interpreting metamemory research. In F. E. Weinert & R. H. Kluwe (Eds.), *Metacognition, motivation, and understanding* (pp. 239–266). Hillsdale, NJ: Erlbaum.

Clark, J. M. & Paivio, A. (1991). Dual code theory and education. *Educational Psychology Review, 3*(3), 149–210.

Chi, M. T. H., Glaser, R. & Farr, M. J. (1988). *The nature of expertise.* Hillsdale, NJ: Erlbaum.

Conrad, R. (1964). Acoustic confusions in immediate memory. *British Journal of Psychology, 55,* 75–84.

Crowley, K., Shrager, J. & Siegler, R. S. (1997). Strategy discovery as a competitive negotiation between metacognitive and associative mechanisms. *Developmental Review, 17,* 462–489.

Demetriou, A., Christou, C., Spanoudis, G. & Platsidou, M. (2002). The development of mental processing: Efficiency, working memory, and thinking. *Monographs of the Society for Research in Child Development, 67*(1, Serial no. 268).

Ericsson, K. A. (1998). The scientific study of expert levels of performance: General implications for optimal learning and creativity. *High Ability Studies, 9,* 75–100.

Ericsson, K. A. (2001). Attaining excellence through deliberate practice: Insights from the study of expert performance. In M. Ferrari (Ed.), *The pursuit of excellence in education* (pp. 21–55). Hillsdale, NJ: Erlbaum.

Flavell, J. (1979). Metacognition and cognitive monitoring: A new area of cognitive-developmental inquiry, *American Psychologist, 34,* 906–911.

Hunt, E. (1989). Cognitive science: Definition, status, and questions. *Annual Review of Psychology, 40,* 603–629.

Joseph, G.-M. & Patel, V. L. (1990). Domain knowledge and hypothesis generation in diagnostic reasoning. *Journal of Medical Decision Making, 10,* 31–46.

Kuhn, D. (2002). A multi-component system that constructs knowledge: Insights from microgenetic study. In N. Granott & J. Parziale (Eds.), *Microdevelopment* (pp. 109–130). Cambridge, UK: Cambridge University Press.

Kuhn, D. & Pearsall, S. (1998). Relations between metastrategic knowledge and strategic performance. *Cognitive Development, 13,* 227–247.

LeFevre, J. A., Bisanz, J. & Mrkonjic, L. (1988). Cognitive arithmetic: Evidence for obligatory activation of arithmetic facts. *Memory and Cognition, 22,* 188–200.

Lesgold, A., Rubinson, H., Feltovich, P. J., Glaser, R., Kopfer, D. & Wang, Y. (1988). Expertise in complex skill: Diagnosing x-ray pictures. In M. T. H. Chi., R. Glaser & M. Farr (Eds.), *The Nature of Expertise* (pp. 311–342). Hillsdale, NJ; Erlbaum.

Miller, G. A. (1956). The magic number seven, plus or minus two: Some limits on our capacity for processing information. *Psychological Review, 63,* 81–97.

Norman, D. A. & Rumelhart, D. E. (1983). Studies of typing from the NLR research group. In W. E. Cooper (Ed.), *Cognitive aspects of skilled typing* (pp. 45–65). New York: Springer-Verlag.

Ornstein, P. A. & Naus, M. J. (1985). Effects of knowledge base on children's memory knowledge. In H. W. Reese (Ed.), *Advances in child development and behavior* (Vol. 19, pp. 113–149). New York: Academic Press.

Paivio, A. (1971). *Imagery and visual processes*. New York: Holt, Rinehart and Winston.

Patel, V. L. & Groen, G. J. (1991). The general and specific nature of medical expertise: A critical look. In K. A. Ericsson & J. Smith (Eds.), *Toward a general theory of expertise* (pp. 93–125). Cambridge, MA; Cambridge University Press.

Robertson, L. J. (1996a). Clinical reasoning, Part 1: The nature of problem solving, a literature review. *British Journal of Occupational Therapy, 59*, 178–182.

Robertson, L. J. (1996b). Clinical Reasoning, Part 2: Novice/Expert differences. *British Journal of Occupational Therapy, 59*, 212–216.

Rogers, J.C. & Holm, M. B. (1991). Occupational therapy diagnostic reasoning: A component of clinical reasoning. *American Journal of Occupational Therapy, 45*(11), 1045–1053.

Schell, B. (2003). Clinical reasoning: The basis of practice. In B. Crepeau, E. Cohn & B.A.B. Schell (Eds.), *Willard and Spackman's occupational therapy*. Philadelphia: Lippincott Williams & Wilkins.

Schmidt, H. G. & Baoshuizen, P. A. (1993). On acquiring expertise in medicine. *Educational Psychology Review, 5*(3), 205–221.

Schneider, W. & D. F. Bjorklund (1992). Expertise, aptitude, and strategic remembering. *Child Development, 63*, 461–473.

Schank, R. C. & Abelson, R. P. (1977). *Scripts, plans, goals and understanding*. Hillsdale, NJ: Erlbaum.

Schoenfeld, A. H. & Herrmann, D. J. (1982). Problem perception and knowledge structure in expert and novice mathematical problem solvers. *Journal of Experimental Psychology: Learning, Memory, and Cognition, 8*, 484–494.

Shepard, R. N. & Metzler, J. (1971). Mental rotation of three-dimensional objects. *Science, 171*(3972), 701–703.

Toglia, J. P. (1998). A dynamic interactional model to cognitive rehabilitation. In N. Katz, (Ed.), *Cognition and occupation in rehabilitation: Cognitive models for intervention in occupational therapy* (pp. 5-50). Bethesda, MD: American Occupational Therapy Association.

Unsworth, C. (1999). Clinical reasoning in occupational therapy. In C. Unsworth (Ed), *Cognitive and perceptual dysfunction: A clinical reasoning approach to evaluation and intervention* (pp. 43–73). Philadelphia: F. A. Davis.

Verhaeghen, P., Cerella, J. & Basak, C. (2004). A working memory workout: How to expand the focus of serial attention from one to four items in 10 hours or less. *Journal of Experimental Psychology: Learning, Memory & Cognition, 30*, 1322–1337.

Waugh, N. C. & Norman, D. A. (1965). Primary memory. *Psychological Review, 72*, 89–104.

Wickens, D. D., Born, D. G. & Allen, C. A. (1963). Proactive inhibition and item similarity in short-term memory. *Journal of Verbal Learning and Verbal Behavior, 2*, 440–445.

Zbrodoff, N. J. & Logan, G. D. (1986). On the autonomy of mental processes: A case study of arithmetic. *Journal of Experimental Psychology: General, 115*, 118–130.

Embodiment: Reasoning with the Whole Body

Barbara A. Boyt Schell and Dana Harris

CHAPTER OUTLINE

The whole body practice
Body, mind, truth, and reasoning
Intelligence and reasoning
  Multiple intelligence
  Bodily-kinesthetic intelligence
  Personal intelligence (intrapersonal and interpersonal)
  Embodiment in language and everyday concepts

Therapists as sensing beings
  Sensitivity and sensibility
  Perceptual acuity and skilled know-how
  Embodied communication
  Sensory preferences
  Sensory chunking
Summary

OBJECTIVES

After reading this chapter, the learner will be able to:

1 Examine how bodily experience fundamentally shapes understanding.
2 Explore the roles that sensation and perception play in professional reasoning.
3 Provide examples of how understanding the embodied mind can help deeper analysis and understanding of professional practice.

KEY TERMS

Embodiment
Sensitivity
Sensibility

I n this chapter, we explore the nature of clinical and professional reasoning as fundamentally grounded in our bodily experiences. At some level, this phenomenon has been recognized for a long time, since occupational therapy education has consistently required students to engage in fieldwork experiences as part of their educational experiences. Fieldwork is seen by some as critical to learning the "art of therapy" and by others as necessary to "apply" theory to practice. Each of these characterizations perhaps misses the point discussed in this chapter: Occupational therapy practice (indeed all practice) occurs through the use of embodied knowledge that develops as an interaction between a person and the environments in which he or she is acting. In other words, practice is personally experienced, and this experience in turn shapes what we expect and in some cases even allow to happen in subsequent therapy encounters. Because each person has individual differences within the commonalities of being human, each person's interpretation of his or her own experience is unique. Because this is a new area of research within occupational therapy, we draw from a wide range of disciplines in framing this discussion. By examining perspectives arising from psychology, cognitive science, linguistics, and philosophy as well as research within the health professions, we can explore implications of the embodied nature of practice for our own reasoning.

Thinking About Thinking 4-1

Human beings are creatures of the flesh. What we can experience and how we make sense of what we experience depend on the kinds of bodies we have and on the ways we interact with the various environments we inhabit. It is through our embodied interactions that we inhabit a world, and is through our bodies that we are able to understand and act within this world with varying degrees of success (M. L. Johnson, 1999, p. 80).

To set the stage for this discussion, the first part of this chapter examines examples of body-based knowledge necessary for effective practice. Historical understandings of body and mind, and the nature of abstract reasoning is discussed next, followed by a closer examination of intelligence and embodied knowledge as it relates to therapy practice. A discussion of Howard Gardner's theory of multiple intelligences provides one way of understanding the differing mix of talents on which therapists base their practices. Recent research looking directly at how therapists use sensory information to inform their clinical actions is presented. In the final sections, we share examples of how embodied practice is described in various health professions. Activities at the end of this chapter are designed to sensitize readers to their own embodied reasoning and its implications for practice.

THE WHOLE BODY PRACTICE

Professional reasoning is a "whole body practice." What does this mean? It means that much of the knowledge that we need and use in the therapy process is knowledge that is obtained from our sensory perceptions and which in turn is expressed in our own motor outputs. It is qualitatively different from the mental processes we use in trying to understand theories of practice. Indeed, as Argyris and Schön (1974) pointed out years ago, because theory is by nature an abstraction of the real world, theory is always too general to fully guide practice. The first author, Barbara, began to appreciate this as a student during her fieldwork experiences. Here are a few examples:

> I remember being told that spasticity was a function of abnormal muscle tone, and could be detected by rapidly stretching the affected muscles. If the person had spasticity you would detect a "clasp-knife type of catch and release." I confess that I had no idea what that meant. It wasn't until I started working with individuals who were recovering from brain injuries that I actually *felt* spasticity (i.e., used my own sense of touch and proprioception to gauge the muscle tension and release of that tension). Then I understood what was meant. Over time I learned to feel the difference between spasticity, rigidity, and other muscle problems, as opposed to tightness in joints due to arthritic changes or other impairments of the joint capsule. This in turn led me to think about activity possibilities and limitations in different ways as I worked with the person to increase his or her functional abilities.
>
> In another fieldwork situation, I was working with a young man who had a high-level spinal cord injury. I remembered from school how to measure muscle strength and what the implications were for decreased muscle strength in terms of the person's ability to perform daily tasks. However, it wasn't until I was working with a person who had no muscle strength in his triceps that I truly "understood" what this meant. I was helping this person get into a sweater, and in the process I raised his arm over his head. Much to my dismay, his forearm flopped forward and his hand hit him on the head! It wasn't until I *saw* and *felt* this happen that I began to truly understand what it meant to have no function in the triceps.

Because Barbara has worked with individuals with physical disabilities during most of her career, these examples focus on the perception of motor impairments. However, once you start appreciating the sensory and perceptual aspects of therapy, it is easy to find examples from all areas of practice. For instance, therapists working with individuals with persistent mental illness will notice if a client has body odor or *smells* as if he is not keeping up with his personal hygiene. This becomes a clue to explore what is going on in terms of his bathing and laundry routines. Therapists working with young children with sensory processing problems and attention deficit syndromes will *see* the child move his body, *hear* the change in the child's rate and quality of speech, and *interpret* from these cues that the child is becoming agitated by sensory overload. This prompts the therapist to introduce calming strategies or to teach parents how to manage the child's environment to avoid sensory overload.

Now that the nature of the whole body practice is somewhat clearer, we turn to some of the dilemmas associated with this aspect of clinical reasoning. One of the first issues is to give careful thought to the nature of truth finding in therapy, particularly with the emphasis on "evidence-based practice" in today's health care arenas. Although this at first seems to be a discussion of mental processes only, it becomes clear that our bodies shape how we think about the world. We will briefly review how our beliefs about knowledge and truth evolved in Western cultures. This review is important to sensitize those of us who come from these cultures about our own beliefs based on these perspectives (see Chapter 10 for a more in-depth discussion of these issues). After that, we will explore some different ways in which we can conceptualize our body–minds (since the English language does not customarily reflect the unitary nature of our bodies and minds, we use the terms *body–mind* or *embodied mind*). In particular, we will explore how we can deepen our understanding of our own body–minds and some of the avenues to consider for improving our body–minds for effective reasoning.

BODY, MIND, TRUTH, AND REASONING

A critical problem for a person engaged in professional reasoning is the discernment of the client's problem (what is *truly* going on) and what is the best (or *true*) way to resolve the problem. At its most fundamental, this requires an understanding of what is truth and how we know something to be true. Philosophers from early Greek times to postmodern eras have evolved different responses to these questions. As summarized by Lakoff and Johnson (1999), there were several key turnings in the evolution of philosophical thought. In early times, Aristotle believed that we knew truth because our minds could "directly grasp the essences of the world" (p. 94). Much later, Descartes postulated a split between the body and the mind: "The body was flesh and of the world; the mind was not" (p. 94). In this understanding, ideas were representations of aspects of the world, but the mind did not directly connect with the world. This view served to underpin much of the sciences developing in the late 1800s and the first part of the 1900s. Scientists attempted to find objective truths, free from the influences of the particular person who was seeking that truth.

In the middle of the 1900s, philosophers began to challenge the separation of mind and body. Merleau-Ponty and John Dewey (Lakoff & Johnson, 1999) both attempted to bring new understandings of physiology and cognitive science to classic philosophical questions. These philosophers brought to the fore the belief that knowledge was constructed by each individual's experience within particular contexts. Truth became more relative. Rather than a fixed reality, they believed that each person's "truth" is an outcome of what that embodied person perceives within a specific context. Similarly, Weiss and Haber (1999) offer a number of essays from different disciplines that "attempt to break down the binary opposition between nature and culture that has all too often been symbolized and reinforced by an association of the body with nature and consciousness with culture." (p. xii). In short, the mind and body were reunited, and knowledge must therefore be understood as a whole bodied phenomenon.

Building on these perspectives, Donald Schön (1983) brought these concepts to the study of professional practice. Indeed, as noted in Chapter 1, it was the American Occupational Therapy Foundation's invitation for Dr. Schön to speak to a group of leaders that launched much of the profession's interest in the nature of clinical reasoning. In his landmark publication, *The Reflective Practitioner* (1983), he challenged the contemporary view of professional practice as being an objective process guided by theory that was instrumentally applied to practice situations. Instead, he proposed that professional knowledge was embedded in the *doing* of the practice, and that professionals both *reflected in* and *on* their experiences to further develop their knowledge.

Picking up on Schön's ideas, the AOTF funded a clinical reasoning study that led to an examination of practitioners in the Boston area over a 2-year period (Mattingly & Fleming, 1994). In this study, Fleming and Mattingly discovered that multiple modes of reasoning appeared to be used by therapists (Fleming, 1994)—a proposition that has received continued support both within and beyond occupational therapy (Schell, 2003; Higgs & Jones, 2002). Fleming's view was informed in part by Gardner's work on the Theory of Multiple Intelligences, which are discussed next. In interpreting the research findings, Mattingly spent considerable time discussing how occupational therapists worked to understand the "lived body" (Mattingly, 1994, p. 71) or phenomenological understanding of the illness experience from the patient's perspective. Ironically, little analysis was provided about the therapist's own lived experience of the therapy process and the embodied nature of clinical reasoning. It is, however, this study, which launched the first author's interest in the nature of clinical and professional reasoning and how it develops.

INTELLIGENCE AND REASONING

If professional knowledge is embedded in the "doing" of practice, as Schön (1983) suggested, then it is reasonable to consider the factors that may influence therapy actions. One of the assumptions guiding this discussion is that therapists have differing constellations of talents and abilities that serve to inform or limit their professional reasoning. Gardner's work on multiple intelligences serves as a useful way to consider the possible explanations of practice variance.

Multiple Intelligences

In the 1980s, Gardner posed a multifaceted approach to understanding intelligence (*Table 4-1*), suggesting that there were at least seven kinds of intelligence, each of which are related to skills used in varying degrees by humans for both finding and solving genuine problems or difficulties (Gardner, 1984/2004). These included linguistic, musical, logical-mathematical, spatial, bodily-kinesthetic, and personal intelligences (intra- and interpersonal). In more recent work, he has suggested an additional possibility of naturalist intelligence (Gardner, 1995). Gardner's research suggests that individuals generally possess some degree of all these forms of intelligence, although traditionally psychologists had attended primarily to linguistic and logical-mathematical intelligence when forming tests of general intelligence, known commonly as IQ tests.

TABLE 4-1
Gardner's Multiple Intelligences*

Intelligence	Characteristics
Linguistic	Enjoys language (including hand symbols) Sensitive to meanings of words and their use Sensitive to sounds of words, phrases and their ordering Learns well listening to others Good at expressing and explaining ideas orally or in writing Often highly developed in novelists, poets, journalists, political leaders, skilled teachers, and scholars
Musical	Enjoys hearing, singing, and making music Discerns meaning and importance in sets of pitches rhythmically arranged Composes or uses music to communicate with others Readily learns and retains tunes and songs Plays musical instruments Often highly developed in composers, musicians, conductors
Mathematical/logical	Likes to solve puzzles and problems Likes logical explanations and can sustain long chains of reasoning Arranges tasks in sensible orderly sequence Recognizes patterns and appreciates connections within and among patterns Often highly developed in scientists, mathematicians
Visual/spatial	Perceives visual world accurately Can remember, reproduce , transform, and modify things observed even when no longer looking at stimulus Observant; sees things others do not Sees clearly with mind's eye Films, slides, videos, help learning Uses charts, diagrams, maps, easily Often highly developed in artists, architects, scientists, chess masters, and peoples dependent on knowing land features for hunting and traveling
Interpersonal	Notices and makes distinctions among other individuals Attends to moods, temperaments, motivations, and intention in others Can help with difficulties among people Enjoys teamwork, discussing and cooperating with others Often highly developed in political and religious leaders, skilled parents, teachers and those in helping professions
Intrapersonal	Able to access one's own feeling life. Discriminates among internal feelings Uses internal feelings to help understand self and guide behavior Ponders on the relevance of what they are doing and learning Often highly developed in novelists, therapists and patients who attain deep knowledge about their inner life and wise elders

(continued)

TABLE 4-1

(continued)

Intelligence	Characteristics
Bodily/kinesthetic	Uses body in highly differentiated and skilled manner
	Can involve body use for either expression (as in dance) or for goal directed movement (as in sports or therapy)
	Likes to deal with problems physically, gets directly involved—hands on
	Demonstrates good timing and sequencing of bodily activities
	Remembers best when they have done it
	Often highly developed in athletes, dancers, some therapists
Naturalistic (proposed)[†]	Able to readily recognize plants and animals
	Makes consequential decisions in natural world
	Uses understanding of natural world productively
	Expected to be highly developed in farmers, hunters, biological scientists, gardeners, ecologists

*Adapted from Gardner (1984/2004).
[†]Adapted from Gardner (1995).

It is likely that occupational therapists must possess solid "IQs," certainly to get into professional programs, but it is also likely that other forms of intelligence are critical for the actual practice of therapy. Of particular interest here are the bodily-kinesthetic and personal intelligences, although a case can be made for the importance of other forms of intelligence in therapy, depending on the practice arena. Gardner himself notes the importance of linguistic intelligence to much of modern life.

Thinking About Thinking 4-2

This essential requirement of any performance that can be called skilled becomes much more plain if we look at a few actual instances. The player in a quick ball game; the operator, engaged at his work bench, directing his machine and using his tools; the surgeon conducting an operation; the physician arriving at a clinical decision—in all these instances and in innumerable other ones that could just as well be used, there is the continuing flow from signals occurring outside the performer and interpreted by him to actions carried out; then on to further signals and more action, up to the culminating points of the achievement of the task, or whatever part of the task is the immediate objective. . .Skilled performance must all the time submit to receptor control, and must be initiated and directed by the signals which the performer must pick up from his environment, in combination with other signals, internal to his own body, which tell him about his own movements as he makes them.

—Sir Frederic Bartlett (1958, pg. 14; quoted in Gardner, 2004, pg. 208).

Bodily-Kinesthetic Intelligence

Bodily-kinesthetic intelligence is reflected in the "ability to use one's body in highly differentiated and skilled ways, for expressive, as well as goal-directed, purposes" (Gardner, 1984/2004, pg. 206). This requires skilled timing, as well as the ability to execute the desired movements. Gronda (1999) describes this sense well in her description of contact dancing:

> **I am dancing with you. My skin is in contact with yours. I feel the weight of my body falling toward the floor, or swept along by a horizontal velocity. I try and feel where you are, where your weight is going. Our pleasure and safety depend on a heightened awareness of our bodies (¶1).**

In similar ways, Fleming shared how observers of videotaped therapy sessions of expert therapists and their patients elicited a common response of "The way the therapist acted with the patient looked so elegant and effortless . . . almost like a dance" (1994, p. 27) (see *Fig. 4-1A* through F). From this description, it is apparent that occupational therapists must have a keen sense of awareness of their bodies in space, and how their bodies are interacting with those of their clients. When practitioners help people with the intimate activities of daily life, there is often a need to touch and provide physical guidance during the therapy process. Therapists working with individuals who have mental illness have to develop an ability to sense when clients are being overwhelmed by environmental demands and need to know how to avoid infringing on each client's personal space while at the same time offering support. Much of this occurs by careful attention to body language of the client, as well as careful positioning of the therapist's body in relation to the client.

Personal Intelligences (Intrapersonal and Interpersonal)

It will be no surprise that therapists are expected to be gifted in the areas of personal intelligence. Gardner (1984, 2004) notes two facets to this form of intelligence, one of which is *intrapersonal*, which refers to the capacity to "access to one's own feeling life" (p. 239) and to use this ability to help understand the self and others, ultimately guiding one's behavior. The companion to this is *interpersonal* intelligence, the "ability to notice and make distinctions among other individuals and in particular, among their moods, temperaments, motivations, and intentions" (p. 239).

Although Gardner focuses on affect and emotion in his discussion, the ability to pick up on quite subtle aspects of one's own bodily responses, as well as those of others, underlie these forms of intelligence. Dr. Linsey Howie, an occupational educator at La Trobe University in Australia, has incorporated therapy techniques from Gestalt psychology (Yontif, 2005) as a way of helping students learn to both recognize and use their own bodily responses as cues to understand their emotions and thereby inform their interactions with patients. She discusses her approach in the Case Study below. Notice how she guides students to use their embodied knowledge and personal intelligences to strengthen the client-therapist relationship. More information about reasoning directed to interacting with clients is discussed in Chapter 9. The point highlighted here is the role that bodily experiences play in this process.

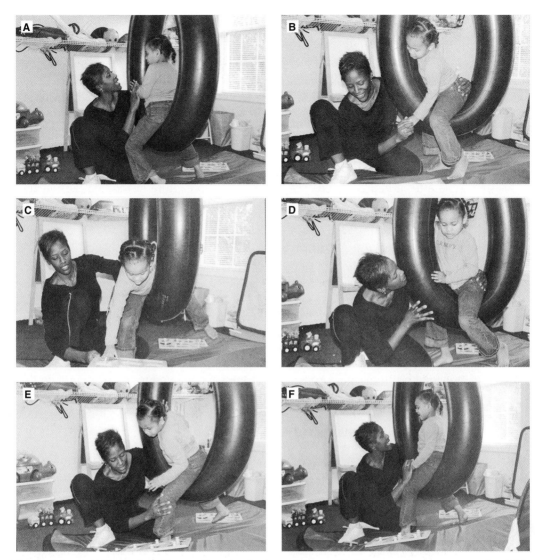

Figure 4-1   A–F. Notice how Dana adjusts her body position and facial expressions to support the child during therapy. (Photos courtesy of Dana Harris. Photographer, Cheryl Rutherford.)

CASE STUDY 4-1

Using Embodied Knowledge to Inform Clinical Practice

As an occupational therapy educator, I have over the years supervised many students during their clinical education placements. The topic of conducting dressing and shower assessments has often arisen during tutorials as a source of concern or embarrassment. Typically, students comment: "I don't know why, but I felt awkward and clumsy and out of my depth"; "I fumbled my way through the assessment and the supervisor was surprised, as I had been doing so well up until that point. I felt dreadful"; "I didn't know where to look, I could feel myself going red in the face, and I could not for the life of me remember what I had to do. I wished the ground had opened up and I could disappear." These comments are replete with indications that the student concerned was experiencing a highly emotional situation that left him or her feeling inadequate, self-conscious, or humiliated. How can we make use of this experience as individuals, supervisors, or educators? Let me share with you an example of how I have worked in this circumstance.

On one occasion, a young male student in the final year of the course brought to the tutorial for discussion a "significant incident" that had occurred in the previous week. Students were familiar with this format whereby they recorded an event, including as much detail as they could recall, as soon as possible after it had occurred. They were asked to capture in the first person, the time of day, who was present and where this event took place, what they observed had happened, what they did, what they were thinking or feeling, and what stood out for them at the end of the event.

One day, late in the afternoon, this student had been told by his supervisor that she would be arriving late the next day and that she would like him to conduct a shower assessment for an older client who was being considered for discharge at a case conference at midday. He described feeling tight in his stomach as she said this but cheerfully said "Yes, I can manage that for you."

He worried most of the night, thinking he should be able to do this—he was, after all, 3 weeks from completing his degree. He felt an acute sense of embarrassment at seeing an older woman naked for the first time in his life. He was aware of his stomach churning. He felt tired and wanted to go to bed. When the time came to conduct the assessment, he observed that his hands were sweating, his heart rate was increased, and he felt inadequate. All he could remember of the assessment was his urge to get it over and done with. He could not recall what he said; the whole event was a "big blur."

In the tutorial, I supported this student to share his narrative, and when he had finished I asked the other male students in the group if they could relate to this experience before asking the female students if they shared similar experiences. We soon had a list of feelings that go with confronting novel experiences or embarrassing situations. Next, we started to look at all the clues this student was given by his "body" and wrote them on the white board for consideration in small groups.

We went on to consider what we can do when our bodies are telling us something. We asked, "how can embodied awareness support professional development and deliver better client care?" We also asked how embodied knowledge could lead to better personal or workplace relationships. Lastly, we wondered how this knowledge might be used to support clinical reasoning and client-centered practice.

—Linsey Howie, June, 2006

Embodiment in Language and Everyday Concepts

Gardner's theory of multiple intelligences has served to reunite the mind and the body, by his inclusion of the various forms of intelligence. Authors Lakoff and Johnson (1999) also have done some very intriguing work on the body-mind. They examine the embodied nature of many of our fundamental concepts, which provides another lens through which to appreciate the interface of our bodies and therapy practice. Lakoff and Johnson draw on cognitive science and linguistics to

TABLE 4-2

Sensorimotor Experience and Concepts

Metaphor	Examples	Sensorimotor Origin
More Is Up (Used to judge quantity)	Gas prices are high	Sense of verticality as it relates to more (i.e., seeing glass fill up with water)
Affection Is Warmth (Used to judge affection)	She greeted me warmly	Temperature (i.e., feeling warm while being held affectionately)
Categories As Containers (Used to judge kinds of objects)	Are tomatoes in the fruit or vegetable category	Space (i.e., things that go together tend to be in same bounded region)
Difficulties Are Burdens (Used to judge difficulty)	She is weighed down by responsibilities	Discomfort of lifting heavy objects

Adapted from Lakoff & Johnson, 1999.

discuss the role of the cognitive unconscious which they describe as "the hidden hand that shapes how we conceptualize all aspects of our experience" (p. 13). This cognitive unconscious is based in bodily experiences and can readily be seen by the everyday metaphors which underlie many typical phrases. A few examples are provided in *Table 4-2* to illustrate how sensorimotor experiences are translated into everyday concepts. These are but a few highlights from their extensive and complex theories about **embodiment**. This discussion of the body, intelligence, and the formation of everyday concepts leads us to look more closely at the role of sensation, and sensory perception in professional reasoning.

THERAPISTS AS SENSING BEINGS

As occupational therapists, we are educated to notice the sensory processing of our clients and how skilled performance is influenced by both the person's body systems and the context in which that person is performing. For instance, in her Eleanor Clark Slagle lecture (2001), Winnie Dunn noted:

> The experience of being human is embedded in the sensory events of everyday life. When we observe how people live their lives, we discover that they characterize their experiences from a sensory point of view (p. 608).

If we focus on therapists themselves as sensory beings (rather than the clients we serve), it opens up a number of issues. For instance, how do the sensory preferences and processes of therapists affect what cues they notice and use in the problem setting phase or evaluation? Going even further, how does a particular therapist's embodied experience of a therapy situation affect the nature of the selection and implementation of interventions? Some of the answers to these questions can be gleaned from incidental information that surfaced while various researchers were focused on other topics. In addition, research from other professions can shed light on the topic of embodiment. Therefore, it is necessary to cast a wider net both within healthcare, as well as from literature and the arts, to gain clues about how the embodied self acts when engaging in the therapeutic process.

Sensitivity and Sensibility

In a lively examination of the role of vision in clinical reasoning, Bleakley and his colleagues address clinical judgment in the visual domains, reflecting ongoing discussions among several medical specialists (a pathologist, a dermatologist, and a radiologist); visual artists; and a psychologist (Bleakley, Farrow, Gould & Marshall, 2003). They draw on Foucalt's distinction between the "gaze" and the "glance" as a part of the clinical reasoning process, describing the gaze as "analytical and technical," and the glance as "appreciative and discriminatory" (p. 546). Bleakley and colleagues note that Foucault did not coin the term himself, but used a 19th century medical textbook, in which the definition included "the frequent, methodical and accurate exercise of the senses" (p. 546).

Bleakley and colleagues agree that clinical reasoning in the visual domain is an "aesthetic, rather than a technical or ethical issue" (p. 544). They elaborate on this by noting that there are two aspects to the aesthetics: **sensitivity** to the phenomenon and **sensibility**, which refers to the discriminative processes that inform clinical reasoning. Applying this idea to an occupational therapy situation, a therapist working with a client who had a hand injury may notice (sensitivity) that the person's skin is changing color and there is increased swelling accompanying the patient's report of pain. She may use this information (sensibility) to consider whether the person is showing signs of complex regional pain syndrome, which is a serious condition requiring effective pain management (Cooper, 2002) to prevent disability and promote normal hand use in daily life. Novice therapists may not even notice the symptoms or may attribute them to typical healing rather than assigning importance to these symptoms as signs of a developing complication. The latter would be an example of how Bleakley and colleagues describe clinical expertise is "a connoisscurship of informational images" (2003, p. 544).

Perceptual Acuity and Skilled Know-How

Benner, well known for her extensive research into clinical reasoning in nursing, notes that one can have the intellectual understanding, but lack the "perceptual acuity" to recognize which issues are important in a particular clinical situation (Benner, Hooper-Kyriakidis & Stannard, 1999, pg. 15). She discusses perceptual acuity in terms of emotional tone as well as in terms of sense-based knowledge, such as visual and tactile information. The role that *skilled know-how* has in critical care nursing is well exemplified in the description of a nurse working with a patient who has just come from cardiac surgery:

> . . .a skilled nurse assesses peripheral rewarming by examining the tem-
> perature change from the thigh down to the foot. She can feel the dif-
> ference in skin temperature, and gain a sense of the degree and extent
> of rewarming. This embodied skill enables the nurse to think-in-action
> about the influence of the warming blanket or the vasoactive drug infu-
> sions on the patient's progressive vasodilation and rewarming (p. 13).

Similarly, in occupational therapy, a therapist working with a child may hold
the child firmly to provide proprioceptive input useful for calming the child. In
doing this, she may notice how rapidly the child's heart is beating and may use
a slowing of the heart rate as an indication that the child is calmer and able to
participate in activity again (Margo, p.c. 2002).

Embodied Communication

In a study of clinical reasoning in physical therapy, Edwards and colleagues noted
that although movement was the most common instrumental procedure observed,
at times the therapist would use his or her hands as a means of communication:

> My hands can actually do more than just about anything and some-
> times . . . most times they're more powerful than what you can say
> anyway . . . putting hands on someone can speak enormous amounts
> (Edwards, Jones, Carr, Braunack-Mayer & Jensen, 2004, p. 325).

In a recent study examining how therapists' own sensory experiences informed
their clinical reasoning, the second author (Harris, 2005) videotaped therapy sessions and interviewed therapists about their sensory processes while reviewing the
video. In the Case Study below, Ila described how she used her body to appraise
the therapy process and communicate with a child during therapy.

CASE STUDY 4-2

Ila

I'm watching all that expression and I'm watching his safety, and his ability to
do what he just chose to do and making split second decisions about 'do I deal
with this or not deal with it?' And at that moment, what he chose to do did-
n't matter and he was safe and I was giving him, probably gave him, a bit of
the eye saying "I know you made a choice different from what I asked you to
do but it was okay." You know that look you can give a kid saying "I'm
acknowledging what you did, don't think that you got away with it, but it
doesn't matter."

Later she says, "I'm watching him carefully at this point. This is one of those
[points] that I wanted him to do something else, and he was defying me so I'm
watching his face to try to decide what I needed to do about that based on his
emotional expressions. Also, when kids are doing that, I try to see if I can do
some of that [intervention] floor time style. Can I take something they are doing
and turn it into something productive?"

Ila explains the messages she is giving: "And based on his behavior I know I'm grading the amount of grasp strength I use, both to tell him something and to control . . . So I'm grading the amount of effort I use and input I give to hold onto him. And that's for . . . that slightly firmer squeeze that says 'I mean business' versus light touch, that in this situation says 'I don't care', or 'You can have control' or holding onto him with a little more firm grasp gives him a message.

Janice Burke, noted occupational therapy scholar, studied the verbal and nonverbal behaviors used by pediatric occupational therapists when they were evaluating young children accompanied by parents. She found that different body positions relative to the client were associated with differing therapy assumptions (Burke, 1997). For example,

> [In the first 10 minutes of an evaluation session] . . . Therapists who used the occupation approaches demonstrated the use of full body orientation to the parents and to the children. . . .In contrast, the therapists using the medical model did not use full orientation to parents or to children during their evaluation interactions (p. 163).

Burke also was able to delineate different bodily behaviors and relate them to responses by the parent. For instance,

> Therapist/parent interaction was more assured when the therapist had direct postural and facial orientation to the parent. When therapists did not coordinate their interactions with direct postural orientation they were not as successful in completing the interaction (Burke, 1997, p. 136).

Although the importance of nonverbal communication is well recognized within occupational therapy, these examples suggest that there is more to be learned. A close examination of embodied aspects of both receiving and imparting messages inherent in the therapy process could help therapists appraise and expand their skills.

Sensory Preferences

In the same study discussed in the previous section, Harris (2005) found that there appeared to be a connection between therapists' own bodily preferences and their approach to therapy in treating children with autism. For instance, Jeff stated:

> I know that deep pressure and activities that involve using the major muscles, pushing activities, jumping activities, activities that involve a lot of joint compression; I find that they help me to calm down and focus, and I find that true with most of the kids that I treat, so I use a lot of deep pressure and heavy work to help them relax and pull it in.

Another example was Maria's discussion about the scent of therapy materials, such as putty with a child: "I avoid that [use of scented therapy objects]. I don't tolerate different smells, so I don't use any scented. . . .I'm intolerant of fragrances." Although therapists may be able to articulate these preferences when asked to reflect directly on videos of their treatment sessions, it is likely that much of the bodily preferences of therapists go unnoticed both in the ways that they inform clinical reasoning and limit therapy options.

Sensory Chunking

Harris (2005) also found evidence that therapists used *combinations* of sensory observations, which both informed their clinical reasoning and in turn guided their therapy actions. These combinations seemed to form sensory patterns or frames, consistent with the discussion of long-term memory discussed in the preceding chapter. For example, Jeff described how he attended to the child's movement in synchrony with his own body movement while at the same time listening to the child's breathing:

> *Jeff*: I watch his head and I can see him bob up and down with me. . . . And I listen to his breathing 'cause that tells me if I'm over-stimulating or under-stimulating him, ...Basically, listening and just feeling the way he moves with me. When he's more relaxed, he makes a different set of sounds, like intake sounds (imitates sounds). So you can tell a lot of where he is by his sounds. When he's getting a lot of stimulation, the sound is really low like (imitates sound). When he's really focusing you don't hear anything from him, he just concentrates on business.
>
> *Dana*: How can you tell that that he's starting to get frustrated?
>
> *Jeff*: His actions become a little less detailed and he tries to use a little more muscle, more force and less movement of the wrist and hand. He reverts to just a quick shove instead of trying to maneuver. I'm watching his eyes because a lot times that tells me when he's about to toss something, when he's about to reach somewhere else and distract and change the subject. . .I'm feeling the actions in his hands, and when he's more relaxed I know that he has an idea of what he's doing, and he continues. When he starts to tense up, I can tell that he's starting to get confused or he's starting to get frustrated . . . When Jonathan has an idea of what he's supposed to do or what he's trying to do, you can feel his body relax—he'll kind of settle into you while he's working. . . . .
>
> *Dana*: When you say settle into you, how do you know?
>
> *Jeff*: He'll relax and you'll feel his back, his body just kind of gently presses into you when he's working, like he's using you for an anchor.

Jeff's appears to have developed an interlinked set of sensory information (rate of breathing, observation of hand movement, observation of eye movement, feel of the child's body). He uses this information to interpret the child's performance and to anticipate when the child may need more active intervention from the therapist to modify the activity challenge so that the child can perform comfortably.

SUMMARY

In this chapter, we have focused closely on the embodied nature of the professional reasoning process. Occupational therapists have long recognized the importance of the body (especially our sensory and motor processing) in the performance of daily occupations. Here, we turn the spotlight on the therapists themselves, attempting to delineate ways in which our bodily make-up, skills, and preferences interface with our problem-finding and preferred intervention approaches. We embrace the notion of the embodied mind and expand on the role that therapists' own bodies play in the therapy process. The ways in which our bodies shape and inform our clinical and professional reasoning process have received little attention in the occupational therapy literature. By attending to the embodied nature of professional reasoning, new avenues for teaching students, as well as improving practice skills, can be explored.

LEARNING ACTIVITY 4-1

Sensory Me

Purpose

The purpose of this activity is to help learners gain insight into their own sensory profiles and to examine the implications for their professional reasoning. It can be used effectively for Level 1 or Level 2 students or for practitioners wishing to examine their own professional reasoning.

Connections to Major Clinical Reasoning Constructs

This activity helps learners operationalize the concept of embodiment described in this chapter.

Directions for Learners

1 Complete the Adult Sensory Profile (Dunn, 1999).
2 Discuss the results with a faculty member, supervisor, or trusted peers.
3 Using the results, consider how your preferences impact the:
   - Choices you make about practice areas to work in
   - Clients you prefer to work with
   - Therapy techniques you choose or avoid
   - Therapy settings and environments you choose or avoid
4 How do your choices impact the effectiveness of the therapy you provide?
5 How might you alter or adapt your therapy practices to improve outcomes and still deal with your own embodied needs and preferences?

LEARNING ACTIVITY 4-2

Observation Guide

Purpose

The purpose of this activity is to help learners attend closely to information they gain from their senses, use that information to observe client skills, make judgments about those skills, and analyze the personal and contextual factors affecting performance. It can be used effectively for Level 1 or Level 2 students, or for practitioners wishing to uncover their embodied reasoning.

Connections To Major Clinical Reasoning Constructs

This activity starts by highlighting the embodied nature of professional reasoning. Involvement in this activity supports the learner in becoming more aware of the sensations they attend to during therapy and how these inform their clinical reasoning.

Directions for Learners

1 Select one therapy task that you either observed or participated in with a client.
2 Using the guide below and the Observation Guide provided (AOTA-COP, 2002; Fisher, 2002), complete the following information:
   ■ Briefly describe the task (i.e., a child with autism was being encouraged to play on a swing)
   ■ Note the sensations you experienced in general (i.e., *skin sensations:* "It was hot and windy, I kept getting sand blown in my face"; *hearing:* "I could hear the other children laughing and yelling as they played nearby"; *smell:* "I could smell flowers from a nearby honeysuckle vine").
3 Using the list of skills provided*, identify three skills that the client seemed to be able to do well, and three that the client appeared to have some difficulty with.
4 Using the analysis grid provided:
   ■ Identify the specific behavior you observed.
   ■ Describe what you sensed that made you identify this behavior.
   ■ Comment on the quality of the performance.
   ■ Identify what personal factors seem to be "causing" the performance observed.
   ■ Identify what environmental factors seem to be affecting the performance observed.
5 Share your analysis with a partner, or in a reflection seminar. Invite comments about alternative implications of the sensory and skill observations you describe.

* The skills listed here are from the AOTA Practice Framework. Other lists from different theories and models may be substituted.

Observation Guide*

Skills Selected	Behavior Observed	Senses Informing Observation	Performance Quality	Personal Factors Affecting Performance	Contextual Factors Affecting Performance
Three skills done well					
1.					
2.					
3.					
Three "problem" skills					
1.					
2.					
3.					

Motor Skills		Process Skills		Communication/ Interaction Skills	
Stabilizes	Moves	Paces	Terminates	Contacts	Expresses
Aligns	Transports	Attends	Searches/Locates	Gazes	Modulates
Positions	Lifts	Chooses	Gathers	Gestures	Shares
Walks	Calibrates	Uses	Organizes	Maneuvers	Speaks
Reaches	Grips	Handles	Restores	Orients	Sustains
Bends	Endures	Heeds	Navigates	Postures	Collaborates
Coordinates	Paces	Inquires	Notices/responds	Articulates	Conforms
Manipulates		Initiates	Accommodates	Asserts	Focuses
Flows		Continues	Adjusts	Asks	Relates
		Sequences	Benefits	Engages	Respects

Behavior observed: Note specifically what you saw, heard, etc (i.e., child screamed each time her feet left the ground).

Senses informing observation: Note what sensory information related to your observation (ie, heard scream, also saw her grip swing chain really hard).

Performance quality: Make a judgment about the quality of the skill performance. Consider effort, efficiency, safety, independence, social appropriateness (i.e., child required moderate assistance to swing, it took her considerable effort, and her negative response was pretty atypical for a child her age).

Personal factors affecting performance: Consider factors instrinsic to the client (i.e., strength, emotional stamina) that appear to be affecting performance (i.e., child appears to have some vestibular problems).

Contextual factors: Consider factors extrinsic to the child that appear to be affecting performance (i.e., swing is too large with no back support, child has no access to swing at home or on nearby playground).

REFERENCES

American Occupational Therapy Association–Commission on Practice (AOTA–COP). (2002). Occupational therapy practice framework: Domain and process. *American Journal of Occupational Therapy, 56,* 609–639.

Argyris, C. & Schön, D. (1974*). Theory in practice: Increasing professional effectiveness.* San Francisco, CA: Jossey-Bass.

Bleakley, A., Farrow, R., Gould, D. & Marshall, R. (2003). Making sense of clinical reasoning: judgment and the evidence of the senses. *Medical Education, 37,* 544–552.

Burke, J.P. (1997). Frames of meaning: An analysis of occupational therapy evaluations of young children. *Dissertation Abstracts International* 58(03), 644. (UMI Number: 9727199).

Cooper, C. (2002). Hand impairments. In C. A. Trombly & M. V. Radomski (Eds.), *Occupational therapy for physical dysfunction (*5th ed., pp. 927–963). Philadelphia: Lippincott Williams & Wilkins.

Dunn, W. (1999). *The sensory profile.* San Antonio: Psychological Corporation.

Dunn, W. (2001). 2001 Eleanor Clarke Slagle Lecture: The sensations of everyday life: Empirical, theoretical and pragmatic considerations. *American Journal of Occupational Therapy, (55)* 608–620.

Edwards, I., Jones, M., Carr, J., Braunnack-Mayer, A. & Jensen, G.A. (2004). Clinical reasoning strategies in physical therapy. *Physical Therapy,* 8(4), 312–335.

Fisher, A. (January 2002). A model for planning and implementing top-down, client-centered, and occupation-based occupational therapy interventions. Manual for OTIPM workshop.

Fleming, M.H. (1994). The search for tacit knowledge. In C. Mattingly & M.H. Fleming (Eds.), *Clinical reasoning: Forms of inquiry in a therapeutic practice* (pp. 22–34). Philadelphia: F. A. Davis.

Gardner, H. (2004). *Frames of mind: The theory of multiple intelligences* (Twentieth anniversary ed.). New York: Basic Books.

Gardner, H. (1995). Reflections on multiple intelligences: Myths and messages. *Phi Delta Kappan,* 77, 200–209.

Gronda, H. (1999). Improvising presence. *Proximity* 2, 2. Retrieved April 17, 2005 from http://proximity.slighty.net/v_four/v2e2alhtm

Harris, D. L.(1995). *Therapist's sensory processing and its influence upon occupational therapy interventions in children with autism.* Manuscript in preparation.

Higgs, J. & Jones, M. (Eds.) (2002). *Clinical reasoning in the health professions.* Woburn, MA: Butterworth-Heinemann.

Johnson, M.L. (1999). Embodied reason. In G. Weiss & H. F. Haber (Eds.), *Perspectives on embodiment: The intersections of nature and culture* (pp. 81–102). New York: Routledge.

Lakoff, G. & Johnson, M. (1999). *Philosophy in the flesh: The embodied mind and its challenge to Western thought.* New York: Basic Books.

Mattingly, C. (1994). Occupational therapy as a two-body practice: The lived body. In C. Mattingly & M.H. Fleming (Eds.), *Clinical reasoning: Forms of inquiry in a therapeutic practice* (pp. 64–93). Philadelphia: F. A. Davis.

Mattingly, C. & Fleming, M. H. (1994). *Clinical reasoning: Forms of inquiry in a therapeutic practice.* Philadelphia: F. A. Davis.

Schell, B. A. B. (2003). Clinical reasoning: the basis of practice. In E.B Crepeau, E. S. Cohn & B. A. B. Schell (Eds.), *Willard and Spackman's occupational therapy* (10th ed., pp. 131–133). Philadelphia: Lippincott Williams & Wilkins.

Schön, D. A. (1983). *The reflective practitioner: How professionals think in action.* New York: Basic Books.

Weiss, G. & Haber, H.F. (1999). *Perspectives on embodiment: The intersections of nature and culture.* New York: Routledge.

Yontif, G.M (2005). Gestalt therapy theory of change. In A.L. Woldt & S.M. Toman (Eds.), *Gestalt therapy: History, theory, & practice* (pp. 81–100). Thousand Oaks, CA: Sage.

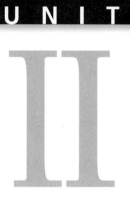

Aspects of Professional Reasoning

5

Scientific Reasoning

George S. Tomlin

OBJECTIVES

After reading this chapter, the learner will be able to:

1 Discuss the nature, history, and present context of scientific reasoning.
2 Differentiate between logical reasoning and the scientific method.
3 Appreciate the scope of scientific reasoning in practice, management, research, and education.
4 Apply scientific reasoning in the occupational therapy process.
5 Appreciate the limitations of scientific reasoning and suggest approaches to deal with these limitations, which avoid "Descartes' error."

KEY TERMS

Scientific reasoning	Syllogism	Procedural reasoning
Generalizable	Empirical	Occupational therapy diagnosis
Logical reasoning	Hypothesis testing	Diagnostic reasoning
Evidence-based practice	Deductive reasoning	Practice errors
Scientific inquiry	Inductive reasoning	Reductionism

Did you go through a **scientific reasoning** process to select occupational therapy as your profession? Did you make careful, systematic observations, collect data from numerous sources, compare alternative professions, and weigh their pros and cons? To what extent was your decision influenced by feelings, related experience, other commitments, prior decisions, or a sudden insight that "this is the right path for me?"

Your selection of a particular occupational therapy educational program may have been similar—part reasoning with factual data, part testing the waters by visiting and attending class, and part relying on overall feelings about a program's distinctive strengths and inescapable drawbacks: a weighing of personal, academic, financial, family considerations, and finally deciding by what means? If you are like most people, you probably underwent a combination of factual or scientific reasoning and drawing conclusions based on feelings, experiences, and the opinions of others close to you for such an important decision. So it seems to be with scientific reasoning in occupational therapy. The decisions therapists make every day are too important to be made without the benefit of careful, systematic, educated thinking, and too important to be made solely that way.

This chapter contains a portrayal and an analysis of what is called scientific reasoning in occupational therapy. My goal is to highlight the unique strengths in this type of thinking, to explore carefully its limitations, and to predict how this type of reasoning may evolve in the future. It is my further intent to argue that splitting off scientific reasoning as something different from our other types of reasoning is actually to reincarnate "Descartes' error," that is, separating the mind from the body in such a fundamental way that it has been difficult ever since, on a philosophical plane, to connect them together again.

Thinking About Thinking 5-1

. . . Now I had before my eyes the coolest, least emotional, intelligent human being one might imagine, and yet his practical reason was so impaired that it produced, in the wanderings of daily life, a succession of mistakes, a perpetual violation of what would be considered socially appropriate and personally advantageous. . . .The instruments usually considered necessary and sufficient for rational behavior were intact in him. . .There was only one significant accompaniment to his decision-making failure: a marked alteration of the ability to experience feelings.

—Damasio, 1994 (pp. xi–xii)

WHAT IS SCIENTIFIC REASONING?

Scientific reasoning is a systematic approach to creating, testing, and using knowledge to make decisions. It follows a prescribed method to compel conclusions that are dependable and **generalizable.** Its reputation is as a "way of deciding" that relies on other than sudden feelings, common sense, practical experience, dogmatic belief, or flights of the imagination. Similarly, its close relative, **logical reasoning,** seeks to establish structured rules for reaching conclusions that are irrefutable.

The derivations of the words "scientific reasoning" provide insights into the evolution of the meaning of the phrase. *Table 5-1* provides the dictionary definitions and etymologies of the pertinent words. From its root origins (science: *skei,* to cut or split; reasoning: *ar,* to fit together [*American Heritage Dictionary*, 4th ed. 2000 pp. 2046, 2021]), one might say that scientific reasoning is derived from a notion that to create knowledge is to "fit together by cutting or splitting."

TABLE 5-1

Sources and Meanings: Science, Scientific, and Reasoning

Science	From Latin *scientia*, from *scire:* to know; akin to Latin *scindere*, to cut or split; Greek *schizein:* to split: (1) The observation, identification, description, experimental investigation, and theoretical explanation of phenomena. . . . (4) knowledge, especially that gained through experience.
Scientific	Of, relating to, or using the methodology of science.
Reasoning	From Latin *ratio*: to consider, confirm, ratify: (1) Use of reason, especially to form conclusions, inferences, or judgments. (2) Evidence or arguments used in thinking or argumentation.

Definitions from the *American Heritage Dictionary,* 4th ed. 2000.

Scientific reasoning is related to similar terms in the following ways: It is said to be one aspect of clinical reasoning, although its applications extend beyond that to the roles of management, research, and education by members of the profession. It is thus one aspect of professional reasoning, the term used in this book to denote comprehensively the types of reasoning used in professional practice. Scientific reasoning also overlaps partly with **evidence-based practice**, in that both are concerned with the evaluation and application of research evidence to clinical practice. In its traditional definition, however, scientific reasoning does not overlap with evidence-based practice on the component of clinical experience and expert opinion, which evidence-based practice includes but scientific reasoning does not. Nor does it (traditionally) include taking into account the wishes, goals, and values of the client, as evidence-based practice in many professions holds that it is crucial to do (Sackett, Straus, Richardson, Rosenberg & Haynes, 2000). Finally, **scientific inquiry** uses many of the same cognitive techniques that scientific reasoning uses, but scientific inquiry is directly focused on the generation of generalizable knowledge, whereas scientific reasoning concerns itself with decision making in practice.

HISTORY AND CONTEXT OF SCIENTIFIC REASONING

The systematic study of logic was first documented in the times of classical Greece (500–400 BC). What has come to be called the scientific method arose between AD 1500 and 1700 during the European Renaissance. The written beginnings of formal logical thought may be found in the works of Plato, Aristotle, and other classical Greek thinkers. Logic was studied for its relationship to rhetoric (to detect when an argument was fallacious). One early codification of the principles of logic was Aristotle's *Organon*, which contained 19 syllogisms of logic, or simple inference rules (Devlin, 1997). An example of a **syllogism** is:

All OTRs are registered with NBCOT.
Gayle is an OTR.
Therefore, Gayle is registered with NBCOT.

Classical philosophy and logic were taken very seriously in Europe's early universities.

> **Bachelors and Masters of Arts who do not follow Aristotle's philosophy are subject to a fine of five shillings for each point of divergence, as well as for infractions of the rules of the _Organum_.**
> —Statutes of the University of Oxford, 14th century (Devlin, 1997, p. 21)

From medieval times to the present, two schools of thought on logic have developed. One school holds that logic is an "objective matter of the relations among propositions, predicates and terms" (Elio, 2002, p. 5). The other school believes that the laws of logic are ". . . suitably generalized accounts of patterns of human thought and reasoning" (Elio, p. 5). Currently, most scholars believe that the syllogisms of logic cannot capture and express the complexity and subtlety of actual daily situations encountered by people. Thus, although they are sometimes useful, syllogisms are not of unlimited value in helping us reason.

The enunciation of modern scientific method came during the early Renaissance in an attempt to shake off the orthodoxy of the Catholic Church controlling legitimate knowledge. Galileo (1638, _Dialogo dei Massimi Sisterni),_ Bacon (1620, _Novum Organum_), Pascal (1670, _Pensees_), and Descartes (1637, _Discourse on Method_) are among the most famous European members of this movement. These Renaissance "men of science" advocated reasoning from **empirical** data via theory and **hypothesis testing,** not analytical reasoning from the prescribed theological ideas of the time (called dialectical reasoning). Their highest standard was a mathematical description of nature, which was claimed to provide certainty about one's conclusions. The essence of logical, mathematical thought is captured in the sequence, "Observation, Abstraction, Understanding, Description, Proof" (Devlin, 1997, p. 22). Once established and accepted, the conclusion of a proof was a justification for feeling certainty; hence, the desirability of using mathematical methods to tackle problems whenever possible. The process of the scientific method, as it has evolved into the 21st century, is found in Box 5-1.

B O X 5 - 1
Scientific Process

Formulating questions based on the current state of knowledge, interests, and
   needs
Defining the approach to gaining insights or answers
Collecting data
Categorizing
Analyzing/synthesizing
Seeking relationships, similarities, differences
Making interpretations
Drawing conclusions and formulating new questions

Adapted from Mosey, 1992 (pp. 124–133)

Logical thinking and the use of the scientific method rely on deductive, inductive, and probabilistic or statistical reasoning. (For a thorough treatment of their application to medical clinical inferencing, see Albert, Munson & Resnik, 1988.)

Deductive Reasoning

The rules for **deductive reasoning** are encapsulated in syllogisms. Does the conclusion follow inevitably from the premises? If so, and if the premises are true, then the conclusion must be true. Deductive reasoning appears to impart certainty to the conclusion (see Case Study 5-1 below).

CASE STUDY 5-1

Clinical Example of Deductive Reasoning

In a mental health setting, a social skills group has taken place. In her own notes, the occupational therapist documents what happened and her conclusion in the underlying form of a syllogism: If a person does not want to have anything to do with a group of people, the person does not interact with them in a sustained way.

Darin said he wanted to have nothing to do with people during the group this afternoon, but he stayed in the room the entire session, often making derogatory comments.

Therefore, Darin actually did want to interact with the group (probably not on the group's own terms).

Deductive reasoning, as here, often has an obvious ring to it. It is said to rearrange knowledge that we already have, not to uncover brand new knowledge.

Inductive Reasoning

Inductive reasoning is said to hold the potential for generating new knowledge. That is, given the empirical evidence available, what can we reasonably infer about a pattern, or predict about a future event? Uncertainty will always reside in our conclusions because no matter how much evidence we have and no matter how persuasive it appears to be, we cannot overcome the limitation of a possible confounding factor (another explanation) somewhere. In addition, there is the unresolved problem—first articulated by the Scottish philosopher David Hume (1748, 1955)—called the problem of induction and the uniformity of nature. That is, even if our inference is correct, our induction holds only if the principles of nature remain uniform into the future. Unfortunately, all we can draw upon in trying to induce that nature will remain uniform in the future is empirical evidence from the present or past. An example of inductive reasoning is found in Case Study 5-2 below.

CASE STUDY 5-2

Clinical Example of Inductive Reasoning

Maria has become more engaged in movement activities most of the time another child also participated.

I want Maria to try out a new activity today, so I will arrange for a playmate to be present so as to promote Maria's task engagement.

Induction has the acknowledged, built-in uncertainty. But deduction is also less than perfect in the certainty that it provides concerning our conclusions. Capturing the complexities of language, not considering for the moment the complexities of reality, in the form of logical syllogism, is usually problematic (Devlin, 1997; Oaksford & Chater, 2002). Take the example of the syllogism in the preceding Case Study 5-1 concerning the young person and the group activity in the mental health setting. Human motivation may not be simple enough to encode properly in syllogisms. When Darin says he wants to have nothing to do with the group, is that really the message behind his speech? Apparently not. He made a statement that could be interpreted as having a hidden or double meaning. Or, he suddenly changed his mind, which people are free to do, after all. Time adds a dimension of dynamism to a situation such that the conditions of the premise or the conclusion may be evolving by the moment. Thus, after the momentary change, the logical impetus of the syllogism is not sustained.

Probabilistic and Statistical Reasoning

To mitigate the uncertainty of induction, scientific inquirers created the mathematical disciplines of probability and statistics (beginning in the 17th and 19th centuries, respectively) (Ferguson & Takane, 1989). These mathematical approaches to uncertainty do not provide solutions of certainty, but rather they allow us to quantify the level of our uncertainty about an inductive conclusion. For example, a statistical analysis of an experimental comparison of splint positions might sustain the conclusion that we can say with 95% confidence that a dorsal forearm splint produced better functional outcomes after a peripheral nerve injury compared to a volar splint, for a particular group of individuals. (This group may or may not be statistically representative of a larger group of people, depending on how they were selected for the study.)

Statistics can never be properly used to "prove" a given statement. Yet, it was readily adopted as a method of analysis by scientific inquirers because it represented the application of precise mathematics to the uncertainty of reasoning in many questions of interest to science. Achieving less uncertainty, or greater confidence, in the outcomes of our reasoning has been one of the main goals of logical and scientific reasoning from very early times (harkening back to Aristotle: reducing the risk of making—or believing—a fallacious argument).

SCIENTIFIC CHALLENGES: LINEAR TO COMPLEX

At first, the Renaissance scientific method was applied to questions in nature that could be addressed through quantification, and where the quantifiable relationships were stable over time. Problems concerning forces, velocities, and sizes of objects encountered on earth (the physical sciences) were indeed eventually amenable to straightforward mathematical solutions. In the 19th and 20th centuries, the scientific method spread from the physical sciences to life sciences (the introduction of statistics was crucial here), to the social sciences, and finally to the sciences of individuals (psychology, anthropology, medicine). The latter part of the 20th century saw a rise in the importance of quantitative, scientific research in occupational therapy (Ottenbacher & Petersen, 1985), just as the profession emulated a narrower (many have used the term *reductionistic*) way of framing challenges in human performance. From the 1980s came the "discovery" and emergence of qualitative research as a legitimate method of scientific inquiry within occupational therapy. (I am using "scientific" here in the sense of a disciplined inquiry to produce knowledge—more the original meaning of the word— and not in the strict way it came to be defined from the 17th to the 20th centuries.) The importance of research findings for the actual practice of the profession has been reinforced by the movement (from the mid-1990s) toward evidence-based practice (Holm, 2000), although there are barriers yet to overcome (Dysart & Tomlin, 2002). Once qualitative research and evidence-based practice become less-hesitant allies (Hammel, 2001), there may even exist the conditions for the profession to have its own recognized distinctive epistemology of practice (Hammel & Carpenter, 2004).

As applied to the practice of a health profession, scientific reasoning is purported to help free us from the errors of surface impression, prejudice, overgeneralization, jumping to illogical conclusions, and the bias of idiosyncratic experience. Its proponents claim that it assists the practitioner in both the original acquisition of professional education and in the later conduct of competent, evidence-based practice.

Scientific reasoning enters into contemporary practice of occupational therapy through many different avenues, perhaps most powerfully in our unquestioned assumptions about "logical thinking," "objective reasoning," "rationality," and "unbiased, scientific approaches" to problems. From ancient Greek until modern times, this mode of thinking has been widely believed to be superior to other modes and even from Renaissance times to possess a separate existence in the mind itself ("I think, therefore I am"), called "Descartes' error" by Damasio (1994). "Rationality versus feelings," and "ruled by passions versus keeping a cool head" are but two examples embedded in our everyday language. The accuracy of these assumptions about objectivity, however, has been challenged in the 20th century from several directions of investigation (of scientific investigation at that): linguistic, empirical, theoretical (qualitative research approaches and assumptions), and the importance of coming to understand "meaning" for people.

Contemporary physical and life sciences, on the other hand, are not standing still, but rather are attempting to describe, understand, and predict phenomena of a complexity far beyond those addressed by classical science (using systems theory, quantum theory, string theory, relativity theory, modern mathematics, chaos theory, complexity theory, fuzzy logic, neural nets). It is similar for advances in modern biology/ecology (Constantz, 1994), with implications and applications rippling outward all the way to the study of human occupation and health. Devlin (1997) among others has voiced a hope that the newer tools of science, created to address far more complex physical problems, may have direct application in the investigation of complex human questions (e.g., Gray, Kennedy & Zemke, 1996; Royeen & Luebben, 2002; attempting to apply dynamical systems [chaos] theory to occupational therapy research questions). These developments reappear in the thesis proposed later in this chapter in discussion of the future of scientific reasoning.

SCOPE OF SCIENTIFIC REASONING

Reasoning in general and scientific reasoning in particular cannot be fully understood outside a context of person–task-environment. What are the embedded occupations of scientific reasoning in the field of occupational therapy?

1. In the creation and testing of disciplinary knowledge through "scientific inquiry" (conducting research).
2. In the systematic use of principles of logic and the scientific method in reasoning about cases in actual practice (professional reasoning in a "scientific" fashion).
3. In the application of the findings of 1 to the actions in 2, or evidence-based practice.

Each of these will be addressed in turn.

Scientific Inquiry

Pure research on human occupation has been conducted by occupational therapists, for example in occupational science (Zemke & Clark, 1996). Occupational science findings contribute to the content knowledge of practitioners in occupational therapy. Specific applied research has been pursued by faculty in academic programs, by practitioners, and by practitioner/faculty teams. Action research is most often conducted by a team of consumers, clinicians, and faculty (Kielhofner, 2004). Research methods range from case studies, normative studies, surveys, and other types of descriptive study through correlational studies and experimental studies (single-case and group studies) to naturalistic, qualitative studies. All methods, as examples of disciplined inquiry, have their own standards of rigor and produce valuable knowledge for the profession. Assigning a single hierarchy to prioritize their value is problematic.

The traditional approach in research put a premium on quantitative measurement and analysis. Recently, there has been greater acceptance of qualitative (linguistic) approaches to address meaning, intent, and context in fields from anthropology to communication to occupational therapy, where the approach lies particularly close to the essential core concerns of the field (Hammel, 2001). In their original forms, quantitative and qualitative research methods entailed very different assumptions about the nature of reality, the role of the researcher, and the nature of "knowledge." In some respects, though, they have been growing closer together. Traditional assumptions about the desirability of "objectivity," or an isolation between the researcher and the research participant, may undermine authentic studies of human behavior, attitudes, cognition, motivation, and meaning—in short, occupation. Some researchers now advocate studies deliberately combining the two approaches to provide the best window into understanding (DePoy & Gitlin, 2005).

Reasoning with Clients

Fleming (1991) identified three interwoven "tracks" of reasoning by occupational therapists: procedural, interactive, and conditional. **Procedural reasoning** "guides the therapist in thinking about the patient's physical performance problems"; interactive reasoning "is used when the therapist wants to understand the patient as a person"; conditional reasoning "is used to project an imagined future condition or situation for the person" (Fleming, p. 1007). Mattingly (1991a) labeled another aspect of reasoning "narrative," whereas Rogers (1983) and Neuhaus (1988) have referred to ethical reasoning. Unsworth (2005) found evidence of a kind of thinking among occupational therapists she named *generalization reasoning*. It appeared in the midst of all other types of reasoning, and entailed the application of outside general or specific knowledge to the problem at hand. Schell and Cervero (1993) coined the term *pragmatic reasoning* to represent the practical framing of possibility, within which other reasoning takes place. These types of reasoning are addressed in detail in Chapters 6, 7, and 8.

Conventional wisdom has assigned scientific reasoning to the procedural reasoning track. In daily professional practice, the decisions during the occupational therapy process that entail sensing problems of occupational performance, identifying problems, and inferring a cause in order to assign the **occupational therapy diagnosis** is referred to as **diagnostic reasoning** (Rogers & Holm, 1991), one aspect of procedural reasoning. In addition, reasoning from biologically based knowledge about humans, injuries, and disease processes to select scientifically established interventions that have demonstrated evidence for their effectiveness is another aspect of procedural reasoning. Scientific knowledge and a structure of rule-based decision making supposedly underlie procedural reasoning. There is presumed to exist a generalizable approach to procedural reasoning, which is systematic and generates findings, conclusions, and decisions that we can have high confidence in and that apply to a variety of people with a similar diagnosis. Later, the argument will be made that the equating of scientific reasoning with procedural reasoning is a misstep, albeit one based on powerful historical precedents (e.g., the mind/body split) dating back at least to the Renaissance.

Evidence-Based Practice

Evidence-based practice is defined as the blending of three sources of information for therapeutic practice: (1) published evidence of an intervention's effectiveness, (2) the clinical experience of the practitioner and the expertise of others, and (3) the values, goals, preferences, and wishes of the client (Sackett et al., 2000). To make use of published research findings in formulating clinical decisions, the practitioner must be adept at analyzing and synthesizing research findings, competent with statistical reasoning, and comfortable in applying generalizations from research to actual practice (Abreu, Peloquin & Ottenbacher, 1998). According to Holm (2000), the individual practitioner must acquire the knowledge outlined by Abreu et al., then infuse into practice the following acts: (1) asking clinical questions, (2) tracking down the best available evidence from literature, (3) appraising the evidence, (4) using the evidence to do the right things right, and (5) evaluating the impact of evidence-based practice through chart audit, patient outcomes, cost-effectiveness, patient satisfaction, and therapist satisfaction studies.

Considering the expected growth in the practice of evidence-based therapy, it is reasonable to predict that the average practitioner will need, obtain, and employ ever more sophisticated research skills in the future, including this type of scientific reasoning.

APPLICATION OF SCIENTIFIC REASONING

Scientific reasoning is applicable throughout the occupational therapy process— from referral to disposition (American Occupational Therapy Association, 2002).

Referral

The moment a referral is received and read, reasoning may begin. Is this referral appropriate for our practice setting? Is this referral appropriate for the occupational therapy service? Is this referral appropriate for me (i.e., do I have the qualifications to intervene in this particular case)? Such questions would arise only if the case is problematic. If it is routine, the application of habit or policy will suffice to reach the decision of whether or not to take the case. If problematic, the practitioner and colleagues would need to consider their qualifications to provide effective therapy for this individual, ideally without regard for their financial interests or professional image. They should consider whether there is evidence that the referred individual may benefit from an occupational therapy intervention. If clinicians use this means of deciding, then their reasoning could be considered more scientific than if they decided for financial reasons only.

Therapeutic Relationship

One could infer from past experience that therapy is more effective, as well as more humane, when the therapist attends to establishing and nurturing a therapeutic relationship with the client. In many situations, a strong therapeutic relation is the *sine qua non* of therapy itself. Rather than leaving therapeutic relation to the whims of personality, manners, and common sense, it is possible to prepare future practitioners to be more aware of how to nurture relationships using established insights and approaches. Although no amount of knowledge would entirely remove the aspect of artistry in human interaction, such knowledge as it exists should be enlisted in the promotion of more effective therapy (see Schwartzberg, 2002, for a thorough treatment of the subject).

Frame of Reference Selection

There exists a spectrum of reasons for selecting a frame of reference:

1. No evidence for its effectiveness has been published in the literature but you, the practitioner, have had one powerful experience that led you to believe in this frame of reference. This experience may have been your attendance at a workshop in which an expert described a successful case outcome using this approach.
2. Some preliminary evidence has been published indicating the effectiveness of this frame of reference. You have used it yourself for a few months with about a dozen clients and with good outcomes for most.
3. You adopted this frame of reference because you found many different studies (some meta-analyses, some qualitative studies) from many different settings in different parts of the world, where it was effective for the type of client you are seeing in therapy. You have used it before and judged it to be effective. Your client agrees with you and wishes to undertake this approach.

For all three of these situations, if that represents the best available evidence, then there is knowledge-based justification for using that frame of reference. To do nothing because persuasive evidence does not exist would be unscientific, as well as unethical.

A nonscientific way of selecting a frame of reference might be if you continued using a once-popular frame of reference, even though the published evidence points to its ineffectiveness, and a better-substantiated, applicable frame of reference exists (or an equally effective, less costly one)—unless, of course, you have a reason to believe this client is exceptional and may experience a better outcome using it or unless your client is adamant about trying it and you are qualified to provide it (and there is an absence of contraindications).

Occupational Profile

To establish the client's occupational profile is the logical thing to do if one is setting out to practice authentic (client-centered, framework-driven) occupational therapy. If done comprehensively (scientifically) the profile would include who (self, family, clan, neighborhood); what occupations are important and why; relevant contexts for the client and caregivers (human/geographic/economic/architectural); history (past and future trajectory of all the above); interests/values/motivations; goals and priorities among goals; and desired and feasible outcomes. This information is deemed necessary to design therapeutic interventions that promote participation in occupational roles.

In most therapy settings, to embark on an intervention without gathering this orienting data would be unscientific: There is a low probability that either (a) these facts about your client don't matter or (b) you will randomly stumble onto just the right approach for him or her without your knowing this information. You might do exactly the right thing in the right way for exactly the wrong reasons (or for no reasons at all), but that would be exceedingly unlikely.

Analysis of Occupational Performance

By far the most material has been published on scientific reasoning and the analysis of occupational performance, or assessment (Barris, 1987; Holm & Rogers, 1989; Mattingly & Fleming, 1994; Rogers & Holm, 1989; Rogers & Holm, 1991; Rogers & Holm, 1997; Rogers & Masagatani, 1982; Schwartzberg, 2002), probably because it is a logical place to start. Assessment is in the early stages of the OT process, and assessing usually involves decision making to identify unknowns. Rogers and Holm (1991) have called this phase "formulating the occupational therapy diagnosis." They have thoroughly elaborated a description of scientific reasoning during assessment that consists of problem sensing, cue acquisition, multiple hypothesis generating, hypothesis testing, and hypothesis elimination or substantiation (Holm & Rogers, 1989; Rogers & Holm, 1989, 1991, 1997). They based their description on the classic hypothetical-deductive model of scientific reasoning (*Fig. 5-1*) and clinical reasoning studies conducted among diagnosing physicians (e.g., Elstein, Shulman & Sprafka, 1978). Mattingly and Fleming (1994) found evidence of this hypothesis-testing type of reasoning among the U.S. occupational therapists they studied in a physical disabilities hospital setting. In other published case studies by occupational therapists (e.g., Canelon, 1993; Labovitz, 2003), there is scant explicit evidence of therapists using hypothesis testing during problem identification.

Most often a finding is simply stated, as in Canelon's case study of an African-American man with a shoulder forequarter amputation after an industrial accident, "In self-care he required minimal to moderate assistance with feeding, bathing, grooming, and upper and lower extremity dressing

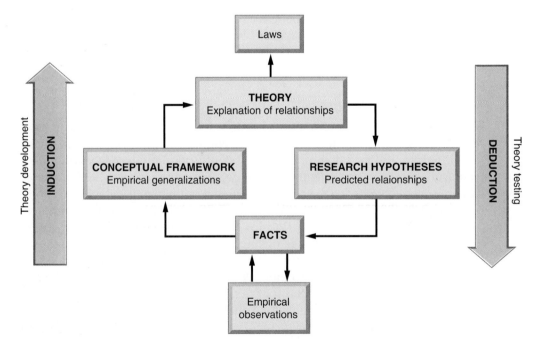

Figure 5-1 Classical hypothetical-deductive model of scientific reasoning. (Used with permission of Portney & Watkins, 2000, p. 23, Prentice Hall.)

because of a mild balance problem resulting from the shift to his center of gravity" (p. 175, emphasis added). A possible exception is the case study by Gillen (2002) in which a task-oriented approach (based on the theory of motor control) was selected to structure the evaluation of a man with multiple sclerosis. Factors increasing and decreasing the man's tremors were investigated to determine whether a powered mobility device was indicated and feasible for him. As reported, however, all the evidence clearly supported the initially chosen approach to evaluation and intervention. No early hypotheses had to be rejected.

It is possible that case studies as typically written leave out the reasoning uncertainty of the therapist for the sake of conciseness, or because it is not deemed important. The following Case Study is taken from the professional experience of my wife, Sybille Tomlin, when she worked as an occupational therapist in skilled nursing facilities. It illustrates how hypothetical-deductive thinking can occur during an evaluation. In this case, however, the logical conclusion was not an occupational therapy diagnosis but that there was a missed medical diagnosis affecting the client's performance.

CASE STUDY 5-3

Hypothesis Testing in Practice

A 72-year-old European-American man received a hip replacement after a fall at home and has been placed in a skilled nursing facility. He was referred for occupational therapy. The OT expected to follow the standard hip replacement treatment protocol. The man claimed he couldn't cook for himself any more, that his self-care was iffy; he had asked his son for help with his finances. The son felt the father was "underperforming" and was opposed to the father moving back to live on his own. The father himself was insecure at the prospect. Since he was already fully weight bearing on the affected side, his physical therapy goals were straightforward: increase strength and endurance. During evaluation, the OT found his UE ROM and strength to be within the expected range, and cognitively he was oriented. When presented with his clothes, he demonstrated independence in upper extremity dressing. He showed no deficits in proprioception or tactile functioning. The OT reflected, "Why does the client report that his son needs to help him with finances, and what does the son mean by 'underperforming'? Why isn't this man independent in all ADL? Is it depression? Dementia? A sensorimotor deficit?" The OT decided to evaluate the client further.

At the next visit an opportunity presented itself. The man hadn't shaved, so the OT asked him to show her how he shaves, thinking, "You don't normally test for hygiene tasks after a hip replacement, but. . ." He retrieved his shaver from the drawer by the bedside table and ambulated to the sink without difficulty. At the sink were a mirror and an electric outlet. The client seemed uncoordinated as he grasped the plug of the shaver cord and tried to plug it in. He was unsuccessful for many attempts, but finally managed it. The OT, thinking she had missed something, asked the client if he needed his glasses. "They don't help" was the response. The client proceeded to shave his face adequately, without cuing from the OT. The OT, suspecting a visual deficit as the cause of the coordination difficulty, held up a finger to the side and asked the client to touch her finger with his finger. He could move his finger immediately to the vicinity of her finger, but had trouble touching it exactly. The OT started to conclude that the client had a focal vision loss, with retained peripheral vision. The OT asked him to write something, and he showed extensive avoidance. Finally, he took a sheet of paper and a pen that was handed to him and wrote, but not in a straight line. The OT showed the client how to locate a signature line on paper, hold that place with a finger of his nondominant hand, and sign along a straight line.

The OT was becoming more certain now of the reason for his difficulties: macular degeneration or a similar condition. The proper response was clear. She referred the client to an ophthalmologist, informed nursing and the physical therapist on the case, and told the son about this condition and its implications. She explained the situation to the client and incorporated an appropriate strategy into the intervention plan.

In this case, there was evidence of alternative hypotheses being held and discounted, and the deliberate seeking of differential confirming/disconfirming evidence. (It also shows how common, efficient, and humane it is to engage in intervention during an evaluation, when indicated.)

For some cases, the cause of an occupational performance deficit may be so obvious (e.g., difficulty with clothing fasteners due to hand flexor tendon laceration and repair) that no alternative hypothesis need be considered. For cases involving neurological, cognitive, or psychosocial difficulties, however, the problems and causes are often not so obvious. When several causes could give rise to the same performance deficit, the occupational therapy detective work becomes important, particularly when different causes would indicate different intervention approaches, as in the Hypothesis Testing in Practice Case Study above. Furthermore, over the course of an intervention different causes of performance deficit could come into prominence as earlier ones recede. Fleishman and Quaintance (1984) noted that during the learning of a complex task, the role of influential factors changes; for example, at the beginning visual-motor skills may be most important, but later in the learning dexterity or a cognitive strategy may rise to the top. To the extent that this applies to re-learning to overcome occupational performance deficits, assessment scientific reasoning may be needed from time to time throughout intervention.

Decision making of the hypothesis generate-and-test type, however, is supplemented by pattern recognition when diagnosticians (physicians or occupational therapists) produce their findings (as described in Chapter 3). Based on extensive experience, "illness scripts" are most often used by doctors to reach a diagnostic conclusion (Schmidt, Norman & Boshuizen, 1990). Embrey, Guthrie, White, and Dietz (1996) found evidence among physical therapists of "movement scripts" acting as diagnostic templates during the assessment and treatment of children with movement disorders. It remains to be discovered whether occupational therapists possess "task scripts" or even "participatory occupation scripts."

Learning scientific, rule-bound processes and procedures allows new therapists to begin functioning as beginners in professional practice. With experience, internalizing patterns, or scripts, allows therapists to make decisions in a more efficient manner. Reasoning out each new step in each new case would take many times longer. Indeed, in a study of the clinical reasoning of occupational therapy students (Tomlin, 2005), I found that for one class cohort, the number of correct decisions per unit of time on a computer-based video case simulation correlated significantly with later fieldwork supervisor ratings of their performance in physical rehabilitation settings. If this finding holds up in future studies, it would indicate that therapists not only need to "do the right things right" for the "right reasons" and be able to articulate those reasons (as evidence-based practice calls for), but also to do them in the "right" amount of time. Accessing scripts instantaneously saves practitioners time.

Curricula may use scientific reasoning, or the principles of scientific reasoning, to impart some of those patterns, processes, and procedures to students (Neistadt, 1992), but once learned academically they must be recast in memory as used in practice (Rogoff & Lave, 1984), after which the responses can become more automatic. Efficiency is the outcome of gaining experience. For this reason, accredited occupational therapy education programs are required to incorporate levels I and II fieldwork in their curricula, and the occupational therapy program at the University of Puget Sound incorporates an on-campus occupational therapy student clinic (Lavelle & Tomlin, 2001). Students thus have a closely supervised opportunity to gain experience as occupational therapy decision makers, even while they are finishing coursework.

Nonscientific ways of performing an evaluation might include failing to collect important data, overlooking data, jumping to conclusions (overinterpreting a supposed symptom or behavior), bending the data interpretation to fit a premature decision, or failing to seek data to confirm a hypothesis, as well as possibly to disconfirm it. Given the inevitability of uncertainty, our expectation for perfection in reasoning should be tempered. Proceeding with a client in the presence of uncertainty in the therapist's mind is not unscientific. Its absence would be unscientific.

Intervention Plan

The analysis of occupational performance results in the identification of strengths and deficits. Formulation of the intervention plan involves the collaborative prioritization of goals between therapist and client/family/caregiver. The selection of intervention approaches, principles, and activities should be in accordance with the tenets of evidence-based practice. A reasonable connection should exist between the proposed therapeutic activities and an expectation of goal achievement (promoting occupational participation). Using a comprehensive approach, the therapist considers person, task, and environmental aspects for the intervention, including adaptive equipment or assistive technology prescription and task or environment modification. Overall, there should be a logical consistency to the plan and feasibility for its success.

No published studies were found in which intervention planning itself was explicitly studied for its logic or scientific virtue. Models of treatment planning in the profession have long advocated scientific consistency (Day, 1973), and the Occupational Therapy Practice Framework (American Occupational Therapy Association, 2002) may be regarded as setting the standard boundaries for planning. One may see in the case study by Canelon (1993) a struggle between the occupational therapist's expertise for promoting rehabilitation in the physical and neurological realms, and the client not experiencing that stage as of prime importance to him. With full hindsight, one might judge that the intervention plan, as described, was unscientifically timed because its implementation was rendered moot by the more pressing psychosocial issues of the client. It could be argued that if our profession is to be occupation-based and client-centered and if therapists have the knowledge so to practice, to do otherwise would be unscientific.

Intervention Plan Implementation

It is with good reason that experienced therapists check on contraindications and safety precautions before approaching a new client. To prevent further harm is one of the fundamental admonitions to healthcare personnel. Thus, it is placed first in the criteria for a scientific implementation of the therapeutic plan (although actually it begins with the first evaluation visit).

Doing No Harm

To avoid undermining their own efforts, therapists maintain vigilance for dangers to the client. Obvious ones are the client falling, harmful objects (sharp tools; caustic materials; hot objects or surfaces; corners of furniture, appliances, or cabinetry), verbal or physical aggression among clients, unnecessary destruction of materials or tools or the intervention environment, overexertion by the client, and dietary restrictions, to name a few. Attention to not-so-obvious dangers is also expected of responsible personnel (keeping a soap container that looks like a drink out of sight of a client with an acute head injury; noticing shampoo spilled on the floor beside the bed as a bed-to-wheelchair transfer is about to be done; seeing early agitation in a client participating in a task group using tools; following protocols for the prevention of blood-borne pathogen transmission). The comfort and personal needs of the client must remain uppermost in the therapist's mind. To do otherwise would be both unethical and unscientific.

Watching for Change

Likewise, it is important for therapists to be on the lookout for changing or new symptoms and behavior by clients and for environmental changes. On any given day in a medical setting, it is more likely than elsewhere that a change in symptoms may occur. In all settings of course, therapists are consistently alert to the signs of improvement or deterioration in performance. Sometimes the signs are subtle (see the Case Study that follows).

CASE STUDY 5-4

Scientific Reasoning During Intervention

An occupational therapy client who is post-CVA [cerebrovascular accident] mentions that since yesterday she has been unable to put on her slippers. That could be caused by deteriorating sitting balance, or diminished range of motion, or fluctuating tone in the affected extremities. In this particular case it was due to quite another cause. After having the client herself try to put on her slippers without success, I attempted to do it for her. Indeed, they no longer fit. Without knowing the significance of that fact, but suspecting it might be important, I mentioned it to the charge nurse. She knew instantly what had happened: the client's blood thinners interfered with her gout medication, and the first metatarsal–phalangeal joint was swelling. The nurse contacted the physician immediately to have the client's medication adjusted.

Because occupational therapists interact with clients in a variety of intimate tasks, they are often the first to have the opportunity to observe such subtle signs. With greater opportunity comes greater responsibility. Greater knowledge about what is a significant finding in a given case provides the ability to uphold that responsibility through acute perception and nimble reasoning.

Effective Activity Sequence

Experienced therapists can build a sequence of therapeutic activities that addresses crucial issues and client priorities in a logical order. Sometimes this means starting with the most important goal first; other times it means starting with the most achievable one first, or the earliest developmentally, depending on client needs and therapist frame of reference. Whichever of these criteria is used in the design process of the plan, the sequence is ultimately based on three sources. First, background knowledge is essential: knowledge of human occupation, injury, and disease, lifespan development, the intrinsic variety of activities, as well as human psychology: occupational science. Second, empirical evidence of therapy effectiveness is urged nowadays. Third, the traits, personality, and goals of the client are equally important. Some add that a theory, a model, a frame of reference, or a school of thought may be required to know how to apply the empirical knowledge to the current new case (Chapporo & Ranka, 1995). One could argue that the scope of occupational therapy demands that scientific reasoning in the profession should be a melding of generalized knowledge and professional knowledge with knowledge of the individual. Fleming and Mattingly (1994) labeled this a combination of a "disease approach" and an "illness experience" approach (p. 338). This combining is rarely described explicitly in case studies, but it may be considered a scientific underpinning of the profession nonetheless, because without all three our stated professional goals cannot be effectively achieved.

Nonscientific reasoning in activity sequencing would be to blend the three realms of knowledge disproportionately: to ignore the client's individuality, to attempt to interact therapeutically while lacking the requisite foundation knowledge, and to approach the client while neglecting common sense. We designate such an approach as unscientific because of the evidence that it results in less effective outcomes. This statement leaves unanswered exactly how the three sources of knowledge are to be balanced as they are mixed together.

Effective Pacing

Decisions about the pacing of therapeutic activities are also inductions based on the therapist's empirical knowledge of task analysis, rehabilitation, and the psychology of the individual client. The therapist must be prepared for the unexpected and be ready to shift gears rapidly when that appears necessary. The signs may be boredom, frustration, agitation, avoidance, activity or group sabotage, or simply no progress for too long, on the negative side, and signs of progress itself, on the positive side.

Adjusting the Plan

A decision to change the sequence or pace of activities may be based on client performance, current stage of progress, or immediate feedback from the client. Knowledge about grading activities and an informed creativity may be drawn upon as well as the application of theory. As during any complex skill acquisition (Fleischman & Quaintance, 1984), one may expect setbacks, progress in fits and starts, and sudden breakthroughs. It would be unscientific to ignore the data one can observe in the client or to discount the client's own testimony about the course of therapy.

Extending Therapeutic Effects

It is recognized that the involvement of others in the intervention (client, family, spouse, case manager, nurse, teacher, hired caregiver) can extend the therapeutic effects. Each new case is an opportunity for the therapist to reason about who should be involved and to what extent. General protocols give guidance, but each case is likely to have unique features. There must be a reasoned balance between the time each person is available and the basic necessities of training.

Ignoring the various sources of knowledge or misapplying them while implementing the intervention could be considered unscientific intervention.

Intervention Review

Knowing that a review eventually happens, therapists use measures in the original evaluation to establish a baseline so that progress (goal achievement) can be determined. Much research has gone into investigating which performance measures address the relevant constructs of occupation and provide the desired sensitivity to actual progress during treatment. A scientific approach to practice includes the careful selection of evaluation instruments, including those that seek to assess context, meaning, and motivation, and that can provide meaningful measures of progress when that has occurred.

Once reevaluation data are collected, a difficult challenge for induction arises: generalizing from "intervention performance" to real life, if services have been provided in a clinic rather than the natural setting. Determining the factors that affect this correlation is key: physical and social context, intrinsic and extrinsic motivation, emotional and cognitive orientation to surroundings, supervision type and amount, and consistency of help available, not to mention physical and architectural matters.

When sufficient evidence accumulates that another professional is likely to be helpful, then a referral is initiated. Knowing one's own boundaries, recognizing them in the instance, and having knowledge of other disciplines and the state of the local scene so as to refer effectively is to practice scientifically.

Outcomes

As with instrument selection for evaluation, careful planning for outcome collection and analysis is the mark of a therapist who is using scientific reasoning (see above on instruments). Such outcome monitoring contributes to evidence-based practice as long as findings are used, published, or presented.

Throughout the OT Process

Even in a routine case, scientific reasoning may be useful. A routine case involves many decisions about (1) shifting from assessment to intervention, as in the Hypothesis Testing in Practice Case Study; (2) shifting between one frame of reference and another and between one problem/deficit/goal and another; and (3) shifting among levels related to occupational performance (participation, task, body structure/function) during assessment and intervention.

Beyond the process of direct client services, scientific reasoning can be used in consultation, population-based approaches, management, research, and educator roles for occupational therapists. Wherever there is a call for knowledge stewardship, scientific reasoning can play a role.

ERRORS IN SCIENTIFIC REASONING

As much as Aristotle's original *Organon* was to help citizens detect flaws in rhetoric, it is useful to enumerate common errors in scientific reasoning. Lists of errors in scientific reasoning come from three sources: studies of medical diagnosticians (cited in Rogers & Holm, 1997), general studies of reasoning errors people make (Gilovich, 1991), and an empirical study of **practice errors** reported by occupational therapy clinicians (Schierton, Mu & Lohman, 2003). A fourth source of reasoning error is the incorrect application of evidence-based practice: either a statistical misinterpretation or a misapplication of existing evidence.

Errors by Diagnosticians

Rogers and Holm (1997) cited four common errors of scientific reasoning, culled from studies of medical diagnosticians.

1. Too few cues observed or too many, leading to confusion
2. Inaccurate interpretation of cues
3. Not generating multiple hypotheses, premature closing of reasoning
4. Favoring the search for confirming evidence, instead of seeking disconfirming evidence of a hypothesis

These errors can lead to a misdiagnosis, which would lead to an incorrect intervention. Specifically, in occupational therapy, the causes of performance deficits could be misidentified, which could lead to the incorrect intervention principles being followed and thus lead to ineffective treatment. Further errors of reasoning committed in clinical practice by psychiatrists, psychologists, social workers, and others are thoroughly described by Gambrill (2005).

General Reasoning Errors

Gilovich (1991, p. v) provided guidelines for avoiding reasoning errors in every-day situations, which are applicable to professional practice. His sources of error consisted of:

1. misperception/misinterpretation of random data
2. misinterpretation of incomplete or unrepresentative data
3. biased evaluation of ambiguous and inconsistent data
4. motivational determinants of belief
5. biasing effects of secondhand information
6. exaggerated impressions of social support

The first two points are similar to those of Rogers and Holm (1997). The next three are concerned with situations of data interpretation in which pre-judgment, wishful thinking, or unreliable related evidence influences interpretation, and each could have a counterpart in therapy practice. The sixth point occurs when the decision maker perceives that there is already social support for a particular conclusion. An example from clinical practice is that when a diagnostic label has already been applied to a client, it is harder to accept evidence to the contrary.

Other general reasoning inaccuracies have been studied by Tversky and Kahneman (1974). They found that when people attempt to make judgments under conditions of uncertainty, they use three heuristics (or reasoning tools):

1. *Representativeness*—how much the situation resembles a known outcome
2. *Availability*—how recent, salient, or dramatic similar cases are
3. *Anchoring*—at what starting estimate reasoning begins

The heuristics can be useful, but each leads to demonstrable biases in decision making, as follows. Representativeness leads the decision maker to overlook background probabilities of the alternative outcome events. Availability to memory strengthens the chances of forming a conclusion based on recent events. Anchoring results in final decisions that are biased toward the initial estimate (Tversky & Kahneman, 1974). The application of these biases to occupational therapy reasoning should be evident.

Empirical Occupational Therapy Error

Schierton et al. (2003) interviewed practicing occupational therapists about their practice errors. The errors identified from physical disabilities practice by therapists talking in focus groups were both physical and psychological. The physical ranged from minor (ripped fingernail, fatigue) to major (falls, bone fractures, contributing to the death of a patient), whereas the psychological consisted of withholding truth from a patient about the prognosis or conveying unrealistic expectations to the patient about the prognosis. The participants also reported treatment management errors, that is, not following standards of practice or the code of ethics in the distribution of therapy. In other words, some people got nonessential treatment because of insurance stipulations, whereas others did not receive what was indicated because of insurance constraints. The causes of errors they cited were inexperience, not listening to the patient, being rushed, or being tired (Schierton et al., 2003).

Inexperienced study participants were described as not knowing what to do as a result of not learning that aspect of practice in their basic professional education program and being relatively new on the job at the time of the error. Other errors were attributed to inattention (patient falling), misjudgment (of weight-bearing status, tolerance level, or comprehension of patient), and communication breakdown (ignoring a statement of the patient).

Of these errors, the following could be considered specifically as errors of scientific reasoning: incorrect anticipation of danger to patient, ignoring data (patient's report of trouble), and overestimating the capacity of the patient. It is hard to say that incorrect treatment planning (too much or too little therapy) is an error in scientific reasoning, since the decision was selected deliberately, but under an external constraint or policy that conflicted with the therapist's best professional judgment (an example of pragmatic reasoning is discussed in Chapter 7). If the outcomes of different types of reasoning clash, as they do here, the practitioner may experience professional distress.

Schierton et al. (2003) concluded that ". . .most of the mentioned causes could likely be avoided by more attentive practice. These findings may have implications for current educational training programs in occupational therapy, including clinical reasoning development related to patient safety. Using case study scenarios about everyday practice that have a potential for error would be one way to address errors in an educational setting" (p. 312).

This is a prudent course, but would case study scenarios have been sufficient to prevent some of the errors described? Errors such as these are committed in the rushed flow of complex, everyday practice, with distractions, pressures, and other concerns that crowd out the crucial opportunity to avoid the injury or mistake. A better learning environment for such challenges might be actual, situated experience, such as an on-campus student clinic (Lavelle & Tomlin, 2001), where students are performing realistic practice, but under close supervision—closer than that often available during level II fieldwork.

Errors of scientific reasoning that occur during intervention review (from grading activities to discontinuing services) have not been explicitly studied, but much secondary material is available in published case studies. Honest accounts may reflect weaknesses in diagnostic reasoning, interactive reasoning, judgment of activity meaning or client context, or undervaluing client goals and priorities. All such weaknesses could be influenced by perception, habit, and awareness, which in turn are ultimately linked to knowledge or the lack thereof. Even inattention leading to decision errors could be said to be unscientific practice if the therapist lacked self-knowledge of such a tendency or chose to ignore such awareness.

Errors in Statistical Reasoning

Common errors in statistical reasoning (not the calculation, but the interpretation) consist of overgeneralizations based on sampling error, extrapolation, interpolation, or misattribution of causation. The contemporary emphasis on evidence-based practice puts a heavier burden on the average practitioner to understand and avoid these errors. Mistakes or implied errors in the occupational therapy literature can be obvious or quite subtle. For example, Case-Smith (1995) studied the correlations among scores in sensorimotor components, fine motor skills, and functional performance in 30 preschool children with motor delays. The correlation coefficients were moderate to strong between sensorimotor components and fine motor skills ($r = 0.4$ to 0.8; $P < .05$ to $P < .005$) but not statistically significant between these two levels and self care, and only sporadically significant between the two and mobility and social function. She concluded that "on the basis of the findings of this study, therapists cannot assume that improvement in foundational sensorimotor abilities will automatically generalize into increased function and success in meeting environmental demands" (Case-Smith, p. 651). Although the statement is technically accurate, its implication is misleading; that is, if the correlations between sensorimotor and functional levels had been high, then practitioners would be justified in believing that causing improvement through therapy in the sensorimotor scores would automatically cause improvement in the functional scores. This unstated implication equates correlation with causation, a common interpretive misstep.

Perhaps the greatest flaw in our use of statistical reasoning, however, is when it gives rise to feelings of certainty, which are not justified. Furthermore, from any scientific study, the question of generalizability cannot be absolutely resolved. How far outward should the scientific conclusions generalize in space? In time? In person? Our reasoning would be better served if we remained open to detecting and correcting errors or weaknesses of interpretation, open to frank discussion of their effects, and open to listening to new perspectives that can change our perceptions of meaning, context, and valued goals (e.g., disability studies, sociocultural awareness) and thus the configuration of our interpretations.

LIMITATIONS OF SCIENTIFIC REASONING

Points of critique of scientific reasoning and of counter-critique are summarized in the following text.

Critique

One critique is of the conceptual basis of traditional scientific reasoning (Damasio, 1994; Devlin, 1997), that is, that the mind–body separation ("Cartesian dualism") at the root of traditional scientific reasoning is ultimately untenable. Thoughts, and therefore reasoning, are inextricably tied to personal and social feelings—Pascal's "reasons of the heart." Some claim that no deductive reasoning, with its seeming certainty, underlies scientific hypothesis testing, only inductive reasoning, with its attendant limitations and uncertainties

(Oaksford & Chater, 2002). Thus scientific reasoning can lay claim to no higher ground of certainty.

Another critique is based on inapplicability: empirically based hypothesis testing derived from medical diagnosing fails to incorporate important realms of meaning, motivation, and intent in human behavior/occupation. For this reason, Fleming and Mattingly (1994) declared that occupational therapy reasoning was different from reductionistic biomedical reasoning. Chapparo and Ranka (1995) have made a similar claim.

A third critique is on the basis of implementation: Therapists rarely use scientific reasoning because they have no time to, and they do not need to, since pattern recognition allows them to short-cut the steps of hypothesis/deduction. "Experts are not people who follow the rules extremely fast and accurately, they do not follow the rules at all, not even subconsciously" (Devlin, 1997, p. 180). Rules exist to help us learn a task. Then with practice, experience, and repetition, we become one with the action.

A further critique of scientific reasoning is based on nongeneralizability: that there is no generalizable scientific reasoning capability. Rather, such reasoning is tied to the content domain within which decisions are being made (an expert early intervention pediatric reasoner is no expert reasoner in adult mental health). Without a general reasoning capacity, the decision making of the field cannot be scientific. Moreover, occupational therapy reasoning with a client is individualized; thus, the process is not generalizable from group to person or person to group. Occupation is too individual with each person, as is the therapeutic interaction between practitioner and client so necessary for successful intervention.

A final critique might be labeled "epistemological," or pertaining to the theory of knowledge. When dealing with knowledge of human beings, how can you (to use an ancient metaphor) step into the same river once—never mind twice—with people? That is, many argue that one cannot step twice—what worked for one person may not work for the next. People differ in too many respects. (The flowing river is always changing; thus, you cannot step into the same river twice.) Others remind us that we cannot even step once: beginning to interact with someone influences that person's behavior (if not their life) immediately. The instantaneous dynamic means that what you just did could not be replicated, even with that person. The flow of time, being, and interaction is ineluctable.

Counter-Critique

There are also many positives to consider in favor of scientific reasoning. Scientific reasoning dictates the knowledge structure of the discipline; it is what professionals profess as a community; it is what bonds us together in the professional therapy enterprise; it forms the basis of our professional education/certification process—that one cannot become an occupational therapy practitioner solely by being an apprentice to an occupational therapy practitioner, no matter how expert the mentor may be. Students are taught professional knowledge in a framework of scientific reasoning (often now as evidence-based practice) so that there is a web of principles in which to embed that knowledge systematically and consistently. It matters not that thought and emotion are deeply conjoined in each person. Professional knowledge is what we share.

Second, empirical knowledge is helpful. Even if we do not use scientific reasoning all the time during therapy and even only occasionally, it still forms the framework of our formal knowledge construction—what the community of practitioners can establish as disciplinary knowledge and agree upon in some generalizable (applicable) fashion. Evidence-based practice stands as the instantaneous state of our scientific knowledge learned to date plus our clinical experience, that is, our own and that of others that is accessible. This empirical understanding of evidence-based practice casts practitioners as knowledge stewards using scientific reasoning, not as scientists in the traditional sense.

Third, there are practical benefits to scientific reasoning. It has been documented as being used in practice when the relevant clinical/occupational pattern cannot be recognized, albeit as an exception rather than the rule in daily decision making. It is far more reliable, dependable, and efficient than truly random trial-and-error efforts to detect performance deficits and uncover their causes. Our goal should be to reason not flawlessly, but more effectively, avoiding common fallacies. Using scientific reasoning and recognizing its limitations allows practitioners to do just that.

A fourth argument is that even some generalizability is useful. The value of scientific reasoning does not stand upon its being universally generalizable; if it contributes to coherent reasoning in one practice realm or setting and there is agreement as to its nature and function in that subfield, then that suffices for it to have prescriptive value. As for group to individual inferencing, some aspects of knowledge about human occupational performance must be generalizable or transferable (otherwise, how could any therapist's experience with people have value?). Overgeneralizing, not generalizing, is the problem. We must keep an open mind about our decisions and be comfortable with uncertainty.

Scientific reasoning itself has evolved and become more sophisticated over time, as knowledge seekers incorporate complex methods that escape reductionism and reflect more closely the types of complexity that are important in human health and occupation (chaos theory, complexity theory, fuzzy logic). Its value should be judged not from an out-dated caricature of science but from the latest brand.

Cartesian dualism is said to have led science into **reductionism,** that a thing can be best understood by taking it apart and studying the individual pieces. Reductionism, however, hardly characterizes innovative contemporary science: general and special relativity theory (Einstein, 1923); general systems theory (Bertalanffy, 1968); the grand "unified theory of everything" in physics (Crease & Mann, 1986); dynamical systems/chaos theory (Gleick, 1987); neural nets (Nelson & Illingworth, 1991); fuzzy logic (McNeill & Freiburger, 1993); complexity theory (Mainzer, 1997); and string theory (Greene, 1999). Even as the original reductionism in physical science began to be applied to the complex questions of individuals and societies (in order to achieve greater quantification and certainty in understanding as well as to secure greater status for those disciplines) and found to be in some important respects wanting, science theory itself had moved far beyond reductionism. It remains for 21st century knowledge stewards to apply these sophisticated systems theories to the manifestly complex realm of the human enterprise.

Someday perhaps, an integrated theory of professional reasoning incorporating many strands will be considered scientific reasoning, because then it would take into consideration all the empirically verified phenomena that contribute to the act (Box 5-2). To do less would be unscientific!

I readily acknowledge that there are aspects of the art of therapy (including therapeutic use of self) that may be forever outside the realm of scientific reasoning (Rogers, 1983). Meanwhile, I see no reason why scientific reasoning could not incorporate much knowledge learned about interactive reasoning, narrative reasoning, conditional reasoning, and pragmatic reasoning. Some have argued that we cannot turn these realms into scientific reasoning because with human individuality we cannot have stable group effects, replicability, and high generalizability. Any findings, however, including those enshrined in solid evidence-based practice, are only relatively generalizable. We need only be somewhat more tentative in the application of principles of, for example, therapeutic use of self, gleaned from past studies or experience, rather than not attempting it at all.

B O X   5 - 2
Directions for Research on Scientific Reasoning

1. Any outcomes research in occupational therapy would contribute to scientific reasoning.
2. The effects on occupational therapy outcomes of the introduction of concerted evidence-based practice into a practice setting; that is, what is the evidence for evidence-based practice in occupational therapy?
3. How to define and systematically measure quantitative aspects of decision making in simulated practice situations (Tomlin, 2005), attempting to overcome the shortcoming of naturalistic clinical reasoning research noted by Rogers and Masagatani (1982).
4. A search for evidence of "cognitive schema" of reasoning for occupational therapists: task scripts or participatory occupation scripts
5. Research on interactive, conditional, narrative, or pragmatic reasoning would contribute to scientific reasoning, broadly defined.
6. How thinking along the multiple tracks is orchestrated: by what principles and by what mechanism is one track elevated into consciousness, while the others recede?
7. How scientific reasoning, narrowly or broadly defined, is being taught in professional education programs (fortunately, unlike 14th century Oxford University, the Accreditation Council for Occupational Therapy Education has no *Organon* standard.)

Is there a difference, ultimately, between this broadest notion of scientific reasoning and humane decision making? I would argue that there is not. If knowledge and reasoning are based on thought and feeling intertwined and if intellect and compassion are what practitioners bring to the therapeutic relation, if it is scientific (i.e., enlightened) to be humane and humane to be scientific, can there be any difference? If some day scientific reasoning is stretched into the dimensions of human thought, motivation, values, goals, and interpersonal communication, where would it lack? Would a lifetime of interactions be stable enough to provide an individual practitioner with the foundation for thorough (multidimensional) scientific reasoning? Perhaps that would be considered wisdom.

If we accept the thesis of Descartes' error, we also need to acknowledge the error of splitting scientific reasoning off from the rest of our thinking, acting, and decision making. Perhaps we need to reconceptualize all types of reasoning so as to reflect their ultimate interconnectivity. Separate existences may merely be our own categorization—convenient but not durable under close examination. Yerxa (1991) wrote, "Persons are authors of their occupational behavior simultaneously as biological, psychological, social, cultural, and spiritual beings" (p. 201). Similarly, occupational therapists may be integrated existentialists as they practice the occupation of occupational therapy (Box 5-3).

BOX 5-3

Recommendations to Therapists (and Future Therapists)

1. Be alert to your own assumptions and background knowledge, to the degree of unreliability in the steps of the occupational therapy process, to the strengths and limitations of your own cognitive and metacognitive foundations, to the uncertainty of your conclusions, and be open to strengthening, and sometimes revolutionizing, the character and content of your thought. Retain a stance of intellectual curiosity and uncertainty, even while presenting a professionally competent persona.
2. Use the best available and applicable evidence (electronic, paper, or human)
   (a) learn and practice how to read, interpret, and appropriately generalize published evidence and
   (b) be mindful of the expertise of others, and of your own, and of its limits and
   (c) knowledgeably collaborate with your clients
3. Learn to use, and be ready, willing, and able to use a deductive approach, logical scientific reasoning, as it were, when confronting a new or atypical case, behavior, or situation. Entertain multiple hypotheses about the cause(s) of performance difficulties and systematically seek confirming and disconfirming evidence for each.
4. Always picture yourself as a holistic professional, without chasms between feeling, sensing, thinking, believing (avoid Descartes' error).

If there are multiple tracks of reasoning in the mind of an occupational therapist, what overseeing function rules which of the tracks we are to be thinking in, at any given time? We have side-stepped an important question of decision making by limiting any professional reasoning model to a set of parallel tracks. To do so throws us right back to the original unknown: how do we decide which problem to reason about?

Just as evidence-based practice is now mandated for those decisions categorized under procedural reasoning, there is no reason why interactive reasoning, conditional reasoning, and narrative reasoning should be exempt from evidence-based practice. Likewise there is no reason why they cannot be subsumed into a broadly conceived, knowledge (thought/feeling)-based, humane, scientific reasoning, with an appropriately sensitive epistemology of human interaction, human occupation, and human narrative. These topics have their own research histories, to which occupational therapy and occupational science have much to add. The sensitive epistemology will need to be accompanied by an appropriately modest level of confidence in the generalization of findings from some people to the situations of other people.

Mattingly (1991b) advocated conceiving of reasoning in occupational therapy as incorporating the reasoning familiar to many on a traditional scientific plane, but transcending it. More of the essence of the field, she wrote, is within the reasoning about meaning in the client's life—how to help the client find it or rediscover it. Although each client is unique, there are patterns and principles to be learned about how these aspects of knowledge interrelate, and how a skilled practitioner can apply past experiences with a new client while keeping an open mind. To articulate a science of therapeutic phenomenology would be to overcome Descartes' error (see Thinking About Thinking 5-2) in separating thought, and thus knowledge, from the lived experience of human life.

Thinking About Thinking 5-2

Descartes' Error

From that I knew that I was a substance, the whole essence or nature of which is to think, and that for its existence there is no need of any place, nor does it depend on any material thing; so that this 'me,' that is to say, the soul by which I am what I am, is entirely distinct from body and is even more easy to know than is the latter; and even if the body were not, the soul would not cease to be what it is.

—Descartes, *Discourse on Method* (in Damasio, 1994, p. 249)

This is Descartes' error: the abyssal separation between body and mind, between the sizable, dimensioned, mechanistically operated, infinitely divisible body stuff, on the one hand, and the unsizable, undimensioned, unpushpullable, nondivisible mindstuff; the suggestion that reasoning, and moral judgment, and the suffering that comes from physical pain or emotional upheaval might exist separately from the body.

—Damasio, 1994 (pp. 249–250)

SUMMARY

Scientific reasoning in occupational therapy entails the use of cognitive tools to aid therapists in their decision making with clients. In the deep nexus of human thought, emotion, value, motivation, and intention, a responsible (i.e., scientific/humane) professional seeks to apply deductive logic, inductive reasoning, probabilistic inferencing about evidence, clinical experience (through pattern recognition and seasoned judgment), and knowledge of the client as a person, in a context-appropriate and effective manner. Opportunities may arise throughout the stages of the occupational therapy process for the use of scientific reasoning for nonroutine decisions. Therapists are serving the client best when they use these cognitive tools to promote an optimal occupational participation.

These thinking tools have evolved through at least 2,500 years of cultural and intellectual sophistication. Their original discovery has probably led to overapplication (e.g., Descartes' error—that the mind is a separate entity from the body, or the approach that knowledge is to be derived by cutting up phenomena until they are reduced to their atomistic parts, studying them individually, and then putting them back together). Recent scientific developments, however, such as dynamical systems theory, ecology, phenomenology, decision-making theories, cognitive science, and the science of human occupation, are providing the tools for occupational therapists to develop an integrated epistemology for our professional practice. This epistemology could unite the "three tracks" of the mind (procedural, conditional, interactive), along with other contextually important paths of thinking, and provide us with a professional foundation that accurately reflects and faithfully sustains the essential nature of our work—an eminently "scientific" undertaking.

LEARNING ACTIVITY 5-1

Case Studies

Purpose

The purpose of this activity is to provide case studies that serve as contexts for understanding elements of scientific reasoning.

Connections to Major Clinical Reasoning Constructs

This activity is related to scientific reasoning.

Directions for Learners

Below are a number of case studies that require particular use of scientific reasoning. For each case study:

1 Read the case.
2 Answer the questions posed.
3 Discuss your answer and your rationale with a partner or your discussion group.
4 Look at the comments at the end to see if you considered the same issues that Dr. Tomlin did in his analysis.

Allow 10 to 15 minutes for each case study analysis, and at least 15 minutes or more for discussion, depending on how many people are involved.

From a Skilled Nursing Facility Setting

1 Walking in the dark, unassisted, causes Mrs. Miller to fall. This morning the charge nurse reported that she fell last night. Therefore last night she was walking unassisted in the dark.

What is the logical fallacy in this example of deductive reasoning?

2 "Every time Mrs. Miller tries to get to the bathroom by herself at night, she falls. Thus we keep the bedrails up when she's in bed. Last night she fell trying to get to the bathroom. Therefore, someone must have left the bedrails down."

Where is the logical fallacy in this example? Comment on any further shortcomings in its accuracy.

From an Ergonomic Evaluation

A person's ability to move a joint against the field of gravity depends on the person generating more torque than the gravitational torque on that joint (torque of muscle > torque of gravity). Torque is calculated by the force involved times the moment arm that force has from the axis of movement.

3 In her aircraft parts supply job, Ms. Phelps has great difficulty lifting the boxes of bearings from the knee-high shelf where they are stored to the customer counter height.

What can you suggest to make it easier for her? How do these steps help?

From a Pediatric Evaluation and Treatment Center Setting

4 Billy, an 8-year-old boy, is being evaluated for extreme behavioral difficulties in school. The occupational therapist asks him to use an empty food can to trace circles onto construction paper, use scissors to cut them out, then to arrange them however he likes on a second large sheet of paper, and glue them down. After some hesitation and coaxing, Billy picks up the can (placed to his left) in his left hand, puts it on the first sheet of paper and lets go of it. He takes the pencil in his right hand with a cylindrical grasp, and with a slight tremor begins to trace around the can. Three times the can moves, and three times Billy pushes the can back into place with the back of his left hand, each time emitting a longer sigh. Finally, he gets five circles traced out. After dropping the scissors twice he manages to cut out all the circles, albeit while uttering sounds of frustration and leaving rough edges. With his right hand, he arranges the circles on the second sheet, adjusting them several times in the process. Leaving them in place he squeezes glue onto one, spreading it with the heel of his right hand, then turns it over with his left hand, makes a fist, and hits it. He does two more circles this way. On the fourth time squirting glue onto a circle Billy realizes when he goes to turn it over that he has already glued that one (that it now has glue on both sides). "Damn, I messed up again!" he cries out, and refuses to continue working.

What problems in occupational performance can you identify? Using the occupational therapy framework what possible causes of these problems can you hypothesize? What data could you point to, or further collect, to confirm or disconfirm these hypotheses? What intervention approaches would you take to address the causes of his difficulties? How much of the treatment could you justify by evidence-based principles?

From an Adolescent Mental Health Setting

5 Kyle, a 15-year–old boy, is undergoing evaluation and treatment after taking his uncle's car without permission and crashing it into a tree (for the third time). He has no siblings and has been raised by his mother for the past 4 years after the alcohol-related departure of his father. Throughout the occupational profile interview with the occupational therapist, Kyle reverts to talk of powerful engines, extolling the virtues of turbo-charging, hemi-headed cylinders, and dual exhaust systems. When asked about his vocational aspirations, he curtly replies, "I'm doing fine in school." He then continues the conversation with references to gear box ratios and anti-lock brakes.

What approach would you try in order to cultivate a real conversation with Kyle? Upon what principles of healthy human interaction and therapeutic use of self would these approaches be based? What signs of response from him would you watch for as you initiated these attempts?

Compare Your Answers to My Ideas

1 This syllogism is of the form, "If A causes B, then if B then A." It is one of the fallacious syllogisms. Just because A causes B does not mean that there aren't other things that could cause B to happen. (A is a sufficient cause for B, but not a necessary cause.) Thus, the existence of B does not allow us to infer A.

2 This one is more complex. It takes the form, "If (if A then B) then C; If B, then not C," where A is trying to get to the bathroom alone, B is falling, and C is putting up the bedrails. Just because C is done if the staff discover A causes B, that doesn't mean that C can totally prevent B. Thus, if B occurs, C still might have been done. For example, Mrs. Miller could have fallen after putting the rails down herself, after climbing over the rails, or after sliding over the end of the bed. She might have also fallen asleep in her chair that night, and fallen while getting up to head to the bathroom.

3 There are four factors involved in the torque contest: force of the muscle, moment arm of the muscle, force of gravity on the box, moment arm of gravity on the box. Taking a person-task-environment approach, we could affect each one of the four. First, we could help her strengthen her elbow and shoulder flexors through activities with a progressive resistive feature. Second, we could have her flex her knees more before lifting the boxes to get the angle of beginning elbow flexion closer to 90 degrees, to increase the moment arm of the muscle; or we could have the shelf raised, or simply store the boxes on a higher shelf. Third, we could have her

store fewer bearings per box to decrease the gravitational pull on the box. Finally, we could have her hold the box closer to her body to decrease the moment arm of gravity. A systematic analysis of factors affecting success in occupation is helpful in providing scientific, effective therapy.

4   Possible problems include difficulty initiating a task, difficulty crossing the midline of the body, difficulty with bilateral hand use, an immature pencil grasp, an intention tremor, inexperience tracing around an object, difficulty manipulating scissors, difficulty monitoring progress through a task (the double-gluing), difficulty using an appropriate amount of force given the materials (pressing circles by fist-hitting, although that could also be adaptive at this point of cumulative frustration), poor confidence and a self-image as commonly failing at tasks—all leading to a brittle engagement in occupation for his age. (His strengths of persisting despite frustration, and his aesthetic standards evident in arranging the circles, should not be forgotten.) In framework terminology, the difficulties could be labeled as problems in areas of occupation (particularly education, play, and leisure), in performance skills and performance patterns, and in client factors. Possible client factor causes of these problems include delayed development of body structure/function (specifically sensory and motor functions). Delayed performance skill and performance pattern development may be caused by a lack of environmental opportunities, and a maladaptive cycle of frustration, overreaction, and disengagement from activities. Further data should be collected in Billy's natural contexts to rule out or confirm a neurological tremor, nervousness causing what appears to be developmental coordination disorder, sequencing and self-monitoring skills, and to determine activity tolerance for other types of tasks. Standardized tests providing data on motor development, visual perception, sensory integration, play and task skills, and school function may be administered. Screening for parental neglect and abuse may be in order. Intervention would probably proceed along several fronts: sequenced sensorimotor activities, strengthening of task behaviors, steady building of self-confidence, and strategizing with teachers and caregivers to enhance therapeutic effects in all Billy's environments. Evidence for the effectiveness of such approaches may be found in the work of Hanft, Polatajko, MacLeod and Nelson, and others.

5   This case is an example of the fusion of interactive reasoning with scientific reasoning. If Kyle's difficulties are to be identified, their causes unearthed, and effective intervention approaches found, it is essential to establish a therapeutic relationship. Much of that relationship will be based on an ability to communicate authentically. How carefully one must balance an acknowledgement of the

ideas and interests that are important to Kyle, with the recognition that conversationally he is using these topics to avoid discussing his real difficulties. A therapist is unlikely to make much headway with him by taking an extreme approach: either by mutually discussing cars and their performance, or by shutting him down by challenging his avoidance tactics. Recognition and re-direction need to be balanced. Schwartzberg (2002) listed numerous therapeutic approaches based on the work of psychologists Frank, Rogers, Maslow, Erikson and others, and of occupational therapists Fidler, Yerxa, Mosey, Howe and Schwartzberg, Reilly, and Kielhofner. Each approach is framed in its own semantics, but what most have in common is the guiding of the client by the therapist toward self-adaptation. Awareness, insight, acceptance, and skill development arise from healthy interactions in discussions and through one-on-one and group activities. One approach would be to engage Kyle in activities and center conversation around the give-and-take of the here-and-now of the tasks themselves. Another would be to give brief but sincere recognition of his automotive interests but gently point out the pragmatics of why he is here for evaluation and what he may need to accomplish in order to be discharged: developing new insights and skills. Task engagement would be a positive sign during the first approach, whereas resistance or silent acknowledgement might indicate progress under the second approach.

REFERENCES

Abreu, B. C., Peloquin, S. M. & Ottenbacher, K. (1998). Competence in scientific inquiry and research. *American Journal of Occupational Therapy, 52,* 751–759.

Albert, D. A., Munson, R. & Resnik, M. D. (1988). *Reasoning in medicine: An introduction to clinical inference.* Baltimore: Johns Hopkins University Press.

American Heritage Dictionary of the English Language (4th ed.). (2000). Boston: Houghton Mifflin.

American Occupational Therapy Association. (2002). Occupational therapy practice framework: Domain and process. *American Journal of Occupational Therapy, 56,* 609–639.

Barris, R. (1987). Clinical reasoning in psychosocial occupational therapy. *Occupational Therapy Journal of Research, 7,* 147–161.

Bertalanffy, L. von. (1968). *General system theory.* New York: Braziller.

Brown, J. S., Collins, A. & Duguid, P. (1989). Situated cognition and the culture of learning. *Educational Researcher, 18*(1), 32–42.

Canelon, M. F. (1993). Training for a patient with shoulder disarticulation. *American Journal of Occupational Therapy, 47,* 174–178.

Chapparo, C. & Ranka, J. (1995). Clinical reasoning in occupational therapy. In J. Higgs & M. Jones (Eds.), *Clinical reasoning in the health professions* (pp. 88-102). Oxford: Butterworth-Heinemann.

Constantz, G. (1994). *Hollows, peepers, and highlanders: An Appalachian mountain ecology.* Missoula, MT: Mountain Press.

Crease, R. P. & Mann, C. C. (1986). *The second creation: Makers of the revolution in twentieth century physics.* New York: MacMillan.

Damasio, A. R. (1994). *Descartes' error: Emotion, reason, and the human brain.* New York: G. P. Putnam.

Day, D. J. (1973). A systems diagram for teaching treatment planning. *American Journal of Occupational Therapy, 27,* 239–243.

DePoy, E. & Gitlin, L. N. (2005). *Introduction to research: Understanding and applying multiple strategies* (3rd ed.). St. Louis: Elsevier Mosby.

Devlin, K. (1997). *Goodbye, Descartes.* New York: John Wiley & Sons.

Dreyfus, H. L. & Dreyfus, S. E. (1986). *Mind over machine: The power of human intuition and expertise in the era of the computer.* New York: The Free Press, Macmillan.

Dysart, A. M. & Tomlin, G. S. (2002). Factors related to evidence-based practice among U. S. occupational therapy clinicians. *American Journal of Occupational Therapy,* 56, 275–284.

Einstein, A. (1923). *The meaning of relativity.* Princeton, NJ: Princeton University Press.

Elio, R. (2002). Issues in commonsense reasoning and rationality. In R. Elio (Ed.), *Common sense, reasoning, and rationality* (pp. 3–36). New York: Oxford University Press.

Elstein, A. S., Shulman, L. S. & Sprafka, S. A. (1978). *Medical problem-solving: An analysis of clinical reasoning.* Cambridge, MA: Harvard University Press.

Embrey, D. G., Guthrie, M. R., White, O. R. & Dietz, J. (1996). Clinical decision making by experienced and inexperienced pediatric physical therapists for children with diplegic cerebral palsy. *Physical Therapy,* 76, 20–33.

Ferguson, G. A. & Takane, Y. (1989). *Statistical analysis in psychology and education* (6th ed.). New York: McGraw-Hill.

Fleishman, E. A. & Quaintance, M. K. (1984). *Taxonomies of human performance: The description of human tasks.* Orlando, FL: Academic Press.

Fleming, M. H. (1991). The therapist with the three-track mind. *American Journal of Occupational Therapy,* 45, 1007–1014.

Fleming, M. H. & Mattingly, C. (1994). Action & inquiry: Reasoned action and active reasoning. In C. Mattingly & M. H. Fleming (Eds.), *Clinical reasoning: Forms of inquiry in a therapeutic practice* (pp. 316–342). Philadelphia: F. A. Davis.

Gambrill, E. (2005). *Critical thinking in clinical practice: Improving quality of judgement and decision-making* (2nd ed.). Hoboken, NJ: John Wiley & Sons.

Gillen, G. (2002). Improving mobility and community access in an adult with ataxia. *American Journal of Occupational Therapy,* 56, 462–466.

Gilovich, T. (1991). *How we know what isn't so: The fallibility of human reason in everyday life.* New York: The Free Press.

Gleick, J. (1987). *Chaos: Making a new science.* New York: Penguin Books.

Gray, J. M., Kennedy, B. L. & Zemke, R. (1996). Application of dynamic systems theory to occupation. In R. Zemke & F. Clark (Eds.), *Occupational science: The evolving discipline* (pp. 309–324). Philadelphia: F. A. Davis.

Greene, B. (1999). *The elegant universe: Superstrings, hidden dimensions, and the quest for the ultimate theory.* New York: W. W. Norton.

Hammel, K. W. (2001). Using qualitative research to inform the client-centred evidence-based practice of occupational therapy. *British Journal of Occupational Therapy,* 64, 228–234.

Hammel, K. W. & Carpenter, C. (Eds.) (2004). *Qualitative research in evidence-based rehabilitation.* Edinburgh, U.K.: Churchill Livingstone.

Holm, M. B. (2000). Our mandate for the new millennium: Evidence-based practice, 2000 Eleanor Clarke Slagle lecture. *American Journal of Occupational Therapy,* 54, 575–585.

Holm, M. B. & Rogers, J. C. (1989). The therapist's thinking behind functional assessment: Part II. In C. Royeen (Ed.), *Assessment of function: An action guide.* Rockville, MD: American Occupational Therapy Association.

Hume, D. (1748|1955). *An inquiry concerning human understanding.* Indianapolis: Bobbs-Merrill.

Kielhofner, G. (2004). *Conceptual foundations of occupational therapy* (3rd ed.). Philadelphia: F. A. Davis.

Labovitz, D. R. (Ed.) (2003). *Ordinary miracles: True stories about overcoming obstacles and surviving catastrophes.* Thorofare, NJ: Slack.

Lavelle, P. & Tomlin, G. S. (2001). Occupational therapy goal achievement for persons with postacute cerebrovascular accident in an on-campus student clinic. *American Journal of Occupational Therapy,* 55, 36–42.

Mainzer, K. (1997). *Thinking in complexity: The complex dynamics of matter, mind, and mankind.* Berlin: Springer.

Mattingly, C. (1991a). Narrative nature of clinical reasoning. *American Journal of Occupational Therapy,* 45, 998–1005.

Mattingly, C. (1991b). What is clinical reasoning? *American Journal of Occupational Therapy,* 45, 979–986.

Mattingly, C. & Fleming, M. H. (1994). *Clinical reasoning: Forms of inquiry in a therapeutic practice.* Philadelphia: F. A. Davis.

McNeill, D. & Freiburger, P. (1993). *Fuzzy logic.* New York: Simon & Schuster.

Mosey, A. C. (1992). *Applied scientific inquiry in the health professions: An epistemological orientation.* Rockville, MD: American Occupational Therapy Association.

Neistadt, M. E. (1992). The classroom as clinic: Applications for a method of teaching clinical reasoning. *American Journal of Occupational Therapy, 46,* 814–819.

Nelson, M. M. & Illingworth, W. T. (1991). *A practical guide to neural nets.* Reading, MA: Addison-Wesley.

Neuhaus, B. E. (1988). Ethical considerations in clinical reasoning: The impact of technology and cost containment. *American Journal of Occupational Therapy, 42,* 288–294.

Oaksford, M. & Chater, N. (2002). Commonsense reasoning, logic, and human rationality. In R. Elio (Ed.), *Common sense, reasoning, and rationality* (pp. 174–214). New York: Oxford University Press.

Ottenbacher, K. & Petersen, P. (1985). Quantitative trends in occupational therapy research: Implications for practice and education. *American Journal of Occupational Therapy, 39,* 240–246.

Rogers, J. C. (1983). Clinical reasoning: The ethics, science and art. *American Journal of Occupational Therapy, 37,* 601–616.

Rogers, J. C. & Holm, M. B. (1989). The therapist's thinking behind functional assessment: Part I. In C. Royeen (Ed.), *Assessment of function: An action guide.* Rockville, MD: American Occupational Therapy Association.

Rogers, J. C. & Holm, M. B. (1991). Occupational therapy diagnostic reasoning: A component of clinical reasoning. *American Journal of Occupational Therapy, 45,* 1045–1053.

Rogers, J. C. & Holm, M. B. (1997). Diagnostic reasoning: The process of problem identification. In C. H. Christiansen & C. M. Baum (Eds.), *Occupational therapy: Enabling function and well-being* (2nd ed., pp. 137–156). Thorofare, NJ: Slack.

Rogers, J. C. & Masagatani, G. (1982). Clinical reasoning of occupational therapists during the initial assessment of physically disabled patients. *Occupational Therapy Journal of Research, 2,* 195–219.

Rogoff, B. & Lave, J. (Eds.) (1984). *Everyday cognition: Its development in social context.* Cambridge, MA: Harvard University Press.

Royeen, C. B. & Luebben, A. J. (2002). Annotated bibliography of chaos for occupational therapy. *Occupational Therapy in Health Care, 16*(1), 63–80.

Sackett, D. L., Straus, S. E., Richardson, W. S., Rosenberg, W. & Haynes, R. B. (2000). *Evidence-based medicine: How to practice and teach EBM* (2nd ed.). Edinburgh, U.K.: Churchill Livingstone.

Schell, B. A. & Cervero, R. M. (1993). Clinical reasoning in occupational therapy: An integrative review. *American Journal of Occupational Therapy, 47,* 605–610.

Scheirton, L., Mu, K. & Lohman, H. (2003). Occupational therapists' responses to practice errors in physical rehabilitation settings. *American Journal of Occupational Therapy, 57,* 307–314.

Schmidt, H. G., Norman, G. R. & Boshuizen, H. P. A. (1990). A cognitive perspective on medical expertise: Theory and implications. *Academic Medicine, 65,* 611–621.

Schwartzberg, S. (2002). *Interactive reasoning in the practice of occupational therapy.* Upper Saddle River, NJ: Prentice-Hall.

Tomlin, G. (2005). The use of interactive video client simulation scores to predict clinical performance of occupational therapy students. *American Journal of Occupational Therapy, 59,* 50–56.

Tversky, A. & Kahneman, D. (1974). Judgment under uncertainty: Heuristics and biases. *Science, 125,* 1124–1131.

Unsworth, C. A. (2005). Using a head-mounted video camera to explore current conceptualizations of clinical reasoning in occupational therapy. *American Journal of Occupational Therapy, 59,* 31–40.

Yerxa, E. J. (1991). Seeking a relevant, ethical and realistic way of knowing for occupational therapy. *American Journal of Occupational Therapy, 45,* 199–204.

Zemke, R. & Clark, F. (Eds.) (1996). *Occupational science: The evolving discipline.* Philadelphia: F. A. Davis.

6

Narrative Reasoning

Toby Ballou Hamilton

CHAPTER OUTLINE

OBJECTIVES

After reading this chapter, the learner will be able to:

1. Define and describe narrative reasoning.
2. Define the role of narrative reasoning in evidence-based practice.
3. Define narrative or story.
4. Identity types of narratives commonly encountered in occupational therapy practice.
5. Identify narratives embedded in conversation or interview.
6. Elicit stories from clients and families to individualize meaningful occupation-based intervention.
7. Classify and interpret narratives told by clients.
8. Use narrative reasoning as part of the evaluation and intervention process.
9. Discuss the significance of narrative reasoning for practice in occupational therapy.
10. Apply narrative reasoning within occupational therapy models of practice.

KEY TERMS

Narrative reasoning	Narrative	Storymaking
Phenomenology	Story	Occupational storymaking
Storytelling	Life story	Volitional narrative
Narrative thinking	Illness narrative	
Plot	Occupational narrative	

W e are as surrounded by narrative as we are by air. We live in narrative. We live out narrative. Universally, throughout time and in all places, humans tell stories. We use stories to explain why we are late, why people act as they do, and why natural phenomena occur. Humans look up at stars, imagine patterns, and invent stories to explain them. Neurologically hard-wired for narrative, even small children differentiate stories from conversation. A Jewish proverb explains the creation and existence of humanity by stating that "God loves stories" (Zeitlin, 1997). To be human is to know, tell, and live stories, prompting some to name our species *homo narrans* (Fisher, 1984).

Thinking About Thinking 6-1

Narrative as the Essence of Practice

The use of narrative and life history method is not a matter of it taking more or less time, it is a matter of being the essence of practice.

—Burke & Kern, 1996, (p. 391)

We live narrative by making occupational choices based on our life stories. We summon, evoke, tell, and make stories as part of our daily lives so that each day is a weaving of the warp and weft of narrative and occupation. Each day's weaving lengthens the tapestry of our own particular life story through occupational choice and performance. We engage in this weaving of occupations and narratives so naturally that we are generally unaware that they relate throughout our day. For example, we may listen to the news (narratives of exceptional recent events) while getting ready for work or school (occupations). We discuss events and experiences either in person or with the technical support of telephones, facsimile machines, copiers, or computers, in the form of stories (narrative). We prepare and eat meals (occupations), perhaps relating the exceptional parts of our day or recording them in a journal (verbal and written narratives). We might engage in leisure (occupation) by experiencing narrative in its many formats by watching drama, comedy, or music videos on television, attending a play, ballet, or movie, viewing art, visiting with friends, or reading fiction or literature (all narrative leisure pursuits). We might include a bedtime story (narrative) as part of our evening self-care routine (occupations), and dream (narrative) to awaken and continue the life story tapestry the next day. Although the particular routines and interactions vary individually, both occupation and narrative intertwine in our daily experiences to structure our time, define ourselves, and make sense of and add meaning to our lives. As a result, all narratives are inevitably about occupation and all occupation can be storied.

Narrative reasoning plays a vital part in health care and science. Appreciation of narrative is evident in occupational therapy literature over the last decade in practice and research across practice models, settings, and clients (Burke & Kern, 1996; Larson & Fanchiang, 1996a). Occupational therapists joined the narrative turn, which began in the 1970s in the social sciences and humanities, building on literary theory (Atkinson, 1997; Bruner, 1991; Charon et al, 1995; Czarniawska, 2004; Molineux & Rickard, 2003). The narrative turn affirmed the importance of narrative as a framework for studying and resolving issues of human existence and the human condition (Brockmeir & Harre, 1997). Throughout the 1980s and 1990s, fields such as political science, psychiatry, psychology, sociology, economics, science studies, history, anthropology, and medical ethics made the narrative turn (e.g., Czarniawska, 2004), and health care has followed. The clinical reasoning study undertaken by the American Occupational Therapy Association and the American Occupational Therapy Foundation used ethnographic and action research methods to study the clinical reasoning of occupational therapists and surfaced narrative reasoning as a major aspect of therapists' thinking (Mattingly & Fleming, 1994).

Consider the relation of narrative to another trend, evidence-based health care practice, defined as "the integration of best research evidence with clinical expertise and patient values" (Sackett, Straus, Richardson, Rosenberg & Haynes, 2000, p.1). Two of the three aspects of the definition explicitly involve narrative reasoning and use of narrative: clinical expertise, "the ability to use our clinical skills and past experience to rapidly identify each patient's unique health state and diagnosis, their individual risks and benefits of potential interventions, and their personal values and expectations" and patient values, "the unique preferences, concerns and expectations each patient brings to a clinical encounter and which must be integrated into clinical decisions if they are to serve the patient" (Sackett et al., 2000, p. 1).

This chapter explores narrative reasoning as a particular type of clinical reasoning, one in which occupational therapists think with narratives or stories. We introduce narrative reasoning and its significance for occupational therapy practice.

REASONING WITH NARRATIVE AND STORY

Once, when my son was about 7 or 8 years old and with me at work, I gave him some money to spend at the snack bar. He told me that he spent all of the money on candy and had eaten it all at once. Not long after he ate the candy, he told me that his stomach began to ache. When we are immoderate, we have to pay the piper and face the consequences. He certainly did not set out to make himself sick, but that is what happened when the candy was so tasty that he ate all of the candy at once. He told me that he did not want to repeat this mistake and even told his younger sister about it. Because of this experience, he has never done it again and I doubt he ever will. Now when he has a stomachache, we look for another cause. Since then, whenever he eats candy, he eats just one bar or a few small candies, except for indulgence that stops short of excess on special occasions. Well, I guess it is just a part of growing up. We have all been greedy and immoderate at some time in our lives, and to tell you the truth, we are all still tempted to overdo it, even on the good things in life. I hope he remembers this story whenever he is tempted to be immoderate again. Now that he is a young adult, he faces temptations a lot more dangerous than too much candy (used with permission of author).

Analyzing the story in short segments illustrates the functions and purposes of narratives. "Once, when my son was about 7 or 8 years old and with me at work, I gave him some money to spend at the snack bar. He told me that he spent all of the money on candy and had eaten it all at once." This simple orienting clause lets you know that I am telling a story because it establishes the characters, time, place, and circumstances that are not present. This information does not have to begin the story (Labov, 1972; Labov & Weletzky, 1967), but often does. You also know the story is told from a point of view gained by my role as a working mother. Note how the organization and shape of this simple beginning shows how subjective and personal narratives are. Where I chose to start telling the story shows my influence as narrator and shows that I omitted details. For example, I do not tell you why my school-age son was at work with me or why I gave him money to spend at the snack bar. Part of the process of shaping narratives into a point or moral is omitting details that narrators think are irrelevant to that point. This shaping or interpretive process makes the narrative mine and tells you not only about my son, but also about me. All narratives do this and as such, all narratives are subjective and intensely personal. This aspect is why narratives are called phenomenological in nature.

Phenomenology tells how an individual experiences phenomena. The way I tell the story tells you a great deal about me and my life, even when I tell a story about someone or something else.

"Not long after he ate the candy, he told me that his stomach began to ache." By introducing the sequence of events that forms the skeleton of the narrative (Labov, 1972; Labov & Weletzky, 1967), it was shaped to show a clear cause-and-effect relationship between candy and stomachache. Part of the shaping or interpretive process is that other events that might have happened in the time between eating the candy and the stomachache were not mentioned, any one of which could be a causal factor. By not suggesting alternatives, my perception of cause and effect shaped the narrative to make the point about the relationship of variables I considered important.

"When we are immoderate, we have to pay the piper and face the consequences." This segment expresses my theme, point, or moral and answers the vital narrative question, "So what?" that explains why I am telling this story. This statement shows how I think the story should be interpreted (Labov, 1972; Labov & Weletzky, 1967) as describing the consequences of immoderation. Note that I expressed it in a saying or axiom that I have internalized from a cultural norm. You might recognize the phrase "pay the piper," which may refer to the 13th-century story of the Pied Piper of Hamelin or the practice of paying musicians after a dance. Another aspect of the phenomenological nature of narrative is that you not only learn about narrators by the points they make, but also by how they make them. You could guess at this point that I grew up hearing European and North American folktales and folklore. In fact, you may learn more about me by the way I tell my stories than by the stories I tell.

"He certainly did not set out to make himself sick, but that is what happened when the candy was so tasty that he ate all of it at once." Now you not only know what I think happened, you also know his intent was not to become ill. By linking his intent to the action and the consequence, I offer my explanation that the taste of the candy overrode the possible consequences of becoming ill.

"He told me that he did not want to repeat this mistake and even told his younger sister about it." Note that my son used narrative to make sense of his experience and to relate his meaning to someone else. Two purposes of narrative are to make meaning and to communicate experience to others, often to teach, caution, or heal. He clearly intended to protect his sister from the same fate and you learn more about him as a result.

"Because of this experience, he has never done it again and I doubt he ever will. Now when he has a stomachache, we look for another cause. Since then, whenever he eats candy, he eats just one bar or a few small candies, except for indulgence that stops just short of excess on special occasions." Now, as the narrative shifts from the past to the present, you see that one outcome is that our family interprets everyday events differently as a result of his experience. It clarifies that narrative concerns change over time and that this experience changed my son's occupational performance with regard to candy, both immediately and subsequently. He changed his behavior because he could prospectively imagine a similar consequence for similar future action. I changed my expectations about his future behavior to look for alternative explanations for his stomachaches. The narrative is coming to a resolution at this point because I tell you the outcome (Labov, 1972; Labov & Weletzky, 1967).

"Well, I guess it is just a part of growing up. We have all been greedy and immoderate at some time in our lives, and to tell you the truth, we are all still tempted to overdo it, even on the good things in life." As the narrative winds down, I place his experience into a universal experience of being human. You might suspect from the telling of this story that I have been immoderate myself, perhaps prompting you to consider your own experiences of immoderation.

"I hope he remembers this story whenever he is tempted to be immoderate again. Now that he is a young adult, he faces temptations a lot more dangerous than too much candy." Here, I not only give you another way to interpret the narrative, I also give it new meaning by applying it to the possibilities of future challenges. Through a hallmark sequence of having a beginning, middle, and end (Bruner, 1990, p. 44), narratives uniquely allow us to reflect on experiences and then project them forward in time and to prospectively imagine the future. In addition, there is a sense that this story represents an episode within my son's larger life story and that this story will prove useful in ways he could not imagine at age 7 or 8. By telling the story, I validate that his life (and all others) "need and merit being narrated" (Ricoeur, 1984, p. 75).

This story is worthy of telling because it makes sense of an experience in which my son learned a vital life lesson. Sometimes we tell stories about ordinary events, but more often we tell about the extraordinary. If my son ate too much candy on a daily basis, it wouldn't be worthy of **storytelling.** We do not tell stories about getting dressed, picking up the mail, or commuting, unless those events form the context or set the scene for a story about an extraordinary experience. No one is ever late without offering an explanation, invariably in the form of a narrative. In fact, we use narratives to make sense of or gain meaning from experience and to help reconcile the ordinary and the extraordinary (Bruner, 1986).

Would you have guessed that motive, intent, desire, conflict, uncertainty, and change could all present in such a short (true) story? Thanks to my now college-age son, Max, I hope that you have a deeper appreciation of narrative and the phenomenological approach it offers. Each of the points shown in Box 6-1 justify why occupational therapists reason through narratives and use them in practice. Collectively, they explain why narrative reasoning is a "central mode" that is fundamental to clinical reasoning in occupational therapy (Mattingly, 1991, p. 998).

BOX 6-1

Narratives in Practice

Practitioners use narratives in practice to:
- make sense of experiences and actions we do not fully understand.
- understand motive, intent, desire, conflict, trouble, uncertainty, and change.
- reconcile differences between the ordinary and the extraordinary.
- make sense of life when change, trouble, or conflict enters.
- place experience within an individual's larger life story and universal human experience.
- explain things to ourselves and others.
- see how others react to gauge their reactions.
- as a means of cautioning, teaching, and healing ourselves and others.
- shape future action by reflecting on experience and living out the life story.
- reflect the grand narratives of culture, like folktale and myth, on an individual scale.
- relate individual experiences to universal human experiences.

(Adapted from Mattingly, 1994.)

NARRATIVE AS A MODE OF THINKING AND KNOWING

Narrative is not only a way to communicate but also a way of perceiving the world (Bruner, 1986; Czarniawska, 2004). **Narrative thinking** deals in subjective, personalized particulars and specifics of lived experience, human intention, and action that connects events across time and defines possibilities. The use of personal experience and concern for the human condition defines its characteristic subjective and personalized position. Although this position helps define possibilities and encourages the consideration of multiple perspectives based on individual interpretations, it is not intended to be generalized beyond particular persons (Bruner, 1986; Czarniawska, 2004; Ricoeur, 1984; White & Epston, 1990). For example, occupational therapists use narrative thinking when considering how a particular person experiences a phenomenon such as falling or how a diagnosis affects that person's life.

A common and inaccurate assumption is that scientific thinking and narrative thinking are opposed to each other or that one has more validity or utility than the other. In Chapter 5, this notion was contested, and further information is provided here. Occupational therapy reasoning blends several types of reasoning (Fleming, 1991). We can illustrate this by examining a coin. We notice that each side contributes different aspects to the coin that we label the "head" and the "tail." Regardless of which side is showing, we recognize the object as a coin.

Similarly, when using a coin to make a purchase, it does not matter how we insert the coin in the vending slot or hand it to the cashier. The coin's validity is apparent regardless of which side of the coin shows. Similarly, occupational therapists reason scientifically, as described in Chapter 5, and through narrative, as discussed in this chapter. Together, scientific and narrative thinking and reasoning help us form perspectives on a single reality and truth, just as the head and tail of a coin show different sides of one coin.

Defining Narrative

The fact that we naturally think in a narrative mode makes narrative surprisingly difficult to define. Another problem is that we already know what a narrative is and no one needs to define it for us. From an early age, humans possess mental schemas for stories made up of conventions and expectations about elements and how stories proceed (Mandler, 1984). This sense of narrative is so strong that we comprehend stories even when causal and temporal details are omitted (Culler, 1997; Gergen & Gergen, 1988; Mandler, 1984). Such findings support our status as *homo narrans* (Fisher, 1984), given our neural network of frontal, temporal, and cingulate areas, Broca's and Wernicke's areas, and the hippocampus, which supports narrative comprehension and production (Bickle, 2003; Mars, 2004; Siegel, 1999). Coherent narratives require both hemispheres—the left, to make sense of and interpret, and the right, to retrieve autobiographical information and create images and narrative themes (Seigel, 1999).

Another obstacle to its definition is narrative's ubiquity or omnipresence; we are surrounded by it and surrounded ourselves with it. Simply, we tell and listen to stories because we need to. This need explains our constant immersion in narrative's myriad forms. Spoken, written, acted, sung, depicted, sculpted, or danced (Barthes, 1977), we not only recognize and think in narrative, we require narrative to understand and make sense of ourselves and our lives.

From the story of my son's experience with candy (see Reasoning with Narrative and Story), you can see that a narrative is a personal cognitive organizational scheme through which the narrator subjectively orders relevant details into a coherent whole. Specific events are linked into the whole through **plot** (Polkinghorne, 1988), the source of narrative's power (Bruner, 1990). The subjectivity and phenomenology of story show when each person tells a unique version of the same experience. Narrative's hallmark is its distinctive temporal sequence of beginning, middle, and end (Bruner, 1990, p. 44), making it much more than a time-ordered list or chronology. Through plot, a narrator organizes, shapes, and structures selected experiences so they build on each other in a way that clarifies how each event contributes individually and as a part of the whole (Bruner, 1986, 1990; Mattingly, 1994, 1998; Polkinghorne, 1988; Ricoeur, 1984). Narrative's capacity to perceive both parts and whole allows us to see the relationship and place a single episode into a larger narrative, like a chapter in a book. Subjective ordering and omission of irrelevance shows causal relationships that give narratives their individualized perspective, point of view, theme, or moral that can be integrated and internalized. The very stuff of story is human belief, desire, and commitment (Bruner, 1990, p. 52); knowledge of intention, motive, and action imparts meaning and makes sense of it (e.g., Bruner, 1990; Mattingly, 1994, 1998; Polkinghorne, 1988). The ability to negotiate and renegotiate meanings through narrative is "one of the crowning achievements" of a person's development and of the development of humanity and culture (Bruner, 1990, p. 67). Because humans possess the capacity to enact a multitude of intentions, narratives provide a variety of differing perspectives that help explain the extraordinary when events deviate from our expectations (Bruner, 1990; Culler, 1997). All that in one simple story.

Obviously, narratives are about an experience or event. Although linked in complex ways, narrative is not a verbalized copy of experience. To tell a story, the narrator attends to particular aspects of the experience and ignores others. By attending to selected aspects of experience from an individually unique perception, narrative reveals the narrator's inner world (Riessman, 1993). Careful listeners learn the narrator's perceptions and interpretations not only from its content but also how the narrative is told (Lieblich, Tuval-Mashiach & Zilber, 1998). In fact, the representation of one's inner life from story is as significant as the expression of the outer reality about experience and tells "what the world does to that someone" (Mattingly, 1998, p. 8). Reciprocally, experience summons narrative, and narrative shapes and structures experience. Particular narratives not only interpret past experience but also shape the future by bringing about the next action that will produce the desired ending (Mattingly, 1998).

For our purposes, **narrative** or **story** is an organizational scheme of subjectively sequenced events that reveals causal relationships, communicates and shapes experience, and creates and expresses meaning (Hamilton, 2001). Although distinguished in literary theory (Culler, 1997; Baldick, 1990), I suggest we use *narrative* and *story* as equivalent terms in occupational therapy practice.

The Life Story: Narrative and Identity

Because occupational performance calls forth the unique capacities of the individual, occupations inherently reflect personal uniqueness and identity. Occupation is the primary way in which we develop and express who we are, set and achieve goals, and develop competence and mastery that shapes identity (American Occupational Therapy Association [AOTA], 1979; Christiansen, 1999; Fidler & Fidler, 1978). We identify ourselves largely by what we do and because we narrate what we do, narratives play a part in the formation and continuity of our personal identities. The social constructivist school of thinking maintains that we construct subjective stories *about* our lives that in turn have profound influence *on* our lives (Czarniawska, 2004).

To understand life, everyone creates a narrative of his or her life, called the **life story.** We create meaning about intentions and actions (ours and those of others) by placing them in story form (Bruner, 1986), the life story particularly (Czarniawska, 2004; Linde, 1993). Because narrative helps us interpret and assign meaning, narratives about ourselves are dynamic interpretations of identity that include experiences, psychological makeup, group membership, personal history, emotional responses, personality traits, and roles (Bruner, 1990; Christiansen, 1999; Polkinghorne, 1996; Riessman, 1993). Narratives contribute to the formation of personal identity by unifying events and showing how each event contributes to the whole life story (Polkinghorne, 1996). Most important, our life stories come to constitute our perception of reality because we tell and retell them and our enactment of them (Kirsh, 1996; Mattingly, 1994). We live our lives according to our life stories by making decisions and occupational choices based on them (e.g., Hamilton, 1999; Helfrich & Kielhofner, 1994; Parry & Doan, 1994; Polkinghorne, 1988). Because narratives are subjective and particular by nature, and created by an interpretive process, we have considerable latitude in creating and revising the life story. However, life stories must include the stories of others (Czarniawska, 2004) and incorporate all major life events without omitting unpleasant experiences or undesirable aspects of one's life (Polkinghorne, 1996); we cannot simply ignore others or leave out parts we do not like. In fact, part of the life story deals with reconciling unpleasant motivations, intentions, and action. Created by a "deeper cognitive process" than the conscious, creative act of writing literary stories (Polkinghorne, 1996, p. 300), our life stories profoundly influence our identity. A personal story from the author is provided as an example in Case Study 6-1.

CASE STUDY 6-1

My Moving Story

> Because of my family's frequent moves as I grew up, my life story was one of inter- rupted studies and friendships. I keep track of my childhood by my grade in school and the states in which I lived. I went to three schools for fifth grade and three high schools; a total of 12 different school in six states. For most of my life, I used the circumstances of frequent moves as an excuse for academic and social short- comings. I lived out the life plot "victim-by-Mayflower-moving-van" until my thir- ties. Through a process of re-examining my life, I revised the story to reinterpret moving as the sacrifice my parents made to provide us with a good living. Now I live out of the "moving-as-bounty" plot instead. Reinterpretation of childhood experience created new meanings that allowed me to revise that part of my life story and enact it in a new way that influenced my life story from that point for- ward (used with permission of author).

Both identity and life stories can be threatened by challenges (Christiansen, 1999). Mattingly proposed that people with chronic illness suffer a "narrative loss" (1998, p. 52), and Frank called the experience of illness and disability a "narrative wreck" (1995, p. 54) in which the life story is interrupted, delayed, and altered. As such, one of the ways to re-form self images and heal the sense of self is by telling stories. Like a mirror reflects our outer being, telling a story about the self allows one to see the inner story reflected on the face of the listener. Telling such narratives helps restore the sense of self by reinforcing the concept that one has a life before and after the health event that segments the life story (Fitzgerald & Paterson, 1995; Frank, 1995). Asking people to tell stories about themselves not only helps the occupational therapist to identify occupations invested with impor- tance and meaning, but also gain perspectives about people's unique perceptions, such as how one perceives experience as ordinary or extraordinary.

Narrative helps us reconcile the ordinary and extraordinary, thriving on their contrast (Czarniawska, 2004). In the cultural context, stories socialize and impart culture by simultaneously defining norms and telling how to deal with deviations from them (Bruner, 1990; Czarniawska, 2004). For example, the folk-tale, *Little Red Riding Hood*, is a cautionary tale that tells us to expect to encounter dangerous strangers if we fail to listen to our mothers and veer off the path, both literally and figuratively. At the same time that narratives remind us that human intentions can cause exceptions to our understanding of the rules, narratives help us make sense when our personal and cultural expectations are not met. Therefore, most of the stories people tell are about exceptions to the usual or ordinary (Bruner, 1990). This tendency not to narrate the ordinary compels occupational therapists to carefully question clients for details about occupational performance that clients assume to be universal, rather than highly individual, routines.

Our natural inclination for narrating the exceptional helps explain why people find it important and satisfying to tell unique narrative accounts about their perceptions and interpretations of extraordinary events. Generations, for example, are defined by their personal stories about what they were doing (occupation) and where they were (context) when they learned of events of international importance. Everyone has an extensive repertoire of personal stories that recount the experience and the meaning of common experiences that serve to unite and remind us of the human condition.

Occupational therapists realize that the deviations from health and occupation experienced by clients and their families are extraordinary exceptions to their expectations of lifelong good health and satisfying, meaningful occupation. Occupational performance problems must be reconciled with personal expectations of "the good life" (Rogers, 1983, p.602).

I once worked with a woman while she was hospitalized during chemotherapy for cancer. As we discussed the occupations that she wanted to resume upon discharge, she told me stories of her home on a small acreage, where she cared for a menagerie of farm animals and pets. Despite a poor prognosis, she told me that she had not asked herself why she had cancer, as many do. Instead, she asked herself, Why not? She made sense of cancer by thinking of it as a disease that happens to people and had unfortunately happened to her. She wondered why she should expect not to have such a condition happen to her. Thus, she reconciled the extraordinary event of having cancer by accepting the potential of illness and disability as part of the human condition that could become a part of anyone's ordinary life story. She had revised her life story to incorporate cancer as a part of her life yet fostered the hope that she could return to former occupations in a modified way and pick up her life story in the process.

The Life Story and Narrative Reasoning

Narrative reasoning is the process through which occupational therapists make sense of people's particular circumstances, prospectively imagine the effect of illness, disability, or occupational performance problems on their daily lives, and create a collaborative story that we enact together in the intervention process (Mattingly, 1994, p. 998). We can symbolize narrative reasoning by a bridge that links the person's past, present and future (McKay & Ryan, 1995). Therapists do this in two ways: by having clients tell us stories about the past and present (storytelling) and by creating stories with them about the future (**storymaking**). Over time, we collect parts of the person's life story. The storytelling and storymaking processes affirm a person's life as a continuous story that links the "pre-illness and the post-diagnosis self" (Fitzgerald & Paterson, 1995, p. 20) in ways that affirm identity.

Narrative reasoning allows therapists to help clients affirm and reform identities, as illustrated by the woman's story above. Despite her illness, this woman affirmed that she is the same person with the same occupational interests as in her "before" life. She reconciled her before and after chemotherapy through desire to continue a meaningful occupation, the same person who loved occupations that even cancer could not keep her from doing. Second, the storytelling process affirms the need for improvisation and revision of the life story (Bateson, 1989), just as people edit and revise stories they write and tell. Seeing the continuity of her before and after identity motivated this woman to accept necessary compensations and imagine improvised solutions for her most important occupations. She connected her postchemotherapy story to her life story by willingness to modify contexts and task demands in order to continue doing what was meaningful to her. Next, therapists use narrative reasoning to discover and incorporate the person's strengths and former adaptations to meet the challenges posed to identity and occupation (e.g., Bateson, 1989; Clark, 1993; Hamilton, 1999; Price-Lackey & Cashman, 1996; Spencer et al., 1996). We built on her strengths to compensate for capabilities she lost by directing her compassion for animals to herself. She could then perceive compensatory techniques such as work simplification and energy conservation positively, as compassionate self-care rather than restrictive self-care. Narratives' temporal sequence allows us to imagine clients in future contexts and time doing meaningful occupations. Envisioning future endings motivates and helps clients develop reasonable hopes for the future (Spencer, Davidson & White, 1997). This woman affirmed her hope that she could continue the most meaningful of her occupations, which helped her reconcile her identity. Together, we used narrative reasoning to imaginatively project her into her desired home context using work simplification and energy conservation techniques to care for her pets. Finally, the storytelling process affirms one as an occupational being (Clark et al., 1996). This story not only illustrates the uses of narrative reasoning to reform identity and revise the life story, but also illustrates that specific aspects of the life story deal with health and deviations from it, called the **illness narrative,** and about occupations, called the **occupational narrative.**

The Illness Narrative

Health professionals elicit information about health conditions and their experiences of it from clients, family members, and others. When health professionals ask questions about symptoms and signs, they use logical, scientific thought and the deductive process to establish a diagnosis. A diagnosis is an abstraction of the conditions that cause a pathological state in general terms that we call *disease*. Use of narrative reasoning reveals the social, psychological, and occupational experience of having disease, which is termed *illness* (e.g., Frank, 1995; Kleinman, 1988). Disease represents the outsider's view of signs and symptoms that results in a medical diagnosis. The insider's perspective of disease as lived experience (Conrad, 1990, p. 1261) is expressed by illness and disability and is unique to each individual, even for those with the same pathology or disease. Only the person can have a disease, but others can share the experience of illness or disability. People tell their experiences of illness in an illness narrative.

The illness narrative is not only the story of the experience of being ill and the problems it poses (Kautzman, 1993; Fitzgerald & Paterson, 1995). The illness narrative expresses the person's fundamental beliefs—both cultural and individual—about health and disease, its causes, care, and potential for treatment (Garro, 1994; Kleinman, 1988). Because the illness narrative lends coherence and meaning to health-related events and even suffering, it helps preserve the sense of self experiencing illness (Fitzgerald & Paterson, 1995; Kleinman, 1988). The illness narrative tells not just the "story of an illness but rather the story of a life altered by illness" (Garro, 1994, p. 775); we learn what it is like for this person to live with this disease (Mattingly, 1991). The illness narrative is the story that shows causal relationships of health, disease, illness, impairment, and disability that communicate the experience, alterations, and individual meaning of living life affected by illness or disability (Hamilton, 2001).

An older rancher from rural Oklahoma who had been diagnosed with a cerebrovascular accident (CVA) told me his illness narrative. He said that he had fallen into a bed of fire ants and that his symptoms were the result of fire ant poisoning from numerous ant bites. Using scientific thinking, we disagreed with the diagnosis. Using narrative thinking allowed the consideration of multiple perspectives and interpretations (Czarniawska, 2004) so that his fall can be interpreted from at least two perspectives: as the cause of his condition (his version) by falling and being bitten and poisoned by the ants or by the result of his condition (medical version) in which the stroke caused his fall. Although I certainly did not understand the reasoning I was using as a relatively new graduate, I eventually abandoned my futile attempts to convince him of his "proper" diagnosis. We worked from the common ground of agreement that the paralysis of his arm and leg interfered with his daily activities, regardless of the cause or cure. He spoke with sadness about being paralyzed and with frustration because he could not imagine how he could continue the occupations he needed to do once back on the ranch. His illness narrative clearly shows how one's beliefs about health, disease, and illness affect the occupational therapy process.

The Occupational Narrative

All health professionals listen to a client's story as an essential facet of clinical practice and interpret it according to their profession's philosophy and intervention methods. Physicians listen to illness narratives to help establish a diagnosis (Kleinman, 1980, 1988; Hunter, 1996), but increasingly some delay questioning patients to allow them to tell their stories first (Ryan, 1999).

In contrast, occupational therapists listen for problems of everyday living to facilitate occupational performance and social participation. Narrative is an ideal medium to express occupational problems, because the details of time, place, and circumstance are embedded in both narrative and occupation. The person may perceive illness as dividing the life story into segments (Fitzgerald & Paterson, 1995) or as repeatedly interrupting the life story in cycles of exacerbation and remission (Helfrich & Kielhofner, 1994). Whether its onset is sudden or insidious, and its duration acute or chronic, disease, injury, trauma, and normative changes such as maturing and aging alter one's perceptions of self, life, health, and occupational performance. Changes in health and occupation necessarily cause revisions in the life story in order to preserve the physical, emotional, and occupational self (Fitzgerald & Paterson, 1995).

Occupational therapists are particularly interested in narratives that focus on the individual's occupational nature, with the primary stories of interest those describing occupational performance (Clark, 1993; Clark, et al., 1996; Molineux & Rickard, 2003). The occupational narrative (Moyers, 1999, p. 16) is a narrative about occupational experience that shows the relationships of health and participation and of illness, disability, or restriction when present; places occupational performance within specific contexts; and expresses the meaning of specific occupations and the relationships of occupations in one's life (Hamilton, 2001). No wonder that Mattingly urged occupational therapists to "take their phenomenological tasks more seriously" (1991, p. 986).

Having defined narrative, examined its functions, and the roles of the life story and illness and occupational narratives, we are ready to examine the two major ways in which occupational therapists apply their narrative reasoning in practice: storytelling and storymaking.

STORYTELLING

Storytelling is a retrospective process that links the past to the present (Mattingly, 1994) and gives a personal interpretation of experiences. Both occupational therapists and clients tell these stories. Therapists tell them to compare one client's circumstances with another's, to determine how health conditions and contexts affect a particular client's occupations, and to describe and explain how clients respond to therapy and how therapeutic processes led to outcomes. Clients and their families tell stories that invite therapists into the life story and link the person's past to occupational therapy in the present (Coe, 1999, p. 77). Storytelling is a bridge from the occupational past to the occupational present and from the actual world of illness, disability, or occupational performance problems to the possible world of occupational wholeness and healing. The very act of telling one's story is therapeutic in itself because it repairs the "narrative wreck" (Frank, 1995, p. 54) by reforming identity, safely re-experiencing events without consequences, and providing hope (e.g., Clark et al., 1996; Mattingly & Lawlor, 2000; Molineux & Rickard, 2003; Spencer, Davidson & White, 1997). Storytelling occurs throughout the occupational therapy process and stories become more complete as therapy continues.

Stories unwind along a temporal axis, with each part adding to the whole story (Mattingly, 1991). Like fiction, additional details give insight into people, contexts, motives, intentions, and actions. In contrast to fiction, which is completely controlled by an author who intentionally metes out details to shed light on the characters or advance the plot, in practice, stories are interrupted, delayed, or otherwise incompletely told. In narrative terms, this adds drama and suspense as a clearer picture emerges bit by bit. Partial stories become dangerous only when we are convinced that we already know the whole story and consider additional details and related stories irrelevant, rather than fitting them into the life story.

Sometimes, therapists need reminders to be patient while storytelling follows its natural course of unwinding over time. With scientific, pragmatic, and ethical reasoning, we seldom have all the information we need or want so that we can make decisions. But with narrative reasoning in particular, we continuously collect details and fit them into the whole to make sense of the story to date, perhaps reasoning, "Okay, now that I know this about her, it makes sense that she wants to do that." This process is like fitting new pieces into a partially completed jig saw puzzle, sometimes matching for shape and sometimes for color, and always knowing that the storyteller is the ultimate authority, like the picture on the front of the puzzle box. Therapists and clients work to piece the story together by checking for accuracy in chronology and honoring the values of occupation expressed in them (Clark et al., 1996).

Stories emerge naturally throughout the entire process of occupational therapy, not just in an evaluation phase. The storytelling process happens during interview and in informal and therapeutic conversations, contributing to what we think we know about people, their contexts, and task demands. New details demand to be fit into the plot so far. Although folktales signal their beginnings and endings by ritual, therapeutic stories are bounded only by the duration and frequency of when therapy enters the person's life story. Therapists must be prepared for the story to be altered or transformed as new information emerges (see Case Study 6-2 below).

CASE STUDY 6-2

Planning Ahead: Mrs. Durley's Story Unwinds

Over the years that I worked at a hospital, Mrs. Durley always contacted me on each admission, so I experienced her story unwinding over several years. She was 89 when we met and I continued as part of her story well into her nineties as she experienced arthritis, cataract surgeries, and a variety of other illnesses. Because she was such an articulate advocate for occupational therapy, I wanted her to speak at a presentation about working with older adults. I telephoned her in November to ask her about a February date. She promised to contact me once she got next year's calendar and transferred her appointments into it. "How awesome," I thought, "to be using a calendar to plan months in advance at 89!" Now I knew something more about her—how organized she was and how well she planned ahead. Knowing this helped me understand her fierce determination to be independent in self-care at discharge when we first met. She refused to allow her daughter, who was recovering from surgery, to help her with activities of daily living at home. She had thought of using her rolling cart, not only to set and clear the table as I suggested, but also to water her houseplants. My picture of this dear woman was more complete as her story unwound over time, especially after I met her daughter, whom I had incorrectly assumed to be my contemporary, not my mother's (used with permission of the author).

Knowing that stories are part of human life and thought, some people are surprised, as I was, to learn that not all human speech is in narrative form. Conversation can contain narratives embedded in description, fact, opinion, and persuasive and technical argument (Czarniawska, 2004). Even talking about one's personal experience or history may not be story (Mattingly & Lawlor, 2000, p. 6). Only by recognizing narratives as they are told can therapists use them in the art and science of occupational therapy practice. Just as we identify folk tales by the presence of culturally stereotyped beginnings and endings, we can attune ourselves to recognize when someone is telling us a story.

Recognizing Narratives

All cultures have a way of cueing listeners that they are about to hear a story so that they know they are entering story time and story reality and can separate themselves from the present moment and suspend their typical disbelief in things mysterious and magical (Livo & Rietz, 1986). Perhaps one familiar cue is "once upon a time." However, all cultures develop specific ritual story openings and beginnings that reflect their beliefs and values (Box 6-2). However, the types of stories we hear in occupational therapy practice do not begin so obviously. Fortunately, we have several cues to recognize storied material embedded in conversation or interview.

B O X   6 - 2

Sample Ritual Folktale Opening and Beginnings

Once there was and once there was not . . . (Armenian, Persian)
We do not really mean . . . We do not really mean . . . That what we say is true (Asanti)
Once upon a time, when bears had tails as big as their heads, and willows bore a fruit juicy and red, there lived . . . (Rumanian)
Somewhere beyond the Red Sea, beyond the Blue Forest, beyond the Glass Mountain, and beyond the Straw Town, where they sift water and pour sand, there was . . . (Russian)
Teller: Cric!
Listeners: Crac! (Haitian)
Teller: I'm going to tell a story.
Listeners: Right!
Teller: It's a lie.
Listeners: Right!
Teller: But not everything in it is false.
Listeners: Right! (Sudanese)

Livo, N. & Rietz, S. A. (1986). *Storytelling process and practice.* Littleton, CO: Libraries Unlimited, Inc.

One approach to story recognition is the list of narrative elements called *Burke's pentad* (1945): actor, action, goal, scene, and instrument (*Table 6-1; Box 6-3*). Although first applied to literature, these elements apply equally well to occupational narratives.

As an imbalance in the other elements, Trouble enters into the life story in a variety of ways. Trouble can appear in the form of pathology, injury, or trauma at any point in one's life, entering with dramatic suddenness, as with injury or conditions with sudden onsets, such as stroke. Or, Trouble may creep insidiously into the scene, as with chronic conditions like Parkinson's disease, chronic obstructive pulmonary disease, or schizophrenia. Trouble might appear briefly in a cameo role, make multiple entrances and exits, or hover in the background, like multiple sclerosis, cancer, or bipolar disorder. Trouble can sneak in during episodes of normative life cycle transitions, such as role change or aging. Regardless of its entrance and appearance, Trouble eventually appears to occupational therapists as an inadequate response to unmet challenges to occupational performance: as problems of caring for oneself or others, working, learning, or participating in leisure or social pursuits. Trouble can be any barrier to occupational goals.

Regardless of how it enters or how long it stays, Trouble is vital to story (Burke, 1945). Occupational therapists would not appear in the story at all without the

TABLE 6-1

Literary and Occupational Therapy Terms

Literary Term	Occupational Therapy Term	Comment
Actor	Person, client, or other term appropriate to the setting	Occupational therapy philosophy views people as intrinsically motivated agents of their own activity and health (e.g., AOTA, 1979; Reilly, 1962). Others, including occupational therapists, play supporting roles in the person's story. Narrative reasoning emphasizes the person, not the diagnosis or impairment (Sacks, 1985).
Action	Occupational performance and social participation in context	Activity and occupation are the actions of everyday life. All storied action is about occupation and activity.
Scene	Environment or contexts	Just as a scene expresses mood and tone and creates forces that forge people and action (Foster, 2003), the contexts in which people work, learn, live, and play shape their occupations (Hamilton, 2003).
Goals	Goals	Actors act with intention and motive to reach goals, just as people do by enacting occupational roles and choices. A person's occupational challenges form their goals and direct the plot of their occupational narratives.
Instruments	Objects and their properties, including tolls, materials, and equipment	To reach goals, people use objects to meet activity demands of occupation and participation. In fairy tales and mythology, actors and instruments may possess magical powers, such as godmothers or beans, a metaphor for powers that actually reside within the person, not the object (Estes, 1992).
Trouble	Occupational challenge	Narratives always imply a struggle to meet challenges or goals. Burke called any imbalance in the previous 5 elements Trouble, which serves as the catalyst for the plot. In practice, the potential for occupational performance problems occurs with imbalances in context, activity demands, and clients' performance skills, patterns, and capacities (AOTA, 2002). Trouble appears as occupational performance problems due to aging, having or being at risk for impairments and disabilities, or contexts that need modification (Moyers, 1999).

Table used with permission of Toby Ballou Hamilton, 2001.
Burke, K. (1945). *A grammar of motives*. Berkeley, CA: University of California Press.
American Occupational Therapy Association. (2002). Occupational therapy practice framework: domain and process. *American Journal of Occupational Therapy* 56, 609-639.
Moyers, P. (1999). *The guide to occupational therapy practice*. Bethesda, MD: American Occupational Therapy Association.

> ## BOX 6-3
> ## Magical Objects: Mythology and Occupational Therapy
>
> The Greek myth of the labors of Psyche (from whose name meaning "soul" we derive the words *psyche, psychology,* and *psychiatry* among others) illustrates the point. Because curiosity led Psyche to disobey the warning of Cupid, her unseen husband/ god, the jealous goddess Venus assigned Psyche three tasks, the first of which was sorting a huge pile of grains and seeds into separate piles—grain by grain and seed by seed—by nightfall. Despairing that such a task could not be accomplished even by Hercules, she saw a black thread moving toward the pile— an army of ants sent by Cupid to sort the seeds (Grant & Hazel, 1993; Hathaway, 2001; Russell, 1989).
>
> Magical? Without a doubt. Symbolic? Most certainly. The ants represent that part of Psyche (and as myth, all our psyches) that is discriminating and capable of sorting details into manageable categories as a first step to making decisions. In therapy, objects and tools that seem quite ordinary to occupational therapists might seem magical to some people. Does enabling someone to use discrimination in forming relationships seem magical to someone bogged down in repeating dysfunctional relationships? Would an offset spoon be magical to someone otherwise unable to eat independently or a communication board for someone who is otherwise unable to express thoughts and needs?
>
> Used with permission of Toby Hamilton, 2005.

presence of Trouble in the form of the person's occupational problem or risk of one. Trouble can appear in several guises: as the affects of impairments on occupation; as pragmatics of practice, such as length of stay, reimbursement, or provision of equipment; as conflict within the team or family (Coe, 1999; Crepeau, 1994). Occupational therapy students and new practitioners often prefer to avoid all conflict. However, conflict is the "impetus required for the spiral of emplotment to continue" in which therapist and client are "waging a war or conflict to overcome adversity" (Coe, 1999, p. 75). Whenever therapists wish (as a form of story magic, perhaps) that Trouble would just go away, they do well to remind themselves that without Trouble, the story would not exist and they would not be in it. The more appropriate wish is that we work with the client and others to make the story end with the best possible outcomes.

Consider the episode in which Trouble causes an occupational performance problem as a chapter in the person's life story, into which occupational therapists enter in a supporting role. The person's life has a continuity that began before we entered the story and continues after our chapter ends. In expressing this idea, Helfrich and Kielhofner said, "the patient does not come to therapy. Rather, therapy comes into the patient's life" (1994, p. 325). Thinking of therapists in supporting roles sets up a therapeutic climate in which clients are in charge of their performance skills, patterns, and client factors, whereas therapists arrange contexts (Schultz & Schkade, 1992). Knowing Burke's pentad and the role of Trouble helps us recognize how and why we appear in clients' stories.

Listening for other elements helps therapists further identify narrative. One is through the structural elements suggested by Labov (1972) and illustrated in *Table 6-2* by excerpts from Nancy Mairs' essay "Taking Care" from *Waist-High in the World* (1996) about her experiences of multiple sclerosis and disability.

TABLE 6-2

Structural Elements of Narrative

Narrative Structure and Function (Labov, 1972; Labov & Weletzky, 1967)	Example (Mairs, 1996)	Practice Application
Abstract Optional structure identifiable as a summary of the story the narrator is about to tell	Mairs began her story of an unexpected change in her activities of daily living by stating, "This morning we've had a breakdown in the Nancy-care apparatus" (1996, p. 64). Explaining that her husband and sister usually help with her morning ADL routine, this phrase indicates the beginning of a story about an extraordinary day.	Mairs' example reminds us that people tell stories about exceptions to the expected (Bruner, 1986).
Orientation clauses Give characters, settings, time, and circumstances of the narrative, similar to Burke's elements. May be at beginning or interspersed throughout narrative	Mairs used orienting clauses by explaining her usual Wednesday morning routine and what made this particular day different, concluding, "Well, no matter how I got this way, I am in a pickle. No one is coming to my rescue, not until George [her husband] returns at 4:30 anyway" (p. 65).	Narrators signal the telling of a story by specifying physical settings, temporal contexts, and people that are not present. Examples: "When I was a little girl growing up on the farm" or "that reminds me of the time when. . . ." People with acquired impairments often divide their life story into before and after segments (Fitzgerald & Paterson, 1995).
Complicating action or plot Sequence of events that forms the skeleton of the plot. The plot is the pattern of events and circumstances that links specific events into the whole story in a way that suggests relationships, such as cause and effect, between events.	The plot begins with Trouble's entry as an alteration of Mairs' usual Wednesday morning ADL routine (1996). The plot is the sequence and the relationship of each occupational response: transferring, showering, dressing; preparing a simple meal and eating; positioning herself in front of the computer ready for a day of work (pp. 65-68).	Challenges to occupation typically begin when Trouble enters, which in Mairs' case is both her chronic medical condition and the day's extraordinary circumstances. The plot tells "what happened" (Labov, 1972) by describing the person's occupational performance in response to challenges.

(continued)

TABLE 6-2

(continued)

Narrative Structure and Function (Labov, 1972; Labov & Weletzky, 1967)	Example (Mairs, 1996)	Practice Application
Evaluation Gives narrator's opinion, point of view, or meaning to convey how to interpret the narrative.	Mairs' shower has concluded with her realization that she is sitting on the only usable towel. She evaluated her adaptation saying, "With the towel under me to protect the [wheelchair] cushions, I can't rub myself dry. I should have brought two towels. Live and learn. Fortunately, it's September, still hot in Tucson, and the air will do the job." (pp. 66-67). She later concluded, "I can hardly wait for George to get home so I can gloat....We both understand that, over time, my competence at even the simplest tasks will decrease rather than increase. But for this moment we can bask in a brief respite from dread" (p. 68).	This element coincides with the integration subprocess of Occupational Adaptation (Hamilton, 2001) as in Mairs' statement "I should have brought two towels. Live and learn" (67). Listen for this summary element as the way the teller wants you to interpret the story, such as "Isn't it pathetic when a grown man can't put on his pants?" or "I never thought I'd end up like this."
Coda The teller shifts back to the present context and time	Mairs concluded "And now here I am in front of the computer, limp but victorious: clean, clothed, and fed" (1996, p. 68). She mused about the continued erosion of her ADLs by her progressive condition and reaffirmed her occupational choice to allow others to assist in her personal care to conserve her limited physical resources for writing, her unique talent.	Listen for the end of the story with the shift to the present. For example, "and that's how I got here" represents the equivalent of "and they lived happily ever after."

Used with permission of Toby Ballou Hamilton, 2001.

Labov, W. (1972). The transformation of experience in narrative syntax. In W. Labov, *Language in the inner city: Studies in the Black English vernacular.* Philadelphia: University of Pennsylvania Press.

Labov, W. & Weletzky, J. (1967). Narrative analysis: Oral versions of personal experience. In J. Helm (Ed.). *Essays on the verbal and visual arts.* Proceedings of the 1966 annual spring meeting of the American Ethnological Society. Seattle, WA: University of Washington Press.

Mairs, N. (1996). *Waist-high in the world: A life among the nondisabled.* Boston: Beacon Press.

Other ways to identify embedded narratives include listening for narrative's relationship to time, such as its characteristic sequence and the location of an event at a specific time (Mattingly & Lawlor, 2000, p. 10). Therapists can identify narrative by its major functions to establish meaning, reconcile the ordinary with the extraordinary, and find identity, as illustrated by the story about my son. Listen for relationships of health, illness, and disability; occupational performance, performance skills and patterns, and contexts; and the experience and meaning of specific occupational performance in relationship to other occupations. Other cues include the alterations in a life affected by disability; the individual meaning of living with disability; and everyday occupational experiences. Listen for recalled or recounted dialogue, a sure sign that a narrative is being told (Mattingly & Lawlor, 2000). With experience, therapists can identify elements of occupational therapy practice models that help establish the most appropriate model to guide intervention with the person. For example, listen for cues to volition and habituation from the Model of Human Occupation; for the person, environment, and interaction elements and adaptation subprocesses from Occupational Adaptation; for the fit between elements of the Person–Environment–Occupation model.

Now that even embedded narratives can more easily be recognized, we turn to the stories themselves: those that occupational therapists tell about clients; the narratives our clients tell us; and the stories occupational therapists tell each other.

Stories Therapists Tell

Therapists tell stories about clients to each other, to other professionals, and, within the ethical obligation of confidentiality, to clients and families. The focus of therapists' storytelling is to understand the unique experience of a person (Crabtree, 1998), what is meaningful and purposeful to this person, and how this person's experience of occupational dysfunction is unique. When therapists tell stories about their clients, they are using the functions of narratives. With recognition of the importance of narrative reasoning, occupational therapy texts feature narratives that therapists tell about clients (e.g., Neistadt & Crepeau, 1998; Crepeau, Cohn & Schell, 2003; Labovitz, 2003; Bruce & Borg, 1997).

Eliciting Stories of Clients

One of my evening routines is to sip Sleepytime tea from my matching mug. The painting on the tea box and mug depicts a family of bears in their nightly routine (Underwood, 1993). A papa bear, smiling, dozes in an armchair near the hearth, while a mama bear carries a sleeping cub nuzzled into her shoulder and holds the paw of an older cub as she leads them off to bed. As I sip my tea, I imagine that they have just finished a bedtime story, perhaps one of a family of humans whose high-rise apartment or house in the suburbs was entered by a too-curious bear cub who raided the refrigerator and broke chairs. But it is the motto on the cup that I love. It reads, "Bread and water can so easily be tea and toast." Although I can think of several meanings, the one that applies to eliciting clients' stories is that even the essentials of life can be made more palatable through small efforts that yield big results.

Limiting evaluation data gathering to asking interview questions or using a standardized interview format is like a diet of bread and water—essential but bland. How much more nourishing it is to ask for stories (tea and toast). Occupational therapists can take advantage of the benefits of stories by eliciting them from clients throughout the course of the occupational therapy evaluation and intervention process.

Eliciting stories has several advantages. The first is their effectiveness and efficiency. We learn so much through stories in such a short time, as illustrated by the clinical stories presented in this chapter. Stories are peopled with significant others who may foster or hinder occupational performance; contextualized with physical, temporal, cultural, social, personal, spiritual, and virtual details; replete with task demands; and prepackaged with occupational challenges that provide motive and intention, and call for action. In addition to learning what is meaningful to a person, stories tell us how the person makes meaning. For example, the woman who wanted to care for her animals made meaning through the spiritual context of caring for others; the rancher through attributing paralysis to something familiar and earthy; Mrs. Durley by organizing and imagining herself in the future. Therapists learn of the challenges people have already faced and, more important, about how those people adapted to previous challenges in ways that build on their strengths and influence dysadaptive patterns (Spencer, Davidson & White, 1996). Finally, eliciting stories sets a therapeutic climate that invites rapport through therapeutic use of self and therapeutic self-disclosure in a natural, familiar way. "The use of narrative and life history method is not a matter of it taking more or less time, it is a matter of being the essence of practice" (Burke & Kern, 1996, p. 391). In other words, the tea and toast.

Therapists elicit stories through familiar means throughout the occupational therapy process. They can ask for stories directly using open-ended questions, with the stock question of describing a typical day often leading to storytelling. Therapists can also direct requests to particular areas of interest, such as the realization of the circumstance or condition or the first moments of experience, and the process of becoming aware of its effect on occupational performance will inevitably invite stories (Hamilton, 2001; Mattingly & Lawlor, 2000; Spencer, Davidson & White, 1996). Therapists can obtain critical information by asking for stories about past challenges and the person's response to them. Comparisons of past and current challenges and responses may lead to interventions leading to mastery of current challenges (Clark, 1993; Hamilton, 1999).

As exemplified by the findings on metaphors by Mallinson, Kielhofner, and Mattingly (1996), narratives can emerge through semi-structured interview format, such as the Occupational Performance History Interview (OPHI-II) (Kielhofner et al., 1998) or the Canadian Occupational Performance Measure (COPM) (Law et al., 1994). Researchers found enhanced prediction of outcomes for adults in physical rehabilitation settings when combining narrative data collected by the COPM with a typical facility evaluation that included items from the Functional Independence Measure (Simmons, Crepeau & White, 2000). The OPHI-II and the COPM support narrative reasoning because they focus on occupations over time.

Client-centered occupational therapy as best practice is clearly linked to narrative reasoning and engagement in storytelling (Burke & Kern, 1996; Mattingly, 1991). Occupational therapists use narrative, whether implicitly or explicitly (Frank, 1996); I encourage a more explicit use. Consider what was learned about Nancy Mairs from her story about one extraordinary morning routine (1994, pp. 64–68). After identifying narratives and eliciting them through storytelling, we turn our attention to listening to them.

Listening to Narratives

Once therapists identify a story, they begin listening for what it tells them. The client's story is like a compass that indicates a direction in which to begin intervention. Storytelling informs about all aspects of occupational therapy: the person (values, interests, performance skills and patterns, client factors); contexts (physical, social, cultural, temporal, personal, spiritual, and virtual); task demands (occupational performance challenges and goals); and the occupation their interactions produce. The story's plot acts like the needle of the compass that indicates a direction to proceed. Plot forms the pattern of events that connect parts of the story to the whole and give stories their cause and effect nature (Baldick, 1990; Polkinghorne, 1988). Plot is familiar in terms of comedy, tragedy, and romance, which may be featured in clients' stories. Although we commonly encounter these types of plots in literature and entertainment, we come across other types of plots in practice (*Table 6-3*).

Listening for plot categories helps structure the interpretation of narratives. When categories are not immediately apparent, they generally reveal themselves as the person's story unwinds over time. Plot classifications help therapists determine patterns in clients' narratives to build on (if helpful) or revise (if not). Recognizing plot categories helps both therapists and clients to determine patterns that facilitate or limit progress.

Gergen and Gergen (1988) suggested that narratives are progressive, stable, or regressive based on the relationship of people to their goals from the beginning to the end of the story. *Progressive narratives* are those in which the person reaches the desired goal, *stable narratives* are those in which little changes over time, and *regressive narratives* are those in which the person is unable to meet goals (1988).

TABLE 6-3

Literary Plot Types

Plot Type	Plot Features
Romance	Idealized characters who have latent potential, such as the hero tale in which the hero symbolizes order and enemies represent disorder or evil
Tragedy	Downfall of a character who is subject to fates beyond human control or has some internal fatal flaw, such as arrogance or unused good qualities, which leads to downfall
Comedy	Amuses through the contrast of flawed and desirable states and a sense of superiority over characters who experience a series of complications due to ordinary human failings
Mystery	Facts presented in such a way that the audience makes incorrect but plausible interpretations of facts
Suspense	Creates tension based on the audience's knowledge not yet known to characters; for example, suspense knows that a character is in danger, although the character does not recognize it

Baldick, C. (1990). *Oxford concise dictionary of literary terms.* New York: Oxford University Press.
Czarniawska, B. (2004). *Narratives in social science research.* Thousand Oaks, CA: Sage Publications.

Examples of progressive narratives in the occupational therapy literature include the transformation of Penny Richardson's self-image and lifestyle after her cerebral aneurysm and stroke (Clark, 1993), Tracey's incorporation of alternative therapies during diagnosis and treatment of Hodgkin's disease (Mostert, Zacharkeiwicz & Fossey, 1996), and Jorge's evaluation that "life doesn't stop because you have AIDS. Now is when I'm going to live" (Braveman & Helfrich, 2001, p. 28). Stable narratives in which the person is not progressing toward the goal may indicate lack of momentum, such as "held back," "unable to get on with life," "life comes to a halt" (Mallinson, Kielhofner & Mattingly, 1996, pp. 341–343) and entrapment, such as "stuck in flypaper" or "trapped" (pp. 343–344). Tom's positive anticipation of the future marred by vague direction on how to enact it created the stability in his narrative (Braveman & Helfrich, 2001, p. 29). A sense of backsliding or deterioration characterizes regressive narratives. The effects of bipolar disorder on the career plans and lives of Tom and Thelma (Helfrich & Kielhofner, 1994; Helfrich, Kielhofner & Mattingly, 1994), Axel's loss of activity and skills one year after his stroke (Knutas & Borrell, 1995), and Mark's perspective that AIDS "turned his life upside down" (Braveman & Helfrich, 2001, p. 30) illustrate this type of plot.

Polkinghorne (1996) suggested categorizing plots based on two constructs familiar to occupational therapists: agency and locus of control (e.g., AOTA, 1979; Breines, 1986; Fidler & Fidler, 1978; Meyer, 1922; Reilly, 1962; Wood, 1996). The influence of a person's locus of control on the life story determines whether the plot is *victimic* or *agentic* (1996). Both plots were exemplified by two men one year after recovering from strokes (Knutas & Borrell, 1995). Axel voiced his victimic stance by stating, "It's this disease that inhibits me from doing what I want to do. It's a shame that I am this ill" (p. 59), echoed by his wife's statement, "We are, of course, afraid of planning anything special now" (Knutas & Borrell, 1995, p. 60). In contrast, Ben's solution for washing dishes one year later was agentic. "I just bought a dishwasher, and that was it" (p. 58).

Frank (1995) suggested that illness narratives can be classified into one of three types (p. 76). Type or motif is a general storyline that underlies plot as a feature of culture (p. 75). Folktales feature motifs such as creation, deception, and reversal of fortunes (MacDonald, 1982). For example, the motif of the folktales Cinderella, Rumpelstiltskin, and the Princess and the Pea is tests: tests of fitting a standard criterion, performing a set task, and proving one's true identity, respectively. Frank suggested three types of clients' illness narratives: restitution, chaos, or quest narratives, relative to underlying relationships with one's body and with other people, control, and desire.

Restitution narratives treat illness as transitory and are most often told by those who are acutely and recently ill. Frank typified the plot as "yesterday I was healthy, today I'm sick, but tomorrow I'll be healthy again" (1995, p. 77), with health defined as the state before the illness and modern medicine as the agent of change. The person seeks a medical cure to curtail the interruption of illness and seeks to regain control of life, body, and occupations. Restitution tales are easy to listen to as long as there is a reasonable hope they are accurate. Therapists must question this type of narrative when the teller's hope for restitution is unreasonable. An example is Russell's continued hope for a complete recovery from a spinal cord injury (Spencer, Young, Rintala & Bates, 1995). After one week of rehabilitation, he stated, "My left leg is still lame, but it's getting stronger. I told the therapist lady as long as I can eventually be able to walk" (p. 57).

On day 33, he stated, "Something's been going on with my legs, my feet these last 2 days. I think they're trying to come back" (p. 56). On the 93rd day, he said, "I just wish my bowels would come back. That's the main thing that bothers me the most" (p. 57).

In stark contrast, *chaos narratives* tell of a hopeless stance in which "nothing will ever get any better" and "no one is in control." These narratives are difficult to listen to and often provoke anxiety in the listener. Frank called it an "anti-narrative" (p. 98) because it does not have a characteristic beginning, middle, and end, often taking the form of a chronology linked by conjunctions. Frank described them as tracing "the edges of a wound that can only be told around" (1995, p. 98). Tellers of the chaos narrative cannot tell a real story because they are stuck in the present without a future, living in pain from which they cannot distance themselves or reflect on. In this excerpt in which a woman describes her arm after a stroke, note both the chaos and dissociation of her shoulder and hand.

> **And the shoulder. I do everything with this cruddy arm . . . and it's been blooming sore . . . . And then I work on my hand all the time. And I try to hold something in this hand and this hand won't work. I can't pick up anything in it and I just get so frustrated (Jongbloed, 1994, p. 1008).**

The person's lack of future or hope for the possibility of resolution makes the chaos narrative difficult to hear. The teller of the chaos narrative fears an indefinite continuation of the present. Many Western societies consider childbirth a severe form of pain. However, it is bearable (or we'd all be only children without siblings or parents of only children) because the pain is mediated by the assurance of its limited duration, the possibility of medically or psychosocially induced relief, the lack of distress, and the reasonable prospect of a happy outcome. However, people in acute or chronic pain may have no such assurances and fear an unremitting continuation of the present physical or psychic pain. Note that the woman in the example above simply linked her complaints using the conjunctions "and" and "and then" without sequence, causal relationship, or overall point or theme. Lived experience organized only by "brute sequence," as in this excerpt, is the "essence of meaninglessness" (Mattingly, 1998, p. 47). This type of narrative is exclusively focused on all that is wrong without any hope of making it right.

People living out chaos narratives may resort to figures of speech to express their pain and hopelessness. Similes and metaphors are figures of speech in which one thing denotes another by suggesting a common quality of both (Baldick, 1990). Wright-St. Clair found that women with multiple sclerosis (MS) used them "where ordinary words seemed inadequate" (2003, p. 50). One woman expressed the difficulty of living with uncertainty when she stated that living with MS was "like living in the twilight zone . . . like having the crew of the Marie Celeste [a ship in pristine condition found floating without crew or passengers in the middle of the Atlantic Ocean in 1872] in your hot water cupboard . . . Who knows when they will pop out and see you?" (p. 50). Similarly, the deep metaphors of lack of momentum and entrapment of people with psychosocial disabilities represented attempts to express what was otherwise inexpressible about the lack of progression and direction of their lives and the disparity of reality and their desires (Mallinson et al., 1996, pp. 341–343).

Therapists who have not yet heard a chaos narrative, surely will sooner or later in practice. As difficult as it is to hear, therapists honor the teller of the chaos narrative by listening and letting the teller know our perception of what is so difficult to express. The use of active or reflective listening techniques that confirm that both the content and the feelings expressed have been heard is powerful. For example, I want to let the woman with the cruddy shoulder know that I hear how frustrated she is feeling, living with an arm and hand that won't let her do the important things she did before the stroke, such as sleeping or picking up things. Be aware, however, that reflective listening often encourages the storyteller to elaborate and continue. Frank cautioned not to hurry the teller of the chaos narrative to "move on" (1995, p. 110) or deny the chaos, because doing so denies the teller. He suggested that practitioners increase their tolerance for the chaos narrative as a part of the life story (p. 111).

Frank's (1995) final type of illness narrative is the *quest narrative*. This type is familiar as the hero's tale, for which mythologist Joseph Campbell outlined requisite steps (1968). Quest narratives always feature someone on a quest, a place to go, a stated reason for going, challenges and trials, and a real reason to go (Foster, 2003). Applied to the illness narrative, the place of the quest may be literal, such as health care, school, shelter, or day treatment, and figurative. Sontag stated that:

> **Everyone who is born holds dual citizenship, in the kingdom of the well and in the kingdom of the sick. Although we all prefer to use only the good passport, sooner or later each of us is obliged . . . to identify ourselves as citizens of that other place (1989, p. 3).**

The quest's challenges and trials vary from contextual factors to impairments of client factors, performance skills, and patterns that cause occupational performance problems. The stated reason for the quest is usually the presenting health or occupational problem. In contrast to the stated reason for questing, the real reason is to gain self knowledge (Foster, 2003). Frank confirmed that tellers of quest narratives perceive illness and suffering as a journey. By facing the suffering "head on" (1995, p. 115), those on the quest become heroes who know more about the self and life and return to share insights with others.

Most published disability narratives are quest narratives. This genre of autobiography focuses on the experience of congenital or acquired disabilities caused by physical, cognitive, and psychosocial impairments or contexts. I extensively studied memoirs (Hamilton, 2001) by neurologist and writer Oliver Sacks, who sustained a severe leg injury while hiking alone on a mountain (1984); essayist and poet Nancy Mairs, who has contended with multiple sclerosis since her diagnosis at age 29 (1996); and publisher and writer Robert McCrum, who had a stroke when he was 42 (1998). Each is a quest narrative, evidenced by the author's acceptance of the challenges of disability and adaptation to it. As a quick search for disability narratives or memoirs illustrates, this subcategory of autobiography has witnessed a tremendous upsurge in the past decade, offering glimpses into lives threatened by a variety of challenges.

Issues in Listening

After investing time and effort reading disability narratives or listening intently to client's stories, you might wonder, "what if they aren't telling the truth?" Perhaps memories fade or become distorted somewhere between experience and relating it. Certainly, memory or perception can be faulty in a variety of health conditions. However, truth in life stories is the truth stated by the narrator (Kohli, 1981) or the narrative truth (Spence, 1982), dependent more on expressing emotional truth and lifelikeness than facts (Barrington, 1997; Bruner, 1986). However, such a subjective approach to truth can mask attempts at reconstruction or revision of truth (Kohli, 1981). Barrington (1997) differentiated between emotional truth and facts, as did novelist Toni Morrison, who positioned the interpretive boundary as not between fact and fiction, but between fact and truth, stating that "facts can exist without human intelligence, but truth cannot" (1987, p. 113). In contrasting the two modes of human thought, Bruner considered verisimilitude or lifelikeness as the best judge of narrative, relegating empirical truth to logic and science (1986). Truth comes from the plot in answer to the essential narrative question, So what? (Bruner,1990). Application of the narrative truth honors storytellers' perceptions of the world, and the more lifelike the narrative, the more convincing and better it is. In her gritty memoir of her childhood, Mary Karr (1995) told of seeing her grandmother standing in the bedroom doorway one night. Her grandmother had returned home after an amputation when Mary was 7 years old and her sister, Lecia, was 9. Note the empirical and narrative truths, verisimilitude, and message from this brief excerpt.

> **. . . with that stump bluntly hanging down under her nightie, her arms spread so she could hold herself up by the doorjamb, and her hair fanned out around her face like white fire. I can see it like yesterday's breakfast, but Lecia claims it never happened (pp. 60–61).**

In the book's acknowledgments, Karr noted that her sister "confirmed the veracity of what I'd written" (1995).

Once convinced that a story is emotionally true, lifelike, and makes a point, I consider them to be true. I rely on my education and experience as a practitioner to judge truth, based on how true the story rings. Sometimes truth is confirmed, but occasionally I am surprised. The three memoirists I studied convinced me of their truth early in their books. Sacks sold me with his raw terror at being chased by the bull and his adaptive responses that allowed him to descend a mountain on three limbs in the face of certain death (1984, pp. 20–21). Mairs invited me to sit next to her wheelchair and experience what life is like when waist-high in the world (1996, p. 18). McCrum persuaded me with his disclosure of unexpectedly urinating on himself while immobilized in bed after his stroke (1998, pp. 10-11).

I once interviewed a man in his thirties who was hospitalized in a locked mental health unit. When I asked about his typical weekday, he told me that he got up, did his personal care, ate breakfast, and walked out the door to board his airplane. "Hmm," I thought, picturing an airplane parked in his driveway, "isn't that interesting?" Given the setting, I wondered if what he was telling me was delusional material. I remained silent, vowing to question him if needed. At the end of his story, neither believing nor disbelieving the information about the airplane, I asked him to clarify that part of his story. He smiled, explaining that he worked as a federal marshal, who accompanied prisoners in transit from one prison to another. He spent the night guarding prisoners at the prison transfer center, located near the airport. So he did walk outside and board an airplane as part of a typical day. By interrupting or disbelieving his story of a typical day,

I could have lost all rapport with him. For the most part, I believe the stories clients tell me until sufficient narrative discrepancies supported by other behavior lead me to ask for clarification and if justified, to question them.

From a colleague, I learned an indicator for questioning truth that I use in both practice and education that I call the rule of three. When I hear a discrepancy or note something out of the ordinary the first time, I think to myself, "Now isn't that interesting?" When I hear it a second time, I wonder, "Could this be a coincidence?" On the third incident, I think, "This could be a pattern" and, depending on the circumstances, either question or confront the person about the situation (Cyndy Robinson, personal communication). Not long ago, a group of students and I talked with clients in a rehabilitation program in a shelter for people who are homeless. A staff member warned us that one of the women might tell us mistakenly that she is pregnant and to consider it as delusional material. The woman, who was quite overweight, stated that she had indeed been pregnant for well over 9 months, an indication of the fervency of belief in delusions. Another client told students that he rented a room at the shelter, which, surprising as it was to me, was later confirmed as true.

Storytelling and Transference

Storytelling as retrospective narrative reasoning links the past and the present across time and physical, social, and cultural contexts. Clients' stories bring therapists into the life story and illness and occupational narratives. Similarly, when therapists tell stories, they fit this unique client into their experiences with other clients. As such, storytelling helps form a powerful therapeutic alliance. However, an unconscious construction of the other person can influence the storytelling process positively or negatively. Transference (client to therapist) and counter-transference (therapist to client) is like an "emotional time warp" that advances emotional and psychological needs from one's past into the present (Conner, 2001, para. 2), projecting them onto people that we do not know well. From psychodynamic theory as described by Freud, transference is a reaction to people, not as they are, but as we construct them based on our past. Transference encompasses thoughts, feelings, fantasies, and actions (Luepnitz, 2002) and often concerns what people want to see or are afraid to see when little is known about another person (Conner, 2002, para. 2). Because it occurs without awareness, therapists need to consider the influence of transference or counter-transference when feeling powerful emotions, such as annoyance, boredom, anger, sexual attraction, or protectiveness toward clients, which are not justifiable to a "reasonable person" (Conner, 2001, para. 7; Luepnitz, 2002). Although usually considered and used therapeutically in psychoanalysis of long duration, transference and counter-transference can occur in therapy of brief duration (Luepnitz, 2002). Because of the subjective and interpretive nature of narratives and the personal and emotionally intimate nature of the storytelling process, occupational therapists need to be especially aware of the possibility of transference and counter-transference when applying narrative reasoning. For example, I may have responded to the rancher as I might to my own favorite rancher, my dear Uncle Yantis, to Mrs. Durley as if she were my maternal grandmother, or to the woman who lived out my childhood dream of having a menagerie of animals. Considering the evocative emotions of both client and therapist helps us determine whether feelings and actions are justified for our relationship in the present and not part of an emotional time warp through storytelling.

Stories Therapists Tell Each Other

Telling stories is a way of transmitting the values of a family, organization, or culture, as illustrated by folktale examples (Box 6-4). Stories socialize one into a culture. The "Three Little Pigs" exemplifies how to, and how not to, make one's way when entering the world of adult responsibilities. The story of "Goldilocks and the Three Bears" warns not to enter the houses of strangers or abuse hospitality. "Little Red Hen" teaches about the value of work by connecting the privilege of eating with the responsibility of working. Notice that these particular stories (and a host of others) include one character at odds to three others. Because three is the culturally sanctioned repeat number in European and some American (not Native American) folktales, other cultures feature different repeat numbers. Such long-lived stories continue to live for a reason, which Czarniawska described as "sediments of norm and practices and, as such, deserve careful attention" (2004, p. 45).

BOX 6-4
Stories of Occupational Therapy Culture

Because stories socialize to bring people into a culture's norms and values, it's not surprising that much of the art of occupational therapy practice comes to us through stories. Kielhofner suggested that ultimately all stories told by occupational therapists about practice are about the paradigm of occupation. Notable examples are Peloquin's use of story to warn about the dangers of depersonalizing clients (1993); from Yerxa's story from her 1967 Eleanor Clarke Slagle lecture telling of a woman reaching for a glass of water illustrating the role of meaning and purpose; Clark's use of story motif to tell of Penny Richardson's recovery from a cerebral aneurysm through occupation and personal narrative (1993); Wood's tale of Betty's bath in which occupation is a respite from dementia (1995).

Used with permission of Toby Hamilton, 2001.

STORYMAKING

Using the rich particulars gathered from the storytelling process, therapists apply inductive reasoning to guide intervention using the second type of narrative reasoning. Storymaking takes in the particulars from storytelling to narrow and shape intervention into a therapeutic plot that helps bring about the story desired by the client. Not all aspects of intervention can be made into stories (Mattingly, 1994). However, working from a therapeutic plot converts preparatory methods into subplots of a larger therapeutic story and motivates by focusing on outcomes and making intervention meaningful, purposeful, and "worth telling stories about" (Mattingly, 1994, p. 245).

Storymaking is prospective narrative reasoning that links the present to the future (Mattingly, 1991; Coe, 1999, p. 77) by imagining the effect of illness,

2. Evoke insights into occupational challenges and threats to identity by finding solutions to occupational problems.
3. Broaden ideas about activities of daily living. In Richardson's case, the emphasis was not on the concrete tasks of getting dressed but on considerations of dressing for a new image. This technique involves themes such as dealing with emotions, friendship and intimacy, and emotional and symbolic dimensions of occupation (pp. 387-389).
4. Focus on image reconstruction, a process in which the client takes "on a persona" that is comfortable and empowering for the future (p. 390).
5. Incorporate as much of the client's physical, cultural, and social contexts as possible into the storymaking process (pp. 390-391).

Richardson's story, along with the others in this chapter, illustrate that occupational therapy is essentially a life editing and narrative revision process. The process of revision begins with storytelling. The discovery of unhelpful narrative patterns, such as regressive narratives (Gergen & Gergen, 1983), unrealistic restitution narratives, chaos narratives (Frank, 1995), or victimic plot patterns (Polkinghorne, 1996) is especially powerful. Through narrative reasoning and the collaborative interventions it produces, clients and therapists create or revise plots and outcomes of the occupational narrative (Doan, 1996; Hamilton, 1999; Mattingly, 1991, 1994, 1998; Parry & Doan, 1994). Collaboratively, therapist and client enact the plot of the occupational narrative through the therapeutic activities and occupations of intervention that lead to the desired outcomes. In fact, storymaking is so effective at motivating and guiding intervention that goals written in official records are subordinate to the prospective treatment story. Acting out the prospective treatment story releases narrative's potential to provide options, inform choices, envision a revised future and ultimately, transform lives (see Case Study 6-3 below) (Hamilton, 1999; Helfrich & Kielhofner, 1994; Larson & Fanchiang, 1996b; Mattingly, 1991, 1994, 1998; Polkinghorne, 1996; Spencer et al., 1996, 1997).

CASE STUDY 6-3

Storymaking: Story Revision

An occupational therapy student and I once used storymaking to revise a problem story in which she was troubled by test anxiety in a neurobiology course (Hamilton, 1999). By mid-semester, she feared that she might not pass the course. The consequences of failure were grave—delaying fieldwork, waiting a year to retake the course, and, if she failed in her second attempt, leaving the occupational therapy program. The stakes were high and her anxiety matched it. She agreed to work on revising the ending of her story.

Using narrative revision techniques (Doan, 1996; Parry & Doan, 1994), I asked Mary (her chosen pseudonym) to tell the story of how Trouble entered her life in the form of test anxiety. Envisioned as a gray mist-like being, Trouble entered as Fear, Frustration, Pressure, and Self-Doubt. Visualization allowed Mary to externalize Trouble so she could be free of living in the problem plot in which Trouble was clearly the bad guy. The process of tearing down or deconstructing the problem plot happened simultaneously with revising the plot to match the desired ending. As we worked back and forth between the problem plot and her dream plot, we recorded keys points on a flip chart sheet. With the two plots side by side, I searched for contradictions to the problem plot to raise Mary's doubts in its truth. She was so entrenched in the problem plot that she ignored contradictions to it: having passed approximately 115 exams to date and failing only two; passing the second exam and course in another science course after failing an exam; passing two other science courses that same semester. We already knew how Fear took exams, so Mary told me how Love would take them. She translated her answers into concrete actions and working from the revised plot, started enacting the ending she wanted. The process of storymaking and plot revision ended happily with Mary making a B in the course, marrying the month before her fieldwork, and graduating as planned a year later (Hamilton, 1999). Mary is a successful occupational therapist and excellent fieldwork educator.

Without editing her life story, Mary could easily have perpetuated the role of failed student by living out the problem plot instead of the one she wanted. Three occupation-based theoretical perspectives inform why and how narrative revision may work. The Occupational Science perspective of occupational story-making already outlined (Clark, 1993; Clark et al., 1996) applied to Mary's revision. The Model of Human Occupation offers the volitional narrative to explain change in personal causation, interests and values (Helfrich & Kielhofner, 1994; Kielhofner, 2002; Kielhofner et al., 1995). The **volitional narrative** is a type of occupational narrative that expresses the person's volition as a "set of ideas, perceptions and values that are assembled into a meaningful account by an investigator through a process of eliciting parts of a person's life story and selectively retelling those aspects which are exemplary of volition . . . and show how volition affects occupational decision making" (Barrett, Beer & Kielhofner, 1999, p. 79). The occupational therapist constructs the volitional narratives from selected parts of a person's life story to show how volition affects the person's occupational choice and decision making (Barrett et al., 1999). The therapist listens to clients' narratives for the personal causation, interests, and beliefs that support or hinder occupational performance. For example, changes in Mary's personal causation empowered her to make occupational choices to achieve her desired outcome by affirming her interests and values in her dream plot. A third perspective is that a new story ending with mastery over occupational challenges occurs through the internal process of Occupation Adaptation (Schkade & McClung, 2001; Schkade & Schultz, 1992, 2003; Schultz & Schkade, 1992, 1997). Comparison of the two plots allowed Mary to generate new adaptive responses, evaluate, and integrate them into a revised story that featured mastery (Hamilton, 1999). My study of the three memoirs confirmed that Occupational Adaptation also occurs naturally without therapeutic intervention and that adaptation always precedes narrative revision (Hamilton, 2001). For example, Mairs showed adaptation when she learned to bring two towels for her next independent shower (1996); Sacks survived by modifying his umbrella into a splint fastened on his leg with strips ripped from his anorak (1984); and McCrum gradually began socializing with colleagues and friends after an initial period of avoidance (1998).

Returning to the story of the rancher and the ants allows us to explore the storymaking process more closely. The rancher's storytelling informed me that Trouble entered his life as hemiparalysis and that his fall into the ant bed segmented his life into before and after stages. Although I did not recognize it at the time, his illness narrative about falling and being poisoned by fire ants was clearly how he made sense of what happened, reconciled the extraordinary circumstance of paralysis, and expressed his beliefs about health, illness, and disability. His was a restitution narrative focused on a complete cure brought about by the passage of time as the poison left his body. His illness narrative explained his victimic role of passive waiting.

Without the storymaking process, I had nothing to offer him. Unfortunately, this was the case, as I recall it. Limping along without a story to guide us, I tried motivating him and myself using impairment-based preparatory intervention approaches. We floundered without the sort of compass that storymaking could have provided us. Although we had agreed to disagree about the cause of his impairments, I simply could not make sense of his seemingly irrational story about the fire ants or its significance in explaining his obstinate lack of cooperation with my efforts. Although this story happened early in my practice before the discussion of clinical reasoning in occupational therapy, reflecting on his story helps me make amends by sharing what I would now do so differently.

Only by projecting him into future contexts and time could occupational therapy offer him hope of resuming his role as a rancher. Although the immediate physical contexts were hospital and therapy rooms, one of the occupational therapist's major roles in the storymaking process is using narrative reasoning to transcend the immediate contexts and occupations for imagined future ones. By accepting the limitations and benefits of the physical space in which we actually intervene with clients, we essentially abandon them and their families to figure out how to perform occupations in other contexts on their own. We avoid this by using narrative's temporal sequence and storymaking to bridge present and future occupational performance.

By helping clients imaginatively project themselves into their own future stories, we use all the elements of Burke's dramatic pentad and narrative's beneficial functions. By eliciting stories and details about his physical, social, cultural, temporal, personal, and spiritual contexts and the task demands of his most important ranching activities, we could have pictured him getting in and out of his pickup, driving it, opening and closing gates, and hauling and distributing feed for the livestock. Through activity analysis of these task demands, I could have estimated more precisely the necessary performance skills and patterns to accomplish his ranching occupations in a way that made sense to us both. The picture of him doing these occupations in context could have guided intervention more effectively than the goals I recorded in his medical chart. Each intervention session could be guided by these imagined stories of future occupations in contexts far beyond the confines of the hospital setting. We could have enacted a story in our sessions in a variety of ways, perhaps devoting the morning sessions to morning ranching tasks and afternoons to the task demands later in the day. By focusing on the essential task demands of his desired occupations, he could have been motivated by knowing that what we did in each session directly related to the occupations he needed and wanted to resume back on the ranch. Engagement in storymaking would have allowed him to connect evaluation and intervention procedures with occupations that brought meaning and purpose to his life and to which he was eager to return. Occupational therapy could have had a positive impact on his life by using his life story to bring meaning to therapy (Crabtree, 1998) if we had only had a story to point in the right direction.

Although all of my examples involve individuals, storymaking can also be applied to working with people in groups, most notably with Madelyn O'Reilly's use of storymaking to transform the boring, problematic Upper Extremity Group into the therapeutic New York Gang group in her story, The New York Subway (Mattingly, 1994, pp. 261-264). Participants in the group looked for excuses not to attend the group, which consisted of rote exercises monitored by an equally unenthusiastic occupational therapist who used the time to catch up on documentation. When O'Reilly assumed the group, she asked participants about their concerns. From their storytelling, she realized that they were all from New York and familiar with the subway system. Creating a therapeutic plot that featured all aspects of therapeutic emplotment (Mattingly, 1994), O'Reilly transformed a treatment room to evoke the contexts of a subway station. Group participants enacted the story in sessions devoted to writing graffiti and suggested future sessions in which they cooked New York pretzels and hot dogs and played stickball. She used the plot of the treatment story to bridge the gap of the present to their past contexts and possible futures. She created drama by dressing as a subway conductor and handing out tokens before the initial session to create suspense. Through storymaking, she transformed a rote chronology of preparatory methods into an enacted therapeutic emplotment that had all participating enthusiastically.

SUMMARY

Occupational therapists use stories in practice either implicitly or explicitly (Frank, 1996). Through narrative reasoning as a central and fundamental mode of reasoning (Mattingly, 1991, p. 998), occupational therapists provide effective, efficient, and satisfying intervention that leads to individualized occupational outcomes that enhance clients' participation and quality of life. Storytelling bridges the client's past to the present and brings therapy into the client's life story at a time when practice demands further "magnify the urgency" to know the client's story (Burke & Kern, 1996, p. 390) in ways that honor the profession's humanistic roots and also contribute to cost-effectiveness (Larson & Fanchiang, 1996b; Wood, 1995). Storymaking structures and guides intervention and motivates clients to edit and revise their life stories. Narrative reasoning is what makes occupational therapy a life editing process. All that from a few simple stories.

LEARNING ACTIVITY 6-1

Daily Tapestry

Purpose

Analyze daily activities to determine the relationship of occupation and narrative.

Connections to Major Clinical Reasoning Constructs

All narratives are inevitably about occupation and all occupation can be storied.

Directions for Learners

Keep a journal for one day, noting your occupations and the narratives you engage in. Record your daily occupations, noting the narrative elements of the day's events. Using the example in the chapter, reflect on (1) how occupation and narrative interweave to form a daily tapestry of your life and (2) how that day's weaving fits into your life story tapestry.

LEARNING ACTIVITY 6-2

Generational Stories

Purpose

Collect stories of extraordinary events from people of several generations. Determine how stories capture details of occupation and context. Determine how these narratives reflect each person's unique perspective of the event.

Connections to Major Clinical Reasoning Constructs

Narrative or story is an organizational scheme of subjectively sequenced events that reveals causal relationships, communicates and shapes experience, and creates and expresses meaning. Narratives inherently capture details of occupation and context for extraordinary events.

Directions for Learners

Generations of people are defined by their stories about what they were doing (occupation) and where they were (context) when they learned of events of international importance. Select an event and collect personal stories from people of several generations. Consider events such as the bombing of Pearl Harbor or London; the assassinations of John Kennedy, Martin Luther King, Jr., or other world leaders; the explosion of the space shuttle Challenger; the 1995 Oklahoma City bombing; the

September 11, 2001 terrorist attacks in the United States; the 2004 tsunami in Southeast Asia; or other internationally known events. How did each person's story subjectively sequence events, reveal causal relationships, communicate and shape experience, and create and express meaning? Compare the collected stories with your story of events that you experienced. Summarize how each story informs about the particular individual while simultaneously capturing the commonality of the event.

LEARNING ACTIVITY 6-3

Illness Narrative

Purpose

Elicit, analyze, and interpret an illness narrative. Compare the constructs of disease and illness from a person's outer and inner perspectives.

Connections to Major Clinical Reasoning Constructs

Narrative reasoning using the illness narrative to show causal relationships of health, disease, illness, impairment, and disability that communicates the experience, alterations, and individual meaning of living life affected by illness or disability.

Directions for Learners

1 Collect an illness narrative.
2 Analyze it using (a) structural elements suggested by Labov or Burke; (b) the functions of narrative; and (c) Frank's plot categories.
3 Summarize what this illness narrative tells about the person's (a) experience of being ill; (b) experience, alterations, and individual meaning of living a life affected by illness or disability; (c) fundamental beliefs, both cultural and individual, about health and disease, its causes, care, and potential for treatment; (d) sense of self within the illness experience; and (e) causal relationships of health, disease, illness, impairment, and disability.
4 Summarize how the illness narrative tells not just the "story of an illness but rather the story of a life altered by illness" (Garro, 1994, p. 775) and what it is like for this person to live with this disease (Mattingly, 1991).
5 Compare the illness narrative with a scientific description of the disease.
6 Discuss the importance of the illness narrative to the practice of occupational therapy and its relationship to the occupational narrative.

LEARNING ACTIVITY 6-4

Occupational Therapy as a Life Story Editing Process

Purpose

Explore occupational therapy as a life story editing and narrative revision process.

Connections to Major Clinical Reasoning Constructs

Occupational therapy is essentially a life story editing process accomplished through the storytelling and storymaking processes of narrative reasoning.

Directions for Learners

1 Select an autobiography (life story to date), memoir (life story focused on a particular time period or theme), or story from the occupational literature of interest, considering whether you want to focus on narratives of illness and disability or not.

2 *Storytelling analysis:* Identify a story, noting the method you used to identify it, about the most critical aspect of occupation that the narrator wants to change. How does this story fit into a chapter within the book of the person's life story? What would you title the story and the chapter? What helpful and unhelpful plot classifications are evident? How was the storytelling process elicited and accomplished (oral or written)? How did the story unwind along a temporal axis? How did storytelling link the occupational past to the occupational present? How did storytelling bridge the actual world and the possible world? In what ways was the telling of this story therapeutic for the narrator?

3 *Storymaking analysis:* Using the same incident, how did the person edit the life story and revise the narrative? What aspects of Mattingly's (1994) steps of emplotment can you identify? How was the storymaking process collaborative and if so, with whom? If the person was not receiving occupational therapy, how might an occupational therapist help with the life editing and revising process? If the person received occupational therapy, how did the therapist use storytelling and storymaking to help the editing and revising process?

4 *Life editing and narrative revision:* How did the storytelling and storymaking processes combine to provide options, inform choices, envision a revised future and ultimately transform this life? How is occupational therapy essentially a life story editing and narrative revision process?

LEARNING ACTIVITY 6-5

Occupational Narrative

Purpose

Elicit and analyze an occupational narrative and use it as the basis for the occupational profile and analysis of occupational performance. Compare the interpretation of an occupational therapist with that of others.

Connections to Major Clinical Reasoning Constructs

Narrative reasoning using the occupational narrative as a unique narrative of interest to occupational therapists that shows the relationships of health and participation; and of illness, disability, or restriction when present; places occupational performance within specific contexts; and expresses the meaning of specific occupations and the relationships of occupations in one's life.

Directions for Learners

1 Collect an occupational narrative.
2 Analyze it using (a) structural elements suggested by Labov or Burke; (b) the functions of narrative; and (c) plot category.
3 Write the occupational profile and analysis of occupational performance based on the story. What does the occupational narrative tell you about (a) the relationships of health and participation; (b) illness, disability, or restriction when present; (c) the specific contexts and task demands of occupational performance; (d) the meaning of specific occupations and relationships of occupations?
4 Discuss how others might listen to and interpret this narrative differently, such as an educator, parent, employer, physician, nurse, physical therapist, or social worker. Discuss the importance of the occupational narrative to the practice of occupational therapy.

LEARNING ACTIVITY 6-6

Scientific and Narrative Thought in Evidence-Based Practice

Purpose

Compare and contrast scientific and narrative modes of thinking and their influence on research and the use of evidence-based practice.

Connections to Major Clinical Reasoning Constructs

Scientific and narrative modes of thinking are complementary ways of understanding phenomena and contribute to the application of evidence-based practice.

Directions for Learners

1 Select a research article of interest. Use the research question(s) to classify the research as using either scientific, deductive reasoning or narrative, inductive reasoning.

2 Rewrite the research question using the other mode of thinking.

3 Compare and contrast how the two research questions would contribute to your understanding of the phenomenon being studied. Consider how the two research questions contribute to evidence-based practice as "the integration of best research evidence with clinical expertise and patient values" (Sackett, Straus, Richardson, Rosenberg & Haynes, 2000, p.1).

LEARNING ACTIVITY 6-7

Taking Your Phenomenology Seriously

Purpose

Incorporate explicit narrative reasoning into clinical writing.

Connections to Major Clinical Reasoning Constructs

Narrative reasoning is an important aspect of the therapists' thinking process. This activity challenges learners to express their narrative understandings in their professional writing.

Directions for Learners

1 Using a piece of your clinical writing, such as a case study, case report, or note documenting the evaluation or intervention process, insert your reasoning by italicizing your thoughts and feelings in appropriate places.

2 Repeat the exercise, underlining sections in which you assume the client's perspective to imagine what the client may have been thinking and feeling in appropriate places.

LEARNING ACTIVITY 6-8

Tea & Toast Exercise

Purpose

Compare storytelling and interview questions as data collection methods for occupational profile and analysis of occupation performance.

Connections to Major Clinical Reasoning Constructs

Eliciting stories from clients is an effective, efficient, and satisfying data gathering method for practice.

Directions for Learners

1 Start with tea and toast as desired. Read Nancy Mairs' story on pages 64–68 (1996) aloud and time how long it took to read it.

2 Using two columns side by side, label the columns "Storytelling" and "Interview Questions". In the storytelling column, write what you know about Nancy (a) as a person (performance skills & patterns and client factors); (b) her contexts (physical, social, cultural, personal, virtual, and spiritual); (c) her unique perspective of the task demands of her morning routine. In the interview column, write the interview questions you would have to ask to obtain the same information. If you work alone, estimate the time for interviewing counting in questions, answers, and time for asking follow up questions. If you work with a partner, have the other person read the section and respond to questions and note the time for questioning, answering, and clarifying.

REFERENCES

American Occupational Therapy Association. (1979). Philosophical base of occupational therapy. *American Journal of Occupational Therapy, 33*, 785.

American Occupational Therapy Association. (2002). Occupational therapy practice framework: domain and process. *American Journal of Occupational Therapy, 56*, 609–639.

Atkinson, P. (1997). Narrative turn or blind alley? *Qualitative Health Research, 17*(3), 325–344.

Baldick, C. (1990). *Oxford concise dictionary of literary terms.* New York: Oxford University Press.

Barrett, L., Beer, D. & Kielhofner, G. (1999). The importance of volitional narrative in treatment: An ethnographic case study in a work program. *Work, 12*, 79–92.

Barrington, J. (1997). *Writing the memoir: From truth to art.* Portland, OR: The Eighth Mountain Press.

Barthes, R. (1966/1977). Introduction to the structural analysis of narratives. In R. Barthes, *Image-music-text* (trans. Stephen Heath). (pp. 79–124). Glasgow: Collins.

Bateson, M. C. (1989). *Composing a life.* New York: Plume.

Bickle, J. (2003). Empirical evidence for a narrative concepts of self. In G. D. Fireman, T. E. McVay, Jr. & O. Flanagan (Eds.), *Narrative and consciousness: Literature, psychology, and the brain* (pp. 195–208). Oxford: Oxford University Press.

Braveman, B. & Helfrich, C. A. (2001). Occupational identity: Exploring the narratives of three men living with AIDS. *Journal of Occupational Science, 8*(2), 25–31.

Brockmeir, J. & Harre, R. (1997). Narrative: Problems and promises of an alternative paradigm. *Research on Language and Social Interaction, 30*, 265–286.

Bruce, B. & Borg, M. A. (1997). *Occupational therapy stories: Psychosocial interaction in practice.* Thorofare, NJ: Slack.

Bruner, J. (1986). *Actual minds, possible worlds.* Cambridge, MA: Harvard University Press.

Bruner, J. (1990). *Acts of meaning.* Cambridge, MA: Harvard University Press.

Bruner, J. (1991). The narrative construction of reality. *Critical Inquiry, 18*, 1–21.

Burke, K. (1945). *A grammar of motives.* Berkeley, CA: University of California Press.

Burke, J. P. & Kern, S. B. (1996). The issue is—is the use of life history and narrative in clinical practice reimbursable? Is it occupational therapy? *American Journal of Occupational Therapy, 50* (5), 389–392.

Campbell, J. (1968). *The hero with a thousand faces.* Princeton, NJ: Princeton University Press. (Original work published 1949).

Christiansen, C. (1999). The 1999 Eleanor Clarke Slagle Lecture. Defining lives: Occupation as identity: An essay on competence, coherence, and the creation of meaning. *American Journal of Occupational Therapy,* 53, 547–558.

Clark, F. (1993). Occupation embedded in a real life: Interweaving occupational science and occupational therapy. *American Journal of Occupational Therapy,* 47(12), 1067–1078.

Coe, R. (1999). Jenny's story: Exploring the layers of narrative reasoning. In S. E. Ryan & E. A. McKay (Eds.), *Thinking and reasoning in therapy: Narratives from practice.* Cheltenham, United Kingdom: Stanley Thornes Publishers, Ltd.

Conner, M. G. (2001). Transference: Are you a biological time machine? *The Source* 2001, June). Retrieved January 6, 2005, from http://www.crisiscounseling.com/Articles/ Transference.htm

Conrad, P. (1990). Qualitative research on chronic illness: A commentary on method and conceptual development. *Social Science and Medicine,* 30, 1257–1263.

Crabtree, M. (1998). Images of reasoning: A literature review. *Australian Occupational Therapy Journal,* 45, 113–123.

Crepeau, E. B. (1994). Three images of interdisciplinary team meetings. *American Journal of Occupational Therapy,* 48, 717–722.

Crepeau, E. B., Cohn, E. S., Schell, B. B. (2003). *Willard and Spackman's occupational therapy* (10th ed.). Philadelphia: Lippincott Williams & Wilkins.

Crestwell, J. W. (1998). *Qualitative inquiry and research design: Choosing among five traditions.* Thousand Oaks, CA: Sage Publications.

Culler, J. (1997). *Literary theory: A very short introduction.* New York: Oxford University Press.

Czarniawska, B. (2004). *Narratives in social science research.* Thousand Oaks, CA: Sage Publications.

Doan, R. E. (1996). *Narratings: Guidelines for narrative therapy.* Unpublished manuscript, University of Oklahoma and Rogers University, Tulsa, OK.

Estes, C. P. (1992). *Women who run with the wolves: Myths and stories of the wild woman archetype.* New York: Ballantine Books.

Fidler, G. S. & Fidler, J. W. (1978). Doing and becoming: Purposeful action and self-actualization. *American Journal of Occupational Therapy,* 32, 305–310.

Fisher, W. R. (1984). Narration as a human communication paradigm: The case of public moral argument. *Communication Monographs,* 51, 1–22.

Fitzgerald, M. H. & Paterson, K. A. (1995). The hidden disability dilemma for the preservation of self. *Journal of Occupational Science: Australia,* 2(1), 13–21.

Fleming, M. H. (1991). The therapist with the three-track mind. *American Journal of Occupational Therapy,* 45, 1007–1014.

Foster, T. C. (2003). *How to read literature like a professor: A lively and entertaining guide to reading between the lines.* New York: HarperCollins.

Frank, A. W. (1995). *The wounded storyteller: Body, illness, and ethics.* Chicago: University of Chicago Press.

Frank, G. (1996). Life histories in occupational therapy clinical practice. *American Journal of Occupational Therapy,* 50(4), 251–264.

Garro, L. C. (1994). Narrative representations of chronic illness experience: Cultural models of illness, mind, and body in stories concerning the temporomandibular joint (TMJ). *Social Science in Medicine,* 38, 775–788.

Gergen, M. M. & Gergen, K. J. (1988). Narrative and the self as relationship. In L. Berkowitz (Ed.), *Advances in experimental psychology* (pp. 17–56). San Diego, CA: Academic Press.

Grant, M. & Hazel, J. (1993). *Who's who in classical mythology.* New York: Oxford University Press.

Hamilton, T. B. (1999). Synergy of Occupational Adaptation and narrative metaphor for student test anxiety. *Innovations in Occupational Therapy Education,* 1, 27–40.

Hamilton, T. B. (2001). Occupational adaptation and relationship to narrative in memoirs of adults with acquired disability. Unpublished doctoral dissertation, Texas Woman's University, Denton.

Hamilton, T. B. (2003). Occupations and places. In C. H. Christiansen & E. A. Townsend (Eds.), *Introduction to occupation: The art and science of living* (pp. 173–196). Upper Saddle River, NJ: Prentice Hall.

Hathaway, N. (2002). *The friendly guide to mythology: A mortal's companion to the fantastical realm of gods, goddesses, monsters, and heroes.* New York: Penguin Books.

Helfrich, C. & Kielhofner, G. (1994). Volitional narratives and the meaning of therapy. *American Journal of Occupational Therapy,* 48(4), 319–326.

Helfrich, C., Kielhofner, G. & Mattingly, C. (1994). Volition as narrative: Understanding motivation in chronic illness. *American Journal of Occupational Therapy,* 48(4), 311–317.

Hunter, K. M. (1996). Narrative, literature, and the clinical exercise of practical reason. *Journal of Medicine and Philosophy, 21*, 303–320.

Jongbloed, L. (1994). Adaptation to stroke: The experience of one couple. *American Journal of Occupational Therapy, 48*, 1006–1013.

Karr, M. (1995). *The liars' club: A memoir.* New York. Penguin.

Kautzmann, L. N. (1993). Linking patient and family stories to caregivers' use of clinical reasoning. *American Journal of Occupational Therapy, 47*, 169–173.

Kielhofner, G., Mallinson, T., Crawford, C., Nowak, M., Rigby, M., Henry, A. et al. (1998). *Occupational Performance History Interview II (OPHI-II) Version 2.0.*

Kielhofner, G. (2002). *The Model of Human Occupation: Theory and Application* (3rd ed.). Baltimore: Williams & Wilkins.

Kielhofner, G., Borrell, L, Burke, J., Helfrich, C. & Nygard, L. (1995). Volitional subsystem. In G. Kielhofner (Ed.), *A model of human occupation: Theory and application* (2nd ed., pp. 39–62). Baltimore: Williams & Wilkins.

Knutas, A. & Borrell, L. (1995). The meaning of stroke in everyday life—A comparative case study of two persons. *Scandinavian Journal of Occupational Therapy, 2*, 56–62.

Kohli, M. (1981). Biography: Account, text, method. In D. Bertaux (Ed.), *Biography and society: The life history approach in the social sciences* (pp. 61–75). Beverly Hills, CA: Sage Publications.

Labov, W. (1972). The transformation of experience in narrative syntax. In W. Labov, *Language in the inner city: Studies in the Black English vernacular.* Philadelphia: University of Pennsylvania Press.

Labov, W. & Weletzky, J. (1967). Narrative analysis: Oral versions of personal experience. In J. Helm (Ed.), *Essays on the verbal and visual arts.* Proceedings of the 1966 annual spring meeting of the American Ethnological Society. Seattle, WA: University of Washington Press.

Labovitz, D. R. (Ed.) (2003). *Ordinary miracles: True stories about overcoming obstacles and surviving catastrophes.* Thorofare, NJ: Slack.

Larson, E. A. & Fanchiang S. C. (1996a). Special issue on life history and narrative in clinical practice [Special issue]. *American Journal of Occupational Therapy, 50*, (4).

Larson, E. A. & Fanchiang S. C. (1996b). Nationally speaking: Life history and narrative research: Generating a humanistic knowledge base for occupational therapy. *American Journal of Occupational Therapy, 50*, 247–250.

Law, M., Baptiste, S., Carswell, A., McColl, M. A., Polatajko, H. & Pollock, N. (1998). Canadian Occupational Performance Measure (3rd ed.). Ottawa, Ontario: Canadian Association of Occupational Therapists.

Lieblich, A., Tuval-Mashiach, R. & Zilber, T. (1998). *Narrative research: Reading, analysis and interpretation. Applied social research methods series* (Vol. 47). Thousand Oaks, CA: Sage Publications.

Linde, C. (1993). *Life stories: The creation of coherence.* New York: Oxford University Press.

Livo, N. & Rietz, S. A. (1986). *Storytelling process and practice.* Littleton, CO: Libraries Unlimited, Inc.

Luepnitz, D. A. (2002). *Schopenhauer's porcupines: Dilemmas of intimacy and the talking cure: Five stories of psychotherapy.* New York: Basic Books.

MacDonald, M. R. (1982). *The storyteller's sourcebook: A subject, title, and motif index to folklore collections for children.* Detroit: Gale Research.

Mairs, N. (1996). *Waist-high in the world: A life among the nondisabled.* Boston: Beacon Press.

Mallinson, T., Kielhofner, G. & Mattingly, C. (1996). Metaphor and meaning in a clinical interview. *American Journal of Occupational Therapy, 50*, 338–346.

Mandler, J. M. (1984). *Stories, scripts, and scenes: Aspects of schema theory.* Hilldale, NJ: Lawrence Erlbaum Associates.

Mars, R. A. (2004). The neuropsychology of narrative: Story comprehension, story production and their interrelation. *Neuropsychologica, 42*, 1414–1434.

Mattingly, C. (1991). The narrative nature of clinical reasoning. *American Journal of Occupational Therapy, 45*(11), 998–1005.

Mattingly, C. (1994). The narrative nature of clinical reasoning. In C. Mattingly & M. H. Fleming, *Clinical reasoning: Forms on inquiry in a therapeutic practice* (pp. 239–269). Philadelphia: F. A. Davis.

Mattingly, C. (1998). *Healing dramas and clinical plots: The narrative structure of experience.* New York: Cambridge University Press.

Mattingly, C. & Fleming, M. H. (1994). *Clinical reasoning: Forms of inquiry in a therapeutic practice.* Philadelphia: F. A. Davis.

Mattingly, C. & Lawlor, M. (2000). Learning from stories: Narrative interviewing in cross-cultural research. *Scandinavian Journal of Occupational Therapy, 7*, 4–14.

McCrum, R. (1998). *My year off.* New York: Broadway Books.

McKay, E. A. & Ryan, S. (1995). Clinical reasoning through story telling: Examining a student's case story on a fieldwork placement. *British Journal of Occupational Therapy,* 58, 234–238.

Molineux, M. & Rickard, W. (2003). Storied approaches to understanding occupation. *Journal of Occupational Science,* 10(1), 52–60.

Morrison, T. (1987). The site of memory. In W. Zinsser (Ed.*),* *Inventing the truth: The art and craft of memoir* (pp. 99–124). Boston: Houghton Mifflin Company.

Mostert, E., Zacharkeiwicz, A. & Fossey, E. (1996). Claiming the illness experience: Using narrative to enhance theoretical understanding. *Australian Journal of Occupational Therapy,* 43, 125–132.

Moyers, P. (1999). *The guide to occupational therapy practice.* Bethesda, MD: American Occupational Therapy Association.

Meyer, Adolph. (1922). The philosophy of occupation therapy. *Archives of Occupational Therapy,* 1, 639–642.

Neistadt, M. & Crepeau, E. B. (1998). *Willard and Spackman's occupational therapy* (9th ed.). Philadelphia: Lippincott Williams & Wilkins.

Parry, A. & Doan, R. E. (1994). *Story re-visions: Narrative therapy in the postmodern world.* New York: Gilford Press.

Peloquin, S. (1993). The depersonalization of patients: A profile gleaned from narratives. *American Journal of Occupational Therapy,* 47, 830–837.

Polkinghorne, D. E. (1988). *Narrative knowing and the human sciences.* Albany: State University of New York Press.

Polkinghorne, D. E. (1996). Transformative narratives: From victimic to agentic life plots. *American Journal of Occupational Therapy,* 50, 299–305.

Price-Lackey, P. & Cashman, J. (1996). Jenny's story: Reinventing oneself through occupation and narrative configuration. *American Journal of Occupational Therapy,* 50, 306–314.

Reilly, M. (1962). Occupational therapy can be one of the great ideas of twentieth center medicine. *American Journal of Occupational Therapy,* 16, 1–9.

Ricoeur, P. (1984). *Time and narrative* (Vol. 1). Chicago: University of Chicago Press.

Riessman, C. K. (1993). *Narrative analysis.* Sage University Paper series on Qualitative Research Methods (Vol. 30). Newbury Park, CA: Sage Publications.

Rogers, J. (1983). Eleanor Clarke Slagle Lectureship—1983. Clinical reasoning: The ethics, science, and art. *American Journal of Occupational Therapy,* 37, 601–616.

Russell, W. F. (1989). *Classic myths to read aloud.* New York: Crown Trade Paperbacks.

Ryan, S. E. (1999). How are narratives being used? In S. E. Ryan & E. A. McKay (Eds.), *Thinking and reasoning in therapy: Narratives from practice* (1–15). Cheltenham, England: Stanley Thornes (Publishers) Ltd.

Sacks, O. (1984). *A leg to stand on.* New York: Touchstone Simon & Schuster.

Sackett, D. L., Straus, S. E., Richardson, W. S., Rosenberg, W. & Hayens, R. B. (2000). *Evidence-based medicine: How to practice and teach EBM.* New York: Churchill Livingstone.

Schkade, J. & McClung, M. (2001). *Occupational adaptation in practice: Concepts and cases.* Thorofare, NJ: Slack, Inc.

Schkade, J. & Schultz, S. (1992). Occupational adaptation: Toward a holistic approach for contemporary practice. Part 1. *American Journal of Occupational Therapy,* 46, 829–837.

Schultz, S. & Schkade, J. (1992). Occupational adaptation: Toward a holistic approach for contemporary practice. Part 2. *American Journal of Occupational Therapy,* 46, 917–925.

Schultz, S. & Schkade, J. (1997). Adaptation. In C. Christiansen & C. Baum (Eds.), *Occupational therapy: Enabling function and well-being* (2nd ed., pp. 459–481). Thorofare, NJ: Slack.

Schkade, J. & Schultz, S. (2003). Occupational adaptation. In P. Kramer, J. Hinojosa & C. B. Royeen (Eds.), *Perspectives in human occupation: Participation in life* (pp. 181–221). Philadelphia: Lippincott Williams & Wilkins.

Siegel, D. J. (1999). *The developing mind: Toward a neurobiology of interpersonal experience.* New York: Guilford Press.

Simmons, D. C., Crepeau, E. B. & White, B. P. (2000). The predictive power of narrative data in occupational therapy evaluation. *American Journal of Occupational Therapy,* 54, 471–476.

Sontag, S. (1990). *Illness as metaphor and AIDS and its metaphors.* New York: Doubleday.

Spence, D. (1982). *Narrative truth and historical truth: Meaning and interpretation in psychoanalysis.* New York: W. W. Norton & Company.

Spencer, J. Davidson, H. & White, V. (1996). Continuity and change: Past experience as adaptive repertoire in Occupational Adaptation. *American Journal of Occupational Therapy,* 50, 526–534.

Spencer, J. Davidson, H. & White, V. (1997). Helping clients develop hopes for the future. *American Journal of Occupational Therapy,* 51, 191–198.

Spencer, J., Young, M. E., Rintala, D. & Bates, S. (1995). Socialization to the culture of a rehabilitation hospital: An ethnographic study. *American Journal of Occupational Therapy,* 49, 53–62.

Underwood, B. (1993). Sleepytime tea logo. Boulder, CO: Celestial Seasonings, Inc.

Ward, J. D. (2003). The nature of clinical reasoning with groups: A phenomenological study of an occupational therapist in community mental health. *American Journal of Occupational Therapy,* 57, 625–634.

White, M. & Epston, D. (1990). *Narrative means to therapeutic means.* New York: Norton.

Wood, W. (1995). Weaving the warp and weft of occupational therapy: An art and science for all time. *American Journal of Occupational Therapy,* 49, 44–52.

Wright-St. Clair, V. (2003). Storymaking and storytelling: Making sense of living with multiple sclerosis. *Journal of Occupational Science,* 10, 46–51.

Yerxa, E. (1967). Authentic occupational therapy. *American Journal of Occupational Therapy,* 21, 1–9.

Zeitlin, S. (1997). *Because God loves stories: an anthology of Jewish storytelling.* New York: Touchstone / Simon & Schuster.

Pragmatic Reasoning

Barbara A. Boyt Schell

OBJECTIVES

After reading this chapter, the learner will be able to:

1 Define pragmatic reasoning.
2 Describe common contextual factors considered by therapists as they plan and implement intervention.
3 Describe how therapists' skills and life situations may affect therapist decision-making.
4 Explore the interface of pragmatic reasoning with other aspects of professional reasoning.

KEY TERMS

Pragmatic reasoning
Practice context
Personal context

Pragmatic reasoning is a term introduced to the occupational therapy literature in the 1990s by myself and Ron Cervero to describe practitioner thinking, which is focused on the everyday realities that affect the delivery of service (Schell & Cervero, 1993). The idea arose from my own experiences as a manager challenged to help practitioners negotiate the practice environment to deliver good care to their clients. Ron had seen similar issues in his work as an adult education professor who researches learning across professions. One of my major motivations for going into management was to try to create environments that supported the delivery of high-quality therapy programs. I was frustrated in my early years of practice by the negative impact of bureaucratic rules. Over the years, I heard others voice concerns over the poor availability of supplies and equipment, size of caseload and payment for services. Since those early days, I learned to accept that all therapy happens in the "real world," rather than some idealized notion of the optimum situation. I have also noticed that the quality of therapy that is actually provided is influenced by far more than either the scientific or narrative reasoning used by the therapist. As important as these perspectives are, they often do little to help therapists negotiate required resources and juggle the competing demands of practice contexts. Indeed, this is an issue in many professions, and one that Ron Cervero continues to pursue in his research on power in the practice of adult education (Cervero, Wilson & Associates, 2001). On the other hand, I continue to explore the range of issues addressed by pragmatic reasoning and the impact of both practice context and the personal life situation of therapists on the therapy that is provided. This chapter explores pragmatic reasoning—that aspect of reasoning that therapists use to attend to the practical realities of service delivery.

Thinking About Thinking 7-1

Our Life's Work

"On some level we are always searching for our life's work, wanting to align our doing and our being with our highest purposes. As such moments of calm we find, to our surprise, that our life's work is here in our hands, at this very moment; it is here as we gaze into another's eyes, it is here with each breath we receive from and give back to the world."

—Simmons, P. (*Learning to Fall*, 2000, p. 129)

PRAGMATIC REASONING DEFINED

In the original introduction of the term to occupational therapy, pragmatic reasoning was suggested as the reasoning therapists use when attending to the contextual factors that inhibit or facilitate therapy (Schell & Cervero, 1993). The word pragmatic was chosen to reflect the notion of practical decisions, or ones that attend to the practical aspects of service delivery. When using pragmatic reasoning, therapists are required to see things as they really are and find ways to deal with them.

There are two aspects of pragmatic reasoning: one that focuses on the **practice context,** and the other that focuses on therapists' **personal context.** Both are important, because each can directly affect the nature of the services that the client receives. Practitioners require effective pragmatic reasoning abilities to deal with the practical realities of providing therapy services. In addition, therapy supervisors, managers, and administrators who want effective therapy programs must grapple with how to create optimum service delivery systems.

Managerial ability to recognize or create options that can be exercised within a practice arena, as well as the willingness to take on the status quo when necessary, can make an important difference in the therapy that occurs. For instance, a manager's ability to develop flexible purchasing approaches can be critical in helping therapists to implement occupation-based approaches, so that therapists can readily obtain needed activity materials. Another example is the importance of thinking about ways to negotiate organizational employment policies and practices for employee retention. Flexible scheduling options can help therapists continue to practice in light of competing family obligations. Careful assignment of support personnel may permit a skilled therapist with health limitations to remain in practice.

In addition to reasoning about the practice context, practitioners also reason about themselves as the service provider. Each therapist has unique preferences and skill sets. Therapists must on occasion take inventory of their capacities relative to therapy demands and may choose to implement, avoid, or alter the therapy process based on these capacities. In addition, life demands, such as child care, may be factors that practitioners consider in choosing when to provide services.

In summation, pragmatic reasoning addresses both the practice context in which therapy is occurring as well as personal factors within each individual practitioner. Both internal and external factors are examined more closely in the following material.

Practice Context

Pragmatic reasoning about the practice context can be characterized as "going beyond the practitioner–client relationship" to address the world in which therapy occurs (Schell, 2003, p. 136). A number of occupational therapists have discussed the impact of a variety of external factors on occupational therapy practice (e.g., Barris, 1987; Howard, 1991). Opacich (1997) summarized the concerns of many home health practitioners in the United States about the "impact of the business of health care delivery. . . . Business strategies are affecting practice in measurement of productivity, in documentation, and in determination of effectiveness . . ." (p. 434). In Australia, Mitchell and Unsworth (2004) found that community health therapists identified both supportive (i.e., relationships with other agencies) as well as detracting factors (i.e., funding, caseload, facilities, driving time) that affected how well they did their work. Until the notion of pragmatic reasoning was raised, the literature within occupational therapy tended to characterize such external pressures as constraints or barriers to clinical reasoning, rather than another focus of what therapists have to consider along with various scientific and narrative concerns.

Once identified, pragmatic reasoning was adopted by others in the profession as another aspect of clinical reasoning. For example, Neistadt and colleagues (Neistadt, Wight & Mulligan, 1998) indicated "pragmatic reasoning considers the treatment environment and the possibilities of treatment within a given setting . . . to meet changing reimbursement requirements and productivity expectations" (p. 126). In their review of the literature, Leicht and Dickerson (2001) included pragmatic reasoning as one of the types of clinical reasoning. More recently, Unsworth (2004) found evidence of pragmatic reasoning in her research, as discussed in more detail later in the chapter.

Skillful reasoning about the practice context has the potential to make a significant impact on the services that clients receive by opening up the possibilities of therapy. If therapists accept physical, organizational, and social constraints as nonnegotiable, then the horizon of options from which to customize a therapy program is necessarily narrowed. Examples of such acceptance are found in Case Study 7-1 that follows. Alternatively, when therapists (and equally important, their managers) are willing and able to negotiate for necessary and desirable resources, then the scope of therapy possibilities opens, as demonstrated in subsequent Case Study 7-2 (What's In the Closet?).

CASE STUDY 7-1

Medicare Won't Pay

This case is a true story involving my mother-in-law. She was a delightful woman who had a variety of avid interests, such as sewing miniature dollhouse items such as bedspreads and rugs. She also loved to read, and even late in her life reread Will and Ariel Durant's *The Story of Civilization*. In the latter parts of her life, she experienced progressive cognitive declines. Fortunately, she was in a life-care community and was able to access increasing support as her abilities changed. Although many of the services provided were excellent in helping her to maintain optimal functioning in her daily life, we ran into problems when she needed to transition from assisted living into the nursing home. At that point, it was clear that she had serious cognitive problems and that environmental cues would become even more critical in helping her to go about her daily routines, such as finding her way to and from her room.

Although we lived quite a distance from her, as the OT daughter-in-law, her sons (including my husband John) relied on me to help coordinate her care and deal with the healthcare staff. As soon as I heard she was being transferred, I ask for orders for OT and PT to help facilitate her transition into this new environment. My thoughts were that the OT could optimize the environment to support her functioning and the PT could check out her ambulation to see if she was using the most effective mobility aid given her changing status. The nurse suggested I also ask for speech therapy, because "they do cognition here." Although I think OT has a big role to play in "doing cognition," I decided not to fight that battle, and agreed to request speech therapy as well. All three services saw her for an initial evaluation, and all three replied that since she had no potential for improvement, Medicare wouldn't pay for services. Consequently, she was discontinued after the evaluations. No one appeared to explore the possibility of improving her performance by focusing on the environment rather than her cognitive skills.

As I reflect on this experience, there were two reasoning factors at play here. The first had to do with framing the problem, as discussed in Chapter 3. From my perspective, the problem was not to improve cognition, the problem was how to adapt the environment to maximize performance with the cognition she had. A second factor related to pragmatic reasoning, in that all the therapists seemed to accept one set of reimbursement rules for guiding their clinical actions. No one even asked us if she could afford the services out of her own pocket (she could) or lacking that if we would be willing to pay (we would).

Whether or not she could have had a more comfortable transition and been more effectively oriented to her new setting is something we will never know, because the therapists in this case *didn't appear to even consider that alternative payment options might be available.*

One of the ongoing challenges that seems to face the profession is how to blend restorative approaches within an occupation-based framework, such that neuromuscular and biomechanical approaches are embedded within activities that are meaningful for the client. Several years ago, I had a great reminder of the importance of available equipment to implementing more naturalistic activities in therapy.

CASE STUDY 7-2

What's in the Closet?

A number of students had completed an intensive seminar with a well-known speaker on the topic of motor control. All of these students had also been deeply immersed in the importance of using occupationally relevant activities throughout their professional education. After the didactic part of the course, the students spent a day with clients at a nearby rehabilitation facility. This field experience was an opportunity for the students to develop skills based on their newly acquired knowledge about motor control.

One small group of students worked with a man who had hemiplegia. They quickly found out that he liked to play golf; therefore, they began to try to figure out ways to encourage upper extremity motor control in the context of golfing. When I looked over at the students, I saw that the man was holding a very long piece of cylindrical foam padding and swinging it like a golf putter. This is a great example of what Fleming called the "willingness to use usual or unusual things in unusual ways" (1994, p. 112). As it happened, I am a golfer and I had my golf clubs in my car. I walked over and offered to go get the clubs when the clinic supervisor overhead me. She said, "Oh, we have clubs in the closet," and proceeded to get a whole set of golf clubs for the students to try with the client. The students then set up an opportunity for the man to try putting using a real golf club and a real golf ball. Not surprisingly, he demonstrated more motor control; even better, several other clients with hemiplegia began to ask to use the putter as well. Soon we had a small "golf clinic" for people recovering from hemiplegia.

There are several things to notice here. First, therapy improved with the use of real, familiar objects when combined with skillful cueing of movements (an example of intertwining both scientific and narrative reasoning). However, these reasoning modes alone were not sufficient to provide the optimal therapy. Initially, the students improvised as best they could with something that is really not very much like a golf club (but better than nothing at all) because *they didn't know how to get what was needed in the time and place that it was needed.* Further, I doubt that it occurred to the students to ask about how to get the needed equipment. The fact that there were golf clubs in the closet reflects a practical resource that made a difference in this therapy session. Obviously, some therapist or manager in this setting knew that golf is a common activity in this region and had arranged to have golf clubs readily available. This is the difference that skillful pragmatic reasoning can bring to therapy.

Personal Context

Another proposed facet of pragmatic reasoning is one that considers personal factors related to the therapist. In the original definition, these were postulated as the "repertoire of therapy skills, ability to read the practice culture, negotiation skills and personal motivation" (Schell & Cervero, 1993, p. 609). Hooper's summary of a therapist's assumptions (see Chapter 2), along with Unsworth's (2004) critique of the personal aspect of pragmatic reasoning raises the question of differentiating between personal pragmatic reasoning and a therapist's worldview. Unsworth's (2004) research into pragmatic reasoning suggested to her that in the "context of everyday practice, it seems unlikely that a therapist's values and beliefs are brought to a conscious level where they can be *reasoned* with" (p. 16). In contrast, Chapparo (1999) offers an explanation of clinical reasoning based on the theory of planned behavior, which she used to analyze cases of therapists' reasoning. Chapparo believes that therapy action is the result of reasoned action within a specific social situation and that it occurs based on therapist *intention*. Therapist intention is in turn influenced by four factors:

1. Attitude
2. Subjective norm
3. Perceived behavioral control
4. Personal norms.

Therapists have favorable or unfavorable attitudes toward the anticipated action (i.e., "I always seem to get good results with this approach" or "I am only doing this because the parent is insisting on it"). They also operate within subjective norms, which are the therapists' internal perceptions of the social pressure relative to the anticipated therapy (i.e., "We are expected to do this with all patients" or "I don't think they like us doing this form of therapy here"). Perceived behavioral control refers to the therapist evaluation of the ease of actually doing the proposed therapy (i.e., "This should work well" or "I'm not really sure I can do this correctly"). The fourth factor that Chapparo proposed is the personal norm, which is comparable to the core beliefs and worldview discussed by Hooper in Chapter 2. Chapparo's work offers another way of looking at how personal pragmatic reasoning might affect therapy action.

Obviously, there is a need for more understanding of the personal aspects of pragmatic reasoning. As a result of this lack of clarity, Carolyn Unsworth and I, along with Barbara Hooper, are engaged in a line of research, which is currently underway. From this research, we hope to understand more about pragmatic reasoning focused on the personal context. Case Study 7-3 (below), drawn from an interview which is part of that research, provides some examples of the sort of therapist thinking which prompted me to think that there are pragmatic issues of a personal nature which require pragmatic reasoning. Readers are cautioned, however, to "stay tuned," since there is much more to explore and no widely accepted explanation of this side of pragmatic reasoning.

CASE STUDY 7-3

Examples from the Field

Natalie (a pseudonym) has provided home health services for many years. She was able to readily provide examples of her own pragmatic reasoning that addressed factors both in the practice context and those that arose from her own personal situation. Below are some examples, some of which are paraphrased for clarity or to protect confidentiality.

Choosing the Therapy Activity

I think that we often make choices about the specific activity based on our own preferences and needs, along with what we know the patient needs. For instance [when seeing a patient who needs training in her homemaking skills], how many times have you had somebody cook because you are hungry? We choose an activity that also suits our personal comfort level. Another example: If it's a nice day outside and you haven't been able to be in the sun much because you work inside, you may decide to do your therapy session outside so you can enjoy some sun, along with your patient.

Scheduling

If I'm really tired today, and if I have a choice in my schedule, I want to schedule somebody at the end of the day who isn't going to take a lot of my energy . . . someone who can do a lot where I'm just monitoring as opposed to somebody where I need to intensely work with them and exert a lot of physical energy.

Finding Time to Eat

I remember working for an agency in a rural county for a couple years. Basically, by the time I left the city there were only two possible places where I could stop and get food. Once you were out there, there was nothing unless you wanted to go in and buy pickled pig's feet at some general store in the middle of nowhere. And so I would need to think as I was scheduling people, "Where am I going to get a chance to stop and eat somewhere?" Sometimes, I would be near a railroad crossing with a lot of freight trains . . . I've sat there and eaten my lunch waiting for the freight trains to go by because that can slow me down.

Compensating for Physical Limitations

[Because I often work alone in home health] I have to think, "What are my physical capabilities here?" and "What's my judgment of risk in this situation?" and "Am I going to try and transfer them?" Or "am I going to need to schedule a session when another practitioner is here?" (Natalie goes on to note that her physical capacities have changed over time due to some health issues.) Even though I know the techniques and even have the skill, that doesn't mean I have the same capabilities.

In the next section, we turn to the evidence about pragmatic reasoning that has been uncovered in studies involving occupational therapy practitioners. As will be seen, most of the evidence to date illustrates pragmatic reasoning about the practice context, although there is one study that shows evidence of personal pragmatic reasoning.

EMPIRICAL EVIDENCE ABOUT PRAGMATIC REASONING

Since the concept of pragmatic reasoning was introduced, research continues to surface that contributes to the understanding of the phenomena, albeit primarily from studies of clinical reasoning in general rather than pragmatic reasoning specifically. Some recurring themes provide insight into the factors that therapists reason about. As Unsworth (2005) noted in her study of pragmatic reasoning, most of the data relate to the practice context. The following list represents a synthesis of factors across studies, which found evidence of pragmatic reasoning (Barris, 1987; Creighton, Kijkers, Bennett & Brown, 1995; Fondiller, Rosage & Neuhaus, 1990; Lyons & Crepeau, 2001; Rogers & Masagatani, 1982; Sladyk & Scheckley, 1999; Schell, 2005; Unsworth, 2005, 2004, 2001; Ward, 2003). The factors are ordered to reflect the frequency with which they were reported across studies, although the reader is cautioned to notice that these studies range widely in terms of the numbers of participants and intensity of the research methodology. *Table 7-1* provides a summary of these factors.

Organizational Norms and Policies

The social expectations associated with practice settings arise in many forms as something that therapists must consider. In the earliest occupational therapy clinical reasoning study, Rogers and Masagatani (1982) noticed the automatic nature of clinical reasoning and how the therapy procedures appeared routine when they examined diagnostic reasoning in medical settings. This suggested that there were normative expectations for therapy routines. Similarly, Barris (1987) noted that the patient population, treatment setting, and department tradition influenced diagnostic reasoning in mental health settings. Therapists in some situations seem to pair pragmatic reasoning with other kinds of reasoning to sort out what is possible within a given set of circumstances. For instance, Unsworth (2004) found more evidence of interactive reasoning in cultures that supported client centered reasoning.

A number of therapists indicated that relationships within the practice setting could either support or hinder the therapy process and had to be considered when deciding on clinical courses of action. Teamwork, such as support from nursing (Creighton et al, 1995), relationship with colleagues (Schell, 2005), staff conflicts and blurred role boundaries (Sladyk & Scheckley, 1999) were all topics of attention. With supportive colleagues, good teamwork, and minimal competition among the disciplines, therapists were freer to implement optimal therapy. Conversely, therapists might not include some aspects of therapy if it would upset another team member or be perceived as encroaching on another's professional territory as it was defined in that setting.

A third aspect of the culture concerning therapists was productivity expectations. Lyons and Crepeau (2001) discussed how productivity expectations were

TABLE 7-1

Factors Requiring Pragmatic Reasoning

Factor	Categories	Examples
Organizational norms & policies	Teamwork	Relations with colleagues Role boundaries Nursing availability to support follow-through
	Perceived organizational expectations	Accreditation requirements Preferred therapy approaches Range of therapy approaches Department tradition Productivity expectations
	Power relations	Physician orders Level of respect for OT
Time	Scheduling	Frequency of visits Availability of special use areas Need to share time with other therapies Being on time or running late
	Treatment duration	Amount of time per session Overall length of stay Number of visits allowed
Physical resources	Space	Access to natural or closely simulated space (i.e., kitchen, apt.) Proximity of therapy spaces
	Supplies & equipment	Availability Quantity
Caseload	Number of clients	Ratio of clients to therapist (1:1, overlapping, group) Overall size of caseload Frequency of turnover in caseload Fluctuations in caseload volume
	Kinds of clients	Similarities of conditions Amount of supervision required
	Prioritization	Deciding who to treat when caseload is too large
Payment for services	Insurance coverage	Whether or not occupational therapy services are covered Rules for coverage of services
	Client ability to pay	What client or family can afford Willingness to pay for services
Discharge options	Place	Number of options Nature of support provided
	Timing	When desired options are open for new clients
Therapists skills	Competence	Weighing therapy skills vs. client needs

This table is based on empirical studies on occupational therapy cited in this chapter.

part of a COTA's clinical reasoning. Additional factors listed next, such as time and caseload may also be proxies for reasoning about productivity.

Time

Therapists have to consider practical concerns regarding time. Fondiller, Rosage, and Neuhaus (1990) discussed the inherent conflicts between the espoused values expressed by their study participants (e.g., holism, multidisciplinary consultation, use of purposeful activity) and the demands of a health care system that packages therapy into 15-minute units. Issues such as length and frequency of therapy sessions provide affordance or barriers to some therapy options (Schell, 2005; Unsworth, 2004; Creighton et al., 1995). These factors may be intertwined with overall length of stay (Schell, 2005; Unsworth, 2005) as well as the need to share time with other health providers (Unsworth, 2004). In addition, decisions about time may be intertwined with other factors, such as resource availability, scheduling of specialty spaces such as a therapy kitchen, or with caseload demands when a therapy schedule can't be followed as planned (Unsworth, 2004).

Physical Resources

The availability of or lack of functionally oriented settings and equipment were considerations in whether therapists used purposeful activities in hospital and rehabilitation in and outpatient settings (Creighton et al., 1995; Schell, 2005). Ward (2003) described a therapist conducting a psychosocial group as having to scan the environment for needed tools in order to keep the group going.

The importance of physical resources in guiding therapy options can be seen in managerial strategies intended to change a practice pattern. For instance, those who advocate a more occupation-based approach in rehabilitation settings often discuss hiding "the pegs and cones" and providing more common objects of daily life in the treatment setting (Schell & Bravemen, 2005). An even stronger acknowledgment of the importance of appropriate physical context can be seen in the trend of providing early intervention services in the natural environment. A tacit understanding underlying all these change strategies is that therapists use the tools and equipment that are readily accessible for daily practice.

Caseload

The number and kinds of clients in therapists' caseloads have already been alluded to earlier as they relate to time and the organizational culture. Therapists working with groups find themselves thinking about how to prioritize who needs services (Ward, 2003). Experts working in inpatient rehabilitation acknowledge that there are limitations to having multiple patients at once (Unsworth, 2001) or at least factors to consider when one has overlapping or waiting patients (Unsworth, 2005).

Payment for Services

Surprisingly, payment and reimbursement issues were raised explicitly in only three studies, although in the United States at least it is a pervasive topic of discussion in the profession. Explicit and perceived rules regarding reimbursement were discussed by close to half of the therapists in my own study (Schell, 2005), and Unsworth (2004) found that insurance, reimbursement, and what the patient can afford were factors considered by therapists in thinking about what services and equipment could or should be provided. Lyons and Crepeau (2001) also found this to be a topic of consideration by the COTA they studied.

Discharge Options

The discharge options for clients appeared to affect both the timing of discharge and the actual discharge recommendation for the therapists that Unsworth studied (2004, 2005). It is not clear whether this is best classified as a pragmatic reasoning issue or whether it fits more with other forms, such as conditional reasoning in which therapists consider possible performance trajectories of their clients.

Therapy Skills

Only one study surfaced an example of the personal context, and in that study the therapist discussed weighing of her therapy skills relative to the therapy need (Unsworth, 2003). Why is the identification of these skills and elements important? If therapists are unaware that they are limiting therapy options for their clients to their own skill set, then they are not likely to seek consultation from others or engage in the professional development required to gain additional skills.

PRAGMATIC REASONING AND OTHER MODES OF REASONING

The interconnections of the various kinds of reasoning have just started to be systematically explored. Fleming's initial proposition about the "therapist with the three track mind" (1991, p. 988) continues to be supported in most of the studies cited here and throughout the book, although the number and naming of the tracks is still up for debate. For instance, Ward's study participant intermeshed pragmatic reasoning with interactive and procedural reasoning when she had therapy group participants help each other. In this way, clients with lower skills received assistance, which she practically couldn't provide to all members at once, whereas those with higher skills verbalized increased self-esteem from being a successful helper (2003, p. 629). This example of pragmatic reasoning contrasts with others in that it reflects a positive use of pragmatic reasoning. Unsworth (2005) noted that the pragmatic reasoning used by therapists in her study "all seemed related to barriers and limitation rather than to opportunities" (p. 36). This observation needs to be interpreted with caution, however, as it has been noticed in the management literature that people tend to credit their own skills, motivation, and so on, when situations turn out well, and to blame external variables when there are problems. As Unsworth appropriately concludes, more explicit study of pragmatic reasoning is required. I will highlight three questions here for discussion.

Is it Ethical or Pragmatic Reasoning?

In their book, *Clinical Reasoning in the Health Professions*, Higgs and Jones (2000) describe "ethical-pragmatic reasoning," about which they write: "It alludes to those less recognized but frequently made decisions regarding morals, political and economic dilemmas which clinicians regularly confront, such as deciding how long to continue treatment" (p. 8). This description makes a connection between what is called ethical reasoning and pragmatic reasoning, perhaps because there are often the tensions raised between practice resources and client needs (see Chapter 8). Although I think they are separate issues—in that not all pragmatic issues involve ethical dilemmas—some issues, such as payment for services, require that therapists draw upon both forms of reasoning to provide therapy services. For example, as I write this chapter there is an active discussion going on via our state occupational therapy association's list serve, in which therapists are trying to figure out what to do about provision of early intervention services in light of a changing payment structure. A new organization has been contracted to manage state funds for this program. They are changing the amount of payment therapists can receive, the number of visits that will be routinely paid for, and the methods required for documentation and billing. Several very experienced clinicians are leading the attempt to clarify these changes and to influence policy so that children can receive necessary services. Another practitioner has researched the company and is suggesting that legal action may be required. Still other therapists are deciding to quit providing services because they are tired of the hassle and do not feel they can earn a living. Many therapists are struggling to figure out how to meet the needs of their children and families while also covering their own costs to deliver services. Clearly, this is an example of both pragmatic and ethical reasoning unfolding.

Thinking About Thinking 7-2

Moral good is a practical stimulus; it is no sooner seen than it inspires an impulse to practise.

—Plutarch (46–120 AD), *Life of Pericles*

Is it Narrative or Pragmatic Reasoning?

In the same book mentioned above, occupational therapists Chapparo and Rankin note: "Clinical reasoning focuses on practical action and therapists are compelled to think about what is achievable within their own or their client's world" (2000, p. 134). Here, there is a subtle blurring between pragmatic reasoning and narrative reasoning, as the client's situation is brought into play. In my original conception, the client's context would be part of their story or narrative reasoning, with pragmatic reasoning referring to that reasoning that attends to factors *beyond* the client's particular health and life situation.

Should it be Personal Context or Underlying Values?

Unsworth's (2004) critique of the construct of personal context described earlier, introduces the question about the distinctions between therapist's underlying worldview and their personal context as a topic of reasoning. Part of her argument is that one's worldview is so tacit as to be beyond reasoning. As we continue to research this topic, we may find that some aspects are tacit (and therefore not available to be reasoned about) and some are available for active reasoning.

These variations are a reflection of the relative newness of the research supporting our understanding of pragmatic reasoning. As discussed in Unit IV of this book, there are a number of constructs within our understanding of clinical and professional reasoning that require further study and refinement. In addition, virtually all authors recognize that forms of clinical reasoning are intertwined in a variety of combinations that help the practitioner to respond to the problems at hand.

SUMMARY

Pragmatic reasoning occurs when therapists are attending to the everyday realities of delivery of therapy services. A small but growing body of research describes the practical concerns that therapists have to consider. These include a range of external contextual factors, such as the amount of time available for intervention, nature of the caseload, and payment rules and regulations. The particular practice culture influences therapy decisions; sometimes therapists must consider factors such as group norms, available tools, and human and nonhuman resources. Speculation continues that therapists' own personal context may also be a factor of consideration, although there is little research yet on that aspect. Skilled pragmatic reasoning holds the potential to unleash the power of occupational therapy, as therapists become more effective in negotiation of optimal conditions for practice.

LEARNING ACTIVITY 7-1

Know Thyself

Purpose

The purpose of this activity is to help learners reflect on their personal abilities and preferences and on how they affect therapy provision.

Connections To Major Clinical Reasoning Constructs

This activity provides the learner with practice in identifying and improving personal pragmatic reasoning skills.

Directions for Learners

1 Complete Part I of the Know Thyself reflection.
2 Discuss your findings with a small group of peers.
3 Using your own thoughts and input from your peers, identify areas in which you need to either develop or improve your personal pragmatic reasoning. Use the action planning grid to formalize your planned development.

Know Thyself Worksheet

Part I Therapy and Me

Think about the therapy that you are currently providing, or have been involved with during field work. With a specific situation in mind, think about your responses to the questions in each topical area. Write down notes to yourself as you go along, so that you can discuss your thoughts with others in your group.

Evaluation: What assessment skills do I have? Are there any assessments that I should be using but am not? Why not? Are there assessments that I overuse? Why?

_____

_____

_____

Intervention approaches: What skills do I have for working with this population? What skills am I lacking? How is my constellation of skills impacting the services my clients receive?

_____

_____

_____

Physical capacities: What abilities do I have that are assets in this therapy situation? What limitations do I have? How is therapy affected by my constellation of physical abilities?

_____

_____

_____

Emotional capacities: What are my feelings about being a therapist in this situation? How do my feelings support or limit the therapy options that I provide to my clients?

_____

_____

_____

Dealing with power: Are there aspects of this therapy situation that are negatively affected by people or circumstances who have power in this setting? Are you aware of your own power within the setting? How effectively do you develop and use your ability to influence situations so as to improve client services?

_____

_____

_____

Dealing with conflict: Are there individuals with whom you have difficulty working? Are there group pressures on you that are inconsistent with your views of how things should be done? How do you characteristically respond to these? How do your responses affect the services that your clients receive?

_____

_____

_____

Life demands: What other demands do you have in your life? How do they affect you as a therapist? Do they support or detract from the services you provide?

_____

_____

_____

Part II Reflection on Findings

Discuss your findings about yourself with a partner or others in a group:

• How do your personal pragmatic abilities support effective provision of therapy?

• How do they detract from therapy?

• What strategies are you using to overcome negative impacts?

• What do you need to work on?

Part III Action plan

Identify three areas that you wish to focus on, and complete the following action grid. Use this to guide your personal development in pragmatic reasoning.

Area of Focus	Action I Will Take	Support Needed	Planned Outcome/Date

LEARNING ACTIVITY 7-2

Pragmatic Reasoning Resource Analysis
Robin Underwood

Purpose

The purpose of this activity is to help learners use their pragmatic reasoning to address the use of occupation-based approaches within a medical environment.

Connections to Major Reasoning Constructs

This activity provides the learner with practice in connecting their pragmatic reasoning skills with one theoretical approach that is recommended by the literature, but not uniformly adopted in practice.

Directions for Learners

1 Select a therapy setting and/or a client situation in which you felt using an occupation-based approach would improve the therapy process.

2 Using the resource analysis guide, consider practical options that could be implemented for each phase of the therapy process.

3 Discuss these with other students or practitioners.

4 Try implementing one or more of your recommended approaches (with appropriate supervision, in the case of students or inexperienced therapists in high risk settings).

5 Based on this experience, identify any realistic changes that could be made in the therapy routines in general to support more occupation-based practice.

Occupation-Based Approach
Pragmatic Reasoning Resource Guide

Review the lists below and check off the issues within your setting that affect your ability to do more occupation-based intervention. For the items selected, suggest at least two realistic ways to deal with these problems in this setting. After you complete that part, consider what ideas might be useful to pursue changing in your practice setting overall or for groups of clients.

During Assessment

☐ Time _____

_____

☐ Space and Equipment to Assess Occupational Performance _____

_____

☐ Room to Document on Assessment Form _____

_____

☐ Responding to Pressures by Peers _____

_____

☐ Responding to Pressures by Bosses/Authorities _____

_____

☐ Dealing with Other Team Members _____

_____

_____

During Intervention

☐ Time to Plan _____

_____

_____

☐ Supplies, Equipment, and Space _____

_____

☐ Intervention Strategies _____

_____

_____

☐ Dealing with Peer Pressure _____

_____

_____

☐ Responding to Pressure by Bosses/Authorities _____

_____

_____

☐ Dealing with Other Team Members _____

_____

_____

Implications for Practice Overall

_____

_____

_____

_____

REFERENCES

Barris, R. (1987). Clinical reasoning in psychosocial occupational therapy: The evaluation process. *Occupational Therapy Journal of Research, 7*, 147–162.

Cervero, R. M., Wilson, A. L & Associates (2001). *Power in practice.* San Francisco, CA: Jossey-Bass.

Chapparo, C. (1999). Working out: Working with Angelica-Interpreting practice. In S. E. Ryan & E. A. McKay (Eds.), *Thinking and reasoning in therapy: Narratives from practice.*

Chapparo, C. & Rankin, J. (2000). Clinical reasoning in occupational therapy. In J. Higgs & M. Jones (Eds.), *Clinical reasoning in the health professions* (2nd ed., pp. 128–137). Oxford, U.K.: Butterworth-Heinemann.

Creighton, C., Kijkers, M., Bennett, N. & Brown, K. (1995). Reasoning and the art of therapy for spinal cord injury. *American Journal of Occupational Therapy, 49*, 311–317.

Fleming, M. H. (1991). The therapist with the three-track mind. *American Journal of Occupational Therapy, 45*, 1007–1014.

Fondiller, E. D., Rosage, L. J. & Neuhaus, B. E. (1990). Values influencing clinical reasoning in occupational therapy: An exploratory study. *Occupational Therapy Journal of Research, 10*, 41–55.

Higgs, J. & Jones, M. (2000). Clinical reasoning in the health professions. In J. Higgs & M. Jones (Eds.), *Clinical reasoning in the health professions* (2nd ed., pp. 3–14). Oxford, U.K.: Butterworth-Heinemann.

Hooper, B. (1997). The relationship between pre-theoretical assumptions and clinical reasoning. *American Journal of Occupational Therapy, 51*, 328–338.

Howard, B. S. (1991). How high do we jump? The effect of reimbursement on occupational therapy. *American Journal of Occupational Therapy, 45*, 875–881.

Leicht, S. B. & Dickerson, A. (2001). Clinical reasoning, looking back. *Occupational Therapy in Health Care, 14*(3/4), 105–30.

Lyons, K. D. & Crepeau, E. B. (2001). Case report. The clinical reasoning of an occupational therapy assistant. *American Journal of Occupational Therapy, 55*, 577–581.

Mitchell, R. & Unsworth, C. A. (2004). Role perceptions and clinical reasoning of community health occupational therapists undertaking home visits. *Australian Occupational Therapy Journal, 51*, 13–24.

Neistadt, M. E., Wight, J. & Mulligan, S. E. (1998). Clinical reasoning case studies as teaching tools. *American Journal of Occupational Therapy, 52*, 125–132.

Opacich, K. J. (1997). Moral tensions and obligations of occupational therapy practitioners providing home care. *American Journal of Occupational Therapy, 51*, 430–435.

Rogers, J. C. & Masagatani, G. (1982). Clinical reasoning of occupational therapists during initial assessment of physically disabled patients. *Occupational Therapy Journal of Research, 2*, 195–219.

Schell, B. A. & Cervero, R. M. (1993). Clinical reasoning in occupational therapy: An integrative review. *American Journal of Occupational Therapy, 47*, 605–610.

Schell, B.A.B. (1994). The effect of practice context on occupational therapy practitioner's clinical reasoning (Doctoral dissertation, University of Georgia, 1994). *Dissertation Abstracts International.*

Schell, B.A.B. (2003). Clinical reasoning: The basis of practice. In E. B. Crepeau, E. S. Cohn & B.A.B. Schell (Eds.), *Willard & Spackman's occupational therapy* (10th ed., pp. 131–139). Philadelphia: Lippincott Williams & Wilkins.

Schell, B.A.B. (2005). *Pragmatic Reasoning: The Role of Practice Context in Occupational Therapists' Clinical Reasoning* (Manuscript in preparation).

Schell, B. & Bravemen, B. (2005). Turning theory into practice: Managerial strategies. In B. Braveman, *Leading and managing occupational therapy services: An evidence-based approach.* Philadelphia: F. A. Davis.

Sladyk, K. & Sheckley, B. (1999). Differences between clinical reasoning gainers and decliners during fieldwork. In P. A. Crist (Ed.), *Innovations in occupational therapy education 1999* (pp. 157–170). Bethesda, MD: American Occupational Therapy Association

Unsworth, C. A. (2001). The clinical reasoning of novice and expert occupational therapists. *Scandinavian Journal of Occupational Therapy, 8*, 163–173.

Unsworth, C.A. (2004). How do pragmatic reasoning, worldview and client-centeredness fit? *British Journal of Occupational Therapy, 67*(1), 10–19.

Unsworth, C. A. (2005). Using a head-mounted video camera to explore current conceptualizations of clinical reasoning in occupational therapy. *American Journal of Occupational Therapy*, 59, 31–40.

Ward, J. D. (2003). The nature of clinical reasoning with groups: A phenomenological study of an occupational therapist in community mental health. *American Journal of Occupational Therapy*, 57, 625–634.

8

Ethical Reasoning

Elizabeth M. Kanny and Deborah Yarett Slater

OBJECTIVES

After reading this chapter, the learner will be able to:

1 Identify the basic ethical concepts and foundational literature relative to the ethical reasoning process.
2 Recognize, discuss, and analyze ethical dilemmas using ethics theories and principles.
3 Apply ethical concepts and a framework for ethical decision making to everyday practice dilemmas/situations.
4 Use learning activities to practice articulating your ethical stances on daily practice challenges.

KEY TERMS

Ethical Dilemma	Beneficence	Fidelity
Ethical Reasoning	Nonmaleficence	Confidentiality
Ethical Principles	Justice	Privacy
Autonomy	Veracity	

E thics, with its foundation in the field of philosophy, may appear too theoretical to have relevance to everyday clinical or educational practice. We believe otherwise; thus, the goal of this chapter is to demonstrate the importance of thinking about, talking about, and, most important, acting on ethics and values in occupational therapy practice.

The goals of this chapter are twofold. First, we hope to provide a foundation for critically thinking about ethical reasoning including the philosophical roots, the writing, and the research done to date. Second, we use structured learning exercises that draw on real-life case studies to provide readers with the opportunity to apply and discuss the ethical reasoning process. This experiential learning calls for reflection and active response to ethical dilemmas that occupational therapists are likely to encounter in daily practice—whether it is in healthcare, schools, or community based settings.

Thinking About Thinking 8-1

People grow through experience if they meet life honestly and courageously. That is how character is built.

—Eleanor Roosevelt, 1941

Clients are at a vulnerable point in their lives and put their trust in their therapists to act in their best interests. This is a moral and ethical imperative as important as specific practice competencies. This chapter accordingly emphasizes action as the critical last step in the ethical reasoning process. Ethical reasoning without action is confined to thinking and intellectualization. True moral character leads the practitioner to go beyond thinking and take action.

HISTORY AND CONTEXT OF ETHICAL REASONING

Theories from philosophy and psychology underpin our discussion of **ethical reasoning.** Seminal psychological development theories include the moral and cognitive development theories of John Dewey, Jean Piaget, Lawrence Kohlberg, and James Rest. Last, Carol Gilligan's feminist theory of moral development identifying justice-based versus caring-based perspectives is presented. Current discussion about ethical reasoning evolves from these theories, and thus they are important to know about and understand.

Philosophical Ethical Theories

Theories provide the rationale behind any course of action or judgment. The use of theoretical frameworks provides a way to look at ethical issues to help clarify the issues. Some focus on the consequences of our actions (teleological) and others focus on the action itself (deontological). As in life, most things are not black or white, but tend to be a blend . . . and so it is for ethical theories.

Focus on Consequences

Teleological or consequentialist theory comes from the school of philosophy that determines right action by its consequences, not by intrinsic features.

Utilitarianism is the most widely known teleological theory, and its origins are in the writings of philosophers David Hume (1711–1776), Jeremy Bentham (1748–1832), and John Stuart Mill (1806–1873) (Beauchamp & Childress, 1989). This theory uses the concept of the greatest good for the greatest number to resolve conflict. The focus is on utility and benefit where the ends justify the means—thus the term "utilitarianism." One has an obligation to act or to avoid action by doing whatever will produce a greater balance of good over evil.

Focus on Action

Deontological theory comes from the school of philosophy that determines right action by examining the duties of individuals to one another. It originates in the writings of Immanuel Kant (1734–1804). An individual is acting rightly when he or she acts according to duties and rights, and the subsequent sense of responsibility one feels. In other words, let your conscience be your guide. The act itself, or the means, are what's important, not the consequence (Beauchamp & Childress, 1989).

Case Study 8-1 below helps illustrate how the two approaches to the same issue result in different actions. You need to examine your own thoughts and feelings about how you decide what is morally right. Is it from the perspective of duty and rights, or is it from the perspective of consequences of the act? Or does it depend on the situation or the severity of the situation for you? Remember that it is common to use a combination of the theories in making ethical decisions.

CASE STUDY 8-1

Means or Ends?

Over the past few weeks, you have provided occupational therapy to Mr. Jones, who has been a patient on the rehabilitation unit since suffering a stroke. He has progressed well and will be discharged home within the next week. His wife will provide assistance and you have done education and training with her. Several days before the actual discharge, Mr. Jones discloses that his wife may not consistently be able to help him as she has a problem with alcohol and periodically gets violent when she drinks. She has physically abused him in the past, yet he insists on going home. You have explored alternate discharge plans, additional help in the house, and alcohol prevention programs for his wife. He has rejected all of them, insisting on returning home with his wife and has asked you not to disclose this situation to anyone. What should you as the therapist do? From a deontological perspective, Mr. Jones' rights to autonomy and confidentiality must be respected. Presumably, he has made an informed decision since the therapist has discussed options for a different, safer discharge and cautioned him about returning to his home environment. From a teleological perspective, the therapist would make the decision based on consequences of action, which in this case would be to prevent harm. She thereby would disclose what Mr. Jones has shared to other members of the team and ask for a more appropriate discharge plan to protect his physical safety.

Moral Developmental Theories

Dewey was one of the first to theorize and write about morality and moral education. In *Moral Principles in Education* (1909), he discussed the moral being as the product of a dynamic interrelationship between self and the social setting. Dewey represented a cognitivist position to moral education, in that he believed morality was linked to reason and intelligence (Chazan, 1985). He believed the aim of education is to provide the optimal conditions in which intellectual and moral development could take place. He also suggested the concept of moral stages as part of the developmental process (Dewey, 1965).

Piaget, like Dewey, suggested that moral reasoning is developed in hierarchical stages (Flavell, 1963; Beilin & Pufall, 1992; Rest, 1994). He conducted extensive research with children, which led him to identify a series of stages of cognitive growth beginning with the inability to distinguish between reality and imagination; use of logical thought with regard to concrete objects (age 7); and use of logic to formulate inferences about abstract ideas (early adolescence). He also studied how children used reasoning to think about moral issues and identified three stages of moral development in children: premoral (no regard for rules), heteronomous (obey rules of those in power), and autonomous (mutually agreed-upon rules). Further, Piaget thought that stages in cognitive development approximated parallel stages of moral development, so the individual developed cognitive structures in order to reason about moral choices and decisions (Flavell, 1963; Beilin & Pufall, 1992; Rest, 1994).

Piaget's view of morality stemmed from his theory of socialization. He saw morality as based on respect for people rather than on tradition or rules. Piaget saw two moralities, one being the morality of constraint and later, as the child developed a general understanding of the social world, the morality of cooperation. He referred to these two moralities as stages that were developmentally sequenced and emphasized peer interaction as crucial for the morality of cooperation. (Rest, 1983)

The principal claims about moral judgment embodied in the cognitive developmental theories are that moral judgment is developmental, is primarily controlled by cognitive processes, and has a role in decision making in real-life situations. The major ideas that are the foundation for applied ethics come from Lawrence Kohlberg's studies on the cognitive developmental theory of moral reasoning (Rest, 1979).

Kohlberg's Stage Theory

Kohlberg's theory focuses on cognition and the sequential stages of moral reasoning. He asserted that people use six problem-solving strategies in a developmental sequence, moving from simple to complex in a logical manner. Kohlberg, like Dewey, emphasized the social nature of morality (Chazan, 1985); like Piaget, he focused on stages of moral development (Rest, 1994).

Kohlberg's research began in the late 1950s and spanned over 30 years, leading to the identification of three levels of moral development, each with two stages (Box 8-1) (Kohlberg, 1984). These six stages represent the reasons people have for choosing moral actions (Rest, 1979). In the *preconventional* level, people respond to what is right and wrong and are primarily driven by consequences of behavior such as avoiding punishment (stage 1) or obtaining rewards (stage 2). At the *conventional level,* people choose to act morally to avoid disapproval of others (stage 3) or to uphold laws and social rules by "doing one's duty" (stage 4). In the *postconventional level*, people use self-chosen principles to guide their reasoning. In stage 5, actions are guided by principles essential to public welfare and to respect peers and self. In stage 6, moral actions are guided by universal **ethical principles** such as justice, dignity, and equality. Development through the six stages is a gradual process occurring in a hierarchical fashion. Kohlberg also found that moral development may cease at any stage, varies from person to person, and is not a function of age (Rest, 1979).

BOX 8-1

Kohlberg's Stages of Moral Development

Level I: Preconventional Morality

Stage 1: Morality of punishment and obedience
Stage 2: Morality to obtain rewards

Level II: Conventional

Stage 3: Morality of mutual interpersonal agreement; avoid disapproval.
Stage 4: Morality of law and social duties.

Level III: Postconventional or Principled

Stage 5: Morality of societal consensus; respect of peers.
Stage 6: Morality of social cooperation.

Adapted from Kohlberg, L. (1984) *The Psychology of Moral Development: The Nature and Validity of Moral Stages.*

The cognitive aspect in each of the six stages is the logic or reasoning pattern individuals use in making decisions about moral problems. Kohlberg saw moral education as focusing on the development of basic problem-solving strategies, rather than on specific content (Rest, 1994).

Four-Component Model of Moral Behavior

James Rest built on and expanded Kohlberg's theory. Rest believes that there is more to ethical behavior than the moral judgment emphasized by Kohlberg. Through extensive research, Rest developed the Four-Component Model (Rest, 1986; 1994), identifying four psychological components that determine moral behavior (Box 8-2). Component 1 is *moral sensitivity*, meaning that a person is able to make an interpretation of a particular situation relative to possible actions, to interpret who would be affected by each action, and to interpret how the people would be affected. Component 2 is *moral judgment*, being able to determine what action is justifiably right or wrong. Social cooperation and fairness are important in this component. Component 3 is moral motivation and involves prioritizing moral values relative to other values. Thus, when other values conflict with moral values, the person must be motivated to put moral values first. Component 4 is *moral character*. A person must have the courage, perseverance, ego strength, and implementation skills to be able to act on his/her moral intentions. Thus, good intentions do not always bring good deeds (Rest, 1986; 1994).

Rest also views Kohlberg's six stages in a somewhat different way, emphasizing that they represent six conceptual ways to organize cooperation (Rest 1994). He asserts that the underlying concept of cooperation leads to moral judgments of right or wrong action. Development is seen as a progressive understanding of the various possibilities in cooperation and how rights and duties are balanced.

BOX 8-2
Four-Component Model of Moral Reasoning

Component 1: Moral Sensitivity

Making an interpretation of a particular situation in terms of the ethical problem, what actions might be taken, and the effects of these actions

Component 2: Moral Judgment

Making a judgment about what course of action is morally right

Component 3: Moral Motivation

Giving priority to moral values; having the motivation to do what is morally right

Component 4: Moral Character

Having the perseverance, ego strength, and skills to do what is morally right

Adapted from Rest, 1994.

Feminist View of Moral Reasoning

Carol Gilligan suggests that there are gender differences in the ways people deal with moral issues. She began her career teaching psychology at Harvard with Erik Erikson and was a research assistant for Lawrence Kohlberg. In her seminal work, *In a Different Voice: Psychological Theory and Women's Development* (1982), she portrays two ways of thinking about morality, one typical of men from the perspective of rules and justice and the other of women from the perspective of caring and relationships. Gilligan says that women will change the rules to preserve relationships, whereas men abide by the rules over relationships.

Gilligan's work is based on extensive interviews with women. She asserts that women speak in a "different" and valuable moral voice, and she identifies three stages of morality with women: orientation to individual survival (preconventional), goodness as self-sacrifice (conventional morality), and responsibility for consequences of choice (postconventional morality) (Gilligan, 1982). In the first stage, women are looking out for their own interests; in the second stage they are caring for and valuing the interests of others; in the third stage, they see caring as universal and take responsibility for others. Relationship is what is important and this requires connection, the ability to listen to and understand others. Gilligan (1993) sees a possibility that justice and care can blend into a postconventional morality and that both genders may have the capacity to view ethical issues from both perspectives.

Summary of Moral Development Theories

In summation, all of these theorists have built and expanded upon the work of each other. Common themes include rights versus consequences, the social nature of morality, developmental stages, cognition and problem solving, and social cooperation. Although controversial, openness to differing ways that men and women approach moral reasoning presents an area for further investigation. There are many ways of looking at moral reasoning and there is still much to be done by researchers in clarifying and describing its dimensions of caring and justice. With this grounding in ethics, we turn next to a discussion of ethical reasoning itself.

BASIC MORAL PRINCIPLES AND THEORIES OF ETHICAL REASONING

The major ethical principles in healthcare include autonomy, beneficence, nonmaleficence, and justice. There are also other ethical principles that relate to relationships between practitioners; veracity, fidelity, privacy, and confidentiality (Purtilo, 2005). An understanding of these eight principles is essential for analyzing and responding to ethical dilemmas. They provide the foundation and terminology needed when discussing cases or situations, giving you a way to articulate your thoughts to others and confidence in your ethical position (Kanny, 2000).

Autonomy

Autonomy is the right of an individual to be self-determining and make independent decisions about his or her life (Hansen, 2003). It is the principle of self-governance and pertains to liberty rights, privacy, individual choice, the right to self-determination, and respect for the wishes of an individual or his/her representative.

Healthcare issues related to autonomy include competency, informed consent, disclosure of information, and acceptance or refusal of medically indicated treatment. Autonomy gives a client the right to make healthcare decisions based on his/her individual goals and values.

Beneficence and Nonmaleficence

Beneficence refers to actions that benefit others, *to do good*. It implies both actively doing good and considering the potential harm of actions. As professionals, we not only strive to do good, but we must avoid doing harm, prevent harm, and remove harm when it is being inflicted (Beauchamp & Childress, 1989). **Nonmaleficence** is inextricably related to the principle of beneficence, but is more specific to "do no harm" (Purtilo, 2005). It is fundamental that occupational therapy practitioners avoid doing harm or creating a situation in which harm could occur. This involves determining the risks and benefits of an action and avoiding actions that could cause harm.

Justice

Justice relates to the issue of fairness and encompasses distributive, procedural, and compensatory justice. When choices need to be made, benefits and harms are distributed fairly. The concepts of human rights, equality, and fair opportunity are all part of this principle. The principle of justice helps us determine priorities in providing our services, determining fees and payments, meeting public aid and private insurance criteria (Veatch & Flack, 1997). *Distributive justice* refers to fairness in allocating healthcare resources, that is, when individuals compete for the same resources. *Procedural justice* is a process for ordering things in a "fair" way. For example, is it fair to treat a patient who arrives at 8:15 AM for his 8:00 AM appointment if it means treating everyone else late that day? *Compensatory justice* is the provision of resources to an individual who is wronged or injured (Purtilo, 2005).

Relationship Principles

Moral principles related to relationships are veracity, fidelity, confidentiality and privacy. They are critical to establishing trust and form the basis for the contract between the client and therapist (Purtilo, 2005).

Veracity is the obligation to tell the truth. This means being honest with a client and in reporting client status and services rendered. **Fidelity** is keeping promises and contracts and meeting the patient's reasonable expectations. These include showing basic respect, being competent, abiding by your professional code of ethics, following policies of your workplace and laws to protect clients' well-being, and honoring agreements such as informed consent, verbal agreements, or serious conversations. (Purtilo, 2005)

Confidentiality pertains to authorized disclosure (or nondisclosure) of personal information; keeping client information within appropriate limits and abiding by rules of consent. Information about a client may be harmful or embarrassing to an individual and needs to be treated with discretion. **Privacy** is linked to confidentiality and means that there are some aspects of a person's life that are not to be intruded upon or shared outside of the healthcare setting (Purtilo, 2005).

FRAMEWORKS FOR ETHICAL DECISION MAKING

Ethical tension may be the first thing that alerts a practitioner to an ethical dilemma in the workplace. Opacich (2003) talks about ethical tensions as affective cues, a visceral response, a sensing of threat to integrity, or feelings of conflict about what action to take. When an occupational therapy practitioner is confronted with an ethical dilemma or ethical stress, it becomes imperative that he/she have a framework with which to think about and come up with a solution. Ethical reasoning is similar to problem solving or scientific reasoning, with more specific details included. In the typical problem-solving processes, a problem situation is recognized, pertinent facts and information are gathered (analysis), key issues are defined, alternative options for action are generated, a decision is made as to the best option, action is implemented, and finally the entire process is evaluated. Numerous frameworks for ethical decision making have been put forth and for our purposes, we will present two of them, one by Purtilo (2005) and the other by Morris (2003). Both have common elements and draw from basic problem-solving strategies.

Purtilo (2005) identifies a "Six-Step Process" for ethical decision making. These five steps include the following:

1. Gather relevant information
2. Identify the type of ethical problem
3. Use ethics theories or approaches to analyze the problem(s)
4. Explore the practical alternatives
5. Complete the action
6. Evaluate the process and outcome

Using your knowledge of the basic ethical principles, the major ethics theories, and the *Occupational Therapy Code of Ethics* (AOTA, 2005), will make this six-step process relatively easy to use. The first step of *gathering relevant information* means examining the facts of the situation as to clinical indications, client preferences, quality of life, and external factors such as policies and reimbursement issues. In step 2, you *identify the type of ethical problem* and decide what moral issues are at stake: autonomy, beneficence, nonmaleficence, justice, veracity, fidelity, confidentiality. You also need to think about the possible consequences. In step 3, you engage in *weighing the moral issues and principles* as they relate to potential consequences, considering the teleological and deontological theories, as well as the *Occupational Therapy Code of Ethics*. Step 4 is where you *explore all strategies and options* as creatively and openly as possible. It helps to be able to discuss this with other students or therapists to identify numerous alternatives that are practical. In step 5 you must *select a solution and develop a strategy* for acting or carrying it out. If you don't act, the whole process is but a mere intellectual exercise. Step 5 is the most difficult, for as you remember with Rest's four-component model, it takes courage, strength, perseverance, and skill to implement ethical actions. In Step 6, it is important to look back and examine the process and action you took in order to learn from the experience. Read through the Case Study below to see an example of how this framework might be applied to a real-life clinical issue.

CASE STUDY 8-2

Who Does Dysphagia?

José is an occupational therapist who works in a pediatric hospital and has met the California advanced practice requirements for dysphagia. Recently, José has noticed that speech language pathologists (SLPs) who do not have specialty or advanced dysphagia training often contradict the OTs in documentation, resulting in embarrassing and sometimes unsafe practices for the children. The newly hired OT manager, who does not have expertise in this practice area, met with the SLP director (without the OT's support) and has agreed to remove OTs from modified barium swallow studies (MBS), and has directed them to discharge dysphagia patients. These patients then got MBS studies and were referred to SLPs.

Applying the Purtilo process for analyzing ethical issues, the first step would be to gather and examine objective facts. This could include the competency and qualifications of both OTs and SLPs in the specialty area of dysphagia, the needs of the patients for these services, frequency of referrals for dysphagia services and response time, reimbursement considerations, etc. Step 2 would identify whether this is an ethical dilemma and what type. In this case, ethical principles at stake might include beneficence (doing good), nonmaleficence, and duty (competence). Are the therapists who provide services competent (or the most competent) to do so to ensure that the patients are likely to benefit and, equally important, not to incur harm? Are there adequate resources (highly competent therapists) available to meet the demand for services in a timely manner to ensure that maximum benefit is achieved? In step 3, consider which ethics approach is most appropriate (teleological, deontological). In this case, the end goal of ensuring appropriate, competent care and protecting patients from harm seems clear. Therefore, step 4 requires identification and consideration of options to achieve that goal. These may include developing or revising dysphagia protocols including clinical competencies for practitioners. It may involve training programs and continuing education to ensure an adequate number of qualified therapists to meet the demand for services in a timely way. If OT and SLP department managers cannot agree on a clinically appropriate plan, it may involve soliciting support from higher levels of hospital administration. The critical step 5 is to select the most appropriate plan for the situation and to act on it. As previously stated, thinking about and analyzing ethical issues is an important exercise but does not bring about a change in behavior without action. Also, keep in mind there may well be additional relevant considerations in each of these steps.

Morris (2003) offers a similar model for ethical decision making but one that emphasizes the achievement of consensus among key players, which is assuring that all involved parties can accept and live with the decision. Again, the most important and difficult piece of the ethical reasoning process is following through on the decision made. "Knowing what is right and doing what is right are two different things" (Morris, 2003, p. 58).

The four major components of the Morris (2003) model for ethical decision making are:

1. Identification of the ethical dilemma
2. Analysis
3. Evaluation
4. Consensus for action

The first component involves identifying the relevant facts, values, and beliefs; the key people involved; and stating the dilemma clearly. The second component, analysis, focuses on possible courses of action and the conflicts that may arise from each, thus, beginning to see what actions are reasonable, practical, or viable. In the evaluation component, one proposes potential courses of action as they relate to ethical principles, the OT Code of Ethics, social roles, and self-interests. Finally, whether to proceed or not depends on whether the selected action leads to consensus. Without consensus, the decision will not be supported and one must return to analysis (Morris, 2003).

If the example in Case Study 8-2 involving dysphagia treatment were analyzed using the Morris model, most of the same elements would be considered. The main difference would be the focus on consensus as the last step in resolution using the Morris process. In this case, if there was no agreement to take on the proposed actions, such as treatment protocol with competencies and competencies to increase the number of qualified personnel, then the practitioners involved would need to re-analyze the situation and seek additional solutions. It is hoped that the group could agree on one of the alternatives to resolve the dilemma. Also, keep in mind that if this is an ethical issue only for the OT with advanced dysphagia training, resolution will be more difficult as he may face a challenging personal decision about whether to continue to work in the setting. See Box 8-3 for a guide to ethical decision making that blends and builds on the Purtilo and Morris models.

BOX 8-3
Guide for Ethical Decision Making

1. Identify the Ethical Dilemma

What are the relevant facts, values and beliefs?
Who are the key people involved?
What key ethical principles are involved?
State the dilemma clearly (legal, ethical, medical).

2. Analyze Options and Conflicts

What are the possible courses of action?
What ethical approach should you use?
What are the conflicts that could arise from each action?

3. Evaluate Proposed Course of Action

Does action address relevant ethical principles?
Is action consistent with the profession's Code of Ethics?
How does action impact social roles and self interests of people involved?

4. Does the Proposed Course of Action Lead to Consensus?

How well is the action supported by those affected?

5. Select A Plan and Implement It

Act on your decision

6. Reflection on Action

What action was taken?
What were the outcomes, both expected and unexpected?
How well did the action address the moral dilemma?

Adapted from Purtilo (2005), Morris (2003), and the authors' perspectives.

ETHICAL REASONING IN PRACTICE

It would be inaccurate to relegate ethical thinking only to the larger societal issues and debates of today like cloning, transplants, stem cell research, and end-of-life issues, to name a few. As work settings for occupational therapy practitioners become increasingly diverse, encounters with realistic implications of societal and policy issues, become more frequent and evident. For example, recall the concerns described in Chapter 7 when state policies and procedures for payment of early intervention services resulted in extensive state-wide discussion of the implications. Based on our experiences working with ethics groups within occupational therapy, questions from clinicians most often, in fact, revolve around the common "day to day" things that elicit ethical tensions. It is important to recognize and use the resources that are available.

Students and practitioners at all levels can benefit from increased education in ethics. Consultation with individuals who can assist in reflecting on issues from a broad range of perspectives and evaluate the options and outcomes that may result from their decisions also helps the practitioner. In facilities where they exist, ethics committees can play a valuable role in clarifying ethical dilemmas and identifying strategies that are viable in that particular setting. In addition to external resources, support and discussion are often available within a department from colleagues and supervisors. More recently, however, the frequent lack of consistent clinical supervision and staffing pattern mix of per diem and part time staff does not lend itself to a cohesive group or environment conducive to such discussions (Horowitz, 2002). Further, practitioners in community-based, private practice, and school systems may have fewer resources for professional feedback. Regardless, the complexity of these issues requires that practitioners seek assistance to ensure that they understand the breadth of the situation and the range of options (and consequences) to address them appropriately.

Thinking About Thinking 8-2

Who can protest and does not, is an accomplice in the act.

—Talmud, 1st through 5th centuries CE

The importance of taking action (and the courage to do so) to be a true moral agent cannot be underestimated. Yet actions have consequences and may have unintended or negative repercussions. A striking example of this may involve *whistleblowers*, or those people who make public unethical conduct in systems and organizations. We have said that ethical practitioners have a moral obligation to do what is best for their patient and prevent or avoid harm. A clinical situation may arise in which the practitioner witnesses harm or at least intervention that does not benefit a patient. From an ethical perspective, adherence to professional ethical standards is an obligation. For example, in the United States, the *Occupational Therapy Code of Ethics*, (AOTA, 2005), the core value of truth (AOTA, 1993), being faithful to facts and reality as they pertain to themselves and recipients of their services, all serve to underpin ethical reasoning. Yet, for whistleblowers, these expectations can be a burden as well and certainly present ethical dilemmas. In the purest sense, whistleblowers attempt to correct a wrong or expose an abuse in the system. In doing so, they may face inappropriate retaliation at many levels including demotion, loss of a job, and harassment. In some cases, laws regarding mandatory reporting of abuse may apply. However, there are also statutory protections for whistleblowers, and when accusations are based on proven objective facts, they may end up being rewarded for their integrity. On the other hand, whistle blowing may be done for self-serving reasons including retaliation for a perceived slight. However, in general, society's attitude toward whistleblowers is positive, acknowledging the personal difficulty and risk of exposing a negative situation (Bailey & Schwartzberg, 2003).

Analysis of ethical dilemmas must consider any and all outcomes and weigh them prior to action. A risk-benefit analysis would be appropriate in many circumstances. In some cases an individual may feel so strongly about an action that he/she is willing to deal with major confrontation and the possible loss of job. This may require great personal soul-searching and weighing of motivations. Other individuals feel most comfortable with a compromise that achieves adequate action to make them and the other parties feel comfortable with consensus—a decision with which the key players can live (Morris, 2003).

In today's practice environments, therapists must consider not only the client's values and their own, but also the culture and values of their organization. Organizations may have a public mission that supports an ethical culture but may enact policies and procedures that reflect a strong business orientation with the heavy influence of reimbursement on clinical decision making. The fiscal realities of capitation and prospective payment systems and regulatory policies cannot be ignored if healthcare institutions are to continue to exist. Therapists often find themselves caught in an ethical no man's land, trying to meet the directives of the organization, the needs of the patient and their own professional ethics and values. In fact, the realities of conflicting priorities often get played out at the clinical staff level on a day-to-day basis. Decisions about how to allocate scarce resources in the most equitable way can challenge clinicians to balance "principles of justice and equity for needy patients, principles of fidelity (faithfulness) to colleagues and employers, and the principles of veracity (honesty) and beneficence (bringing about good) in relationships with patients and families" (Horowitz, 2002, p. 10). This can create a great source of angst and frustration. An example may be in an inpatient rehabilitation facility (IRF) where admissions must consist of 75% patients who fall into one of 13 diagnostic categories. To keep beds full and maintain status as an IRF, the facility admits many patients from an acute care referral hospital who are already independent. Therapists are instructed to "be more creative" and define goals for these patients who would more appropriately be serviced in home care settings. In this situation, therapists know they are not providing a skilled service that benefits the patient and therefore stand to violate Medicare rules, ethical principles, and legal statutes with potential fraudulent billing.

In addition to ethical dilemmas resulting from questionable administrative directives, which do not benefit clients but may in fact do harm (nonmaleficence), other dilemmas can arise from ambiguities around scope of practice.

Licensure laws often do not contain specific language to provide guidance in these situations. Sometimes, an occupational therapy practitioner is directed to provide an intervention that he/she may not be competent to perform or does not relate to the occupational performance focus of the profession or that is not appropriate for the client's clinical status but is reimbursable. In some cases, the fact that a practitioner "can" do something does not mean it "should" be done. The practitioner may not have the knowledge and skills, or the intervention itself may be inappropriate for the patient clinically or otherwise. Any number of reasons may apply. Official documents including standards of practice, licensure laws, and ethical codes, such as the *Occupational Therapy Code of Ethics* (AOTA, 2005) may provide objective language to support decisions.

Confusion sometimes exists between the ethical and legal aspects of a particular dilemma. Actions may be legal, but may not be ethical. Legal precedents may render some decisions right, but from an ethical standpoint, they may not be the best decision to meet the client's interests or needs. For example, in many states occupational therapy practitioners may use physical agent modalities as part of their legal scope of practice. However, these modalities are not generally part of the OT curricula, so practitioners who use them must, according to the ethical principle of duty, obtain continuing education to achieve clinical competence.

A different example may involve work relationships. For instance, consider a small therapy company that contracted therapists out to a local skilled nursing facility (SNF). The owner of the practice was notified that the SNF was ending their contract. Shortly thereafter, an employee of the contract company resigned and the owner found out that she had taken a job as an employee of the SNF. Since the practice owner did not have an employment contract with a non-compete clause, the employees were legally free to leave and work for the competition, even though this would not be perceived as professional.

Some situations have both legal and ethical implications. For example, a school-based occupational therapist signed a contract for the 9-month school year. Four months into the school year, the therapist got a terrific job offer. She decided to resign and take the new job. Because of the shortage of therapists, the school is unable to find an OT to replace her; consequently, the children at the original school do not receive the therapy services they are legally entitled to in their IEP. Although it is legal in the state to break a contract, there are ethical implications related to veracity and nonmaleficence, as well as professional duty.

The law is based on the principle of justice, and there is no scientific right or wrong answer; rather, one must weigh the equities of each argument. Society is governed by rules and regulations compiled through court decisions, state and federal statutes, and regulations and procedures. Thus, interpretations of laws may lead to different conclusions in what appear to be similar situations, depending on the circumstances of the case and the views of the judge (Bailey & Schwartzberg, 2003). Laws tell us what we shouldn't do; ethics give us standards to live by. Careful understanding of the difference between ethical and legal actions thus becomes important to occupational therapists.

Another tool that can be helpful to students and practitioners is a framework for reasoning around ethical and scope of practice questions or directives (Slater, 2004). See Box 8-4 for self-reflection questions that can help one decide whether therapy options are within your scope of practice.

> **BOX 8-4**
> ## Reflections on Scope of Practice: Is This Something I Should Do?
>
> - Was this body of knowledge part of my educational curriculum?
> - Am I competent to provide this intervention based on my entry-level education or current or continuing education?
> - Is my knowledge in this area current and adequate to provide competent services?
> - Is this intervention or practice usual and customary among occupational therapy practitioners, and would most of them agree? If not, is it defensible and consistent with the occupational therapy scope of practice?
> - Have I sought clarification from the state licensure board in interpreting less well-defined areas of the occupational therapy scope of practice?
> - Have I sought official resources from my professional organization, such as position papers or official documents relating to this area of practice?
> - Have I done a literature search on this topic and does it provide evidence for my practice interventions?
> - Is this occupational therapy? How does this relate to the philosophy of occupational therapy? Am I using occupation to promote engagement in meaningful activities and participation in life roles?
>
> From Slater (2004). Used with permission of AOTA.

In practice, situations of ethical unease can arise quickly and need resolution just as quickly. Students or practitioners may be challenged or observe an uncomfortable event, demanding they use their ethical reasoning at an accelerated pace. They will then need to take action and anticipate and be prepared for any number of outcomes. Good decision making requires that the practitioner has anticipated these scenarios, has played out alternatives and their likely results, and has the language and objective facts to support choices for action.

STUDIES IN APPLICATION OF ETHICAL REASONING

There are numerous descriptive articles related to methods for teaching ethics and ethical decision making in occupational therapy practice (Barnitt, 1993); Haddad, 1988; Horowitz, 2002; Kanny & Kyler, 1999; Kyler, 1998; Wood et al., 2000). There have also been several studies related to ethics education in occupational therapy, which surprisingly found no significant increases in the level of ethical reasoning of occupational therapy students as a result of their professional education (Barnitt, 1993; Dieruf, 2004; Greene, 1997; Hansen, 1984; Kanny, 1996; Wittman, 1990). However, no research found to date specifically addresses how occupational therapists apply ethical reasoning effectively to actual practice dilemmas. Therefore, we will discuss research on applied ethical reasoning in other professions and offer suggestions for future research within occupational therapy.

Rest and Narvaez (1994) describe and summarize results of applied ethics studies conducted in the professions of college teaching, nursing, school teaching, counseling, accounting, dentistry, medicine, veterinary medicine, and journalism. This research demonstrates that gains in ethical reasoning are most affected by formal education (Rest & Narvaez, 1994). Rest (1988, 1994; Rest & Narvaez, 1994) hypothesizes that the reason for this is that individuals who go on for higher education love to learn, enjoy intellectual stimulation, are more involved in their communities, and take more interest in larger societal issues. He cautions, however, that reasoning at a higher Kohlberg stage should not be interpreted to mean that these individuals have more intelligence, but rather that they have better conceptual tools for making sense out of the world and decision making. Thus, individuals who demonstrate higher levels of moral reasoning abilities may be more able to think critically (problem solve) and see what might be best for individuals and society as a whole (Rest, 1994).

Physical therapy (PT) research has addressed how therapists make moral decisions. In 1992, Davis conducted qualitative research with thirteen physical therapists ranging in age from 29 to 59 years and with 3 to 30 years experience in various practice settings (Davis, 2005). Participants were asked to talk about a time when they felt "stopped" from moving forward in their work, which facilitated talk of a moral dilemma. Taped interviews were transcribed and analyzed. It was found that before taking action, half of the therapists used the utilitarian approach to ethical reasoning ("do what is best for the patient") and the other half considered ethical principles. What Davis (2005) found to be most surprising was that the therapists did not consult the PT Code of Ethics or colleagues, but rather used their own inner values to decide what was best to do. In another study conducted by Wise in 2000, 10 physical therapists were interviewed about how they solved ethical dilemmas (Davis, 2005). Analysis revealed a process that included identifying the problem, weighing the contextual factors, gathering and sharing information with colleagues and APTA Code of Ethics, problem solving, deciding and acting, and then reflecting. Subjects in this study also made decisions based on their values and morals learned early in life. Wise (2000) emphasized the use of an "ethics of care" over reasoning, going on to describe this as having a basis in emotional and relationship reasons for acting. Davis (2005) concludes from both these studies that data show that when making ethical decisions, physical therapists "tend to emphasize the importance of an ethic of care over rule-based problem solving, and also that they tend to place highest emphasis on values instilled in them at a young age" (p. 222). Thus, she sees engagement as the key to developing moral behaviors in adults. Educators "must commit not just to influencing our students to act with moral courage, we must inspire them to it. . .it must be modeled" (Davis, 2005, p. 224).

A study was conducted to describe and compare how occupational and physical therapists describe ethical dilemmas (Barnitt & Partridge, 1997). Eight OTs and eight PTs were asked to analyze transcripts of interviews involving ethical dilemmas. Results showed differing reasoning styles in physical therapists and occupational therapists. Physical therapists were more likely to use a diagnostic or procedural style and occupational therapists the narrative style. The reasoning style of therapists was affected by the context of the dilemma, where it occurred, the work group, the patient group, and the hierarchical relationships within the organization. Factors identified by therapists as having a negative influence on solving ethical dilemmas included uncertainty of outcome, emotional aspects of event, and social pressure from peers to behave in a certain way. Factors identified as having a positive influence on dealing with ethical dilemmas were experience with similar dilemmas, time for reflection, and peer support (Barnitt & Partridge, 1997).

So what kind of research is needed in helping us to understand the process that occupational therapists use in ethical reasoning? We think it is useful to go back to Rest's Four-Component Model and recommend studies that address how moral sensitivity, moral judgment, and moral motivation impact an individual's moral character (the ability and courage to act on moral decisions). This means studying each component as a predictor of behavior. We need qualitative and quantitative studies focusing on practitioners thinking and processing (sensitivity, judgment), as well as their motivation and ability to take action. We also need to know what learning experiences result in effective ethical reasoning and lead to moral action. This provides information that will help us educate both occupational therapy students and practitioners in their role as moral agents. After all, what benefit is ethics education if it does not bring about gains in real-life behavior?

SUMMARY

Fulfilling the moral imperative of acting in our clients' best interest requires competency in the ethical reasoning process. Ethical dilemmas can be challenging to identify and complex to analyze. In some cases, the options to resolve them may be less than optimal so evaluation of likely consequences is an important part of the process. Knowledge and skills acquired through relevant literature, ethics committees, professional resources and documents, and members of the healthcare team are essential to attain these competencies. Skill in ethical reasoning helps a therapist be more reflective, thus enhancing thinking and decision making in all aspects of professional reasoning. The process of developing these skills is one of maturation, professional growth, experience, and, in the end, having the moral courage to take action (see the quotation from Eleanor Roosevelt earlier in the chapter). During this lengthy process, focusing on the client as the central figure in this process will help ground ethical decision making. Finally, the link between thinking and taking action is critical. Growth in knowledge and skills is meaningful only if higher-level ethical reasoning is used to bring about a positive change in behavior.

LEARNING ACTIVITY 8-1

Explaining Clinical Reasoning

Purpose

To clarify one's personal values affecting ethical reasoning, and to explore the impact of these on actual common ethical dilemmas which may be encountered in practice

Connections to Major Clinical Reasoning Constructs

Provides opportunity for using ethical reasoning framework and practicing ethical reasoning

Directions for Learners

1 Divide into groups of three to five to discuss each case study.
2 Using the Guide for Ethical Decision Making provided in this chapter as a resource, answer all of the questions and come to a decision as to the action to be taken. Then select two people in your group to role play; one will take the role of the person taking ethical action and talking directly to the other person regarding his/her ethical stance. The other group members will be observers and provide feedback. Feel free to switch roles and practice role-playing ethical action dialogue as each of you may have different approaches for talking it through.

CASE STUDY 8-3

Sure You Can Do It!

Josh is an occupational therapist working in an outpatient clinic. The physical therapist certified in lymphedema management has resigned and there is no plan to replace her. Josh's manager has requested that he start treating patients who require lower extremity lymphedema treatment. Josh took a continuing education course related to lymphedema about 5 years ago and has used the techniques occasionally with upper extremity patients who present with this condition. However, he is not certified and has never worked with patients who need lower extremity lymphedema management. Josh is being pressured to "step up to the plate" since, in his manager's eyes, he has skills and the manager sees upper extremity and lower extremity interventions as interchangeable.

Questions

1 What factors are important to consider in making this decision?
2 With whom should Josh discuss this?
3 What resources should he use?
4 What ethical principles are at stake?

CASE STUDY 8-4

Creativity or Fraud?

Susan is an employee of a contract therapy service who works for a skilled nursing facility (SNF). The SNF is reimbursed under the Prospective Payment System (PPS). The contract therapy company always promises the facility that they will maximize revenue through provision of rehabilitation services. In fact, the program manager (not a therapist), has instructed Susan to categorize all patients into the high and ultra-high RUGS (resource utilization group) category. This requires that patients receive a certain number hours of therapy and frequency between OT, PT and speech therapies per 7-day period. This arbitrary categorization may be based solely on the patient's diagnosis and the company's revenue targets. Susan is finding that many patients are elderly and have been discharged from the acute care setting after 3 days and are unable to tolerate intensive therapy on a daily schedule. In addition, she is challenged about discharging patients when they have achieved their goals, even if they are independent. Therapists are being told to be "more creative" and find reasons to keep patients in therapy until the rehabilitation manager approves discharge orders. Susan is conflicted by these directives. She thinks these decisions may not be in the patients' best interests based on appropriate professional judgment, but rather based on administrator desires to maximize reimbursement.

Questions

1 What ethical principles may be violated in the AOTA Occupational Therapy Code of Ethics and why? (Note, for readers outside the United States, substitute appropriate professional code.)
2 Are there other legal or ethical issues that may be relevant to this situation?
3 What strategies might Susan use to address these situations that will benefit her patients, reflect her professional ethics, and allow her to feel comfortable?

CASE STUDY 8-5

She's Cheating. . . I Think

Three students are having lunch together, and the topic of the test in one of their occupational therapy classes comes up. After some hesitation, one of the students says she thinks she saw Jennifer, one of her classmates, looking at another student's test. The other two chime in, with sighs of relief, saying "I've seen the same thing, but have been afraid to mention it to anyone." As they continue talking, they begin to feel uncomfortable and even a bit angry. Melissa says, "maybe someone should know about this and do something about the situation." Christine wonders if maybe they should talk to Jennifer and ask her about it. All three students are becoming more uneasy and conflicted about the situation as they talk about what to do. They don't want to report a fellow student, but at the same time think this could be serious and that something should probably be done. However, they share that maybe they are misjudging her and should just watch to see if it happens again. But what are the future implications for her career as an occupational therapist?

Questions

1 What are the ethical issues here?
2 Should the students talk to their classmate they suspect of cheating, or should they go to a faculty member about the situation?
3 What options for action do the students have?

CASE STUDY 8-6

Can We Date?

Megan is a fieldwork II student at a psychiatric outpatient clinic in a small town. She is an excellent student and is working independently as a therapy group leader by the second month in the placement. She and her occupational therapy supervisor get along quite well and she is comfortable in being open about her feelings with her supervisor.

Matthew, a 25-year-old weather announcer from a local television station is admitted for acute situational depression related to several crises in his life. In the last 6 months, both his grandfather and mother died, his grandfather of a long-term illness and his mother from acute leukemia. He has been experiencing increased stress on the job and feels overwhelmed at work. Matthew was placed in the therapy group in which Megan is co-leader with the psychologist.

After about 2 weeks, Megan confided to the supervising occupational thera-pist that she was very attracted to Matthew and that he has been flirting with her. They discussed the importance of upholding a professional client–therapist rela-tionship and nothing more was said. During the next 2 weeks, Matthew continues to progress well in therapy and was scheduled to be discharged in a week. At this time, Megan decides to go out with him to a local movie, at which the supervising OT sees her. Megan has 3 more weeks remaining on her fieldwork placement.

Questions

1 What are the ethical issues here?
2 What should the occupational therapy supervisor do?
3 Are the actions of the student within professional boundaries?

REFERENCES

American Occupational Therapy Association (2005). Occupational therapy code of ethics. *American Journal of Occupational Therapy, 59,* 639–641.

American Occupational Therapy Association (1993). Core values and attitudes of occupational ther-apy practice. *American Journal of Occupational Therapy, 47,* 1085–1086.

Bailey, D. M. & Schwartzberg, S. L. (2003). *Ethical and legal dilemmas* (2nd ed.). Philadelphia: F. A. Davis.

Barnitt, R. E. (1993). Deeply troubling questions: The teaching of ethics in undergraduate courses. *British Journal of Occupational Therapy, 56,* 401–406.

Barnitt, R. & Partridge, C. (1997). Ethical reasoning in physical therapy and occupational therapy. *Physiotherapy Research International, 2*(3), 178–194.

Beauchamp, T. L. & Childress, J. F. (1989). *Principles of biomedical ethics.* New York: Oxford University Press.

Beilin, H. & Pufall, P. (1992). *Piaget's theory: Prospects and possibilities.* Hillsdale, NJ: Lawrence Erlbaum Associates.

Chazan, B. (1985). *Contemporary approaches to moral education: Analyzing alternative theories.* New York: Teachers College Press.

Davis, C. M. (2005). Educating adult health professionals for moral action: In search of moral courage. In Purtilo, R. B., Jensen, G. M., & Royeen, C. B. (Eds.), *Educating for moral action: A sourcebook in health and rehabilitation ethics.* Philadelphia: F. A. Davis.

Dewey, J. (1909*). Moral principles in education.* Boston: Houghton Mifflin.

Dewey, J. (1965). Reflective morality and ethical theory. In R. Ekamm (Ed.), *The nature of moral theory,* New York: Charles Scribner's.

Dierf K. (2004). Ethical decision-making by students in physical and occupational therapy. *Journal of Allied Health,* 33(1), 24–30.

Flavell, J. H. (1963). *The developmental psychology of Jean Piaget.* New York: D. Van Nostrand.

Gilligan, Carol (1982). *In a different voice: Psychological theory and women's development.* Cambridge, MA: Harvard University.

Gilligan, Carol (1993). *In a different voice: Psychological theory and women's development.* Cambridge, MA: Harvard University.

Greene, D. (1997). The use of service learning in client environments to enhance ethical reasoning in students. *American Journal of Occupational Therapy,* 51(10), 844–852.

Haddad, A. M. (1988). Teaching ethical analysis in occupational therapy. *American Journal of Occupational Therapy,* 42, 300–304.

Hansen, R. A. (1984). Moral reasoning of occupational therapists: Implications for education and practice. Doctoral dissertation. Detroit, MI: Wayne State University.

Hansen, R. A. (2003). Ethics in occupational therapy. In E. B. Crepeau, E. C. Cohn & B. A. Boyt Schell (Eds.), *Willard and Spackman's occupational therapy* (10th ed., pp. 953–961). Philadelphia: J. B. Lippincott.

Horowitz, B. P. (2002). Ethical decision-making challenges in clinical practice. *Occupational Therapy in Health Care,* 16(4), 1–13.

Kanny, E. M. (2000). Guiding ethics for professionalism. In J. Kasar & N. Clark (Eds.), *Developing professional behaviors.* Thorofare, NJ: Slack.

Kanny, E. M. (1996). Occupational therapists' ethical reasoning: Assessing student and practitioner responses to ethical dilemmas. (Doctoral dissertation, University of Washington, 1996). University Microfilms, 1490 Eisenhower Place, P.O. Box 975, Ann Arbor, MI, 48106.

Kanny, E. M. & Kyler, P. L. (1999). Are faculty prepared to address ethical issues in education? *American Journal of Occupational Therapy,* 53(1), 72–74.

Kyler, P. (1998, April 2). The merger of clinical and ethical competence. *OT Week,* 12, 22–23.

Kohlberg, L. (1984). *Essays on moral development, volume II: The psychology of moral development.* San Francisco: Harper & Row.

Morris, J. F. (2003). Is it possible to be ethical? In J. B. Scott (Ed.), *Reference guide to the occupational therapy code of ethics.* Bethesda: AOTA Press.

Opacich, K. J. (2003). Ethical dimensions of occupational therapy management. In McCormack, Jaffe, Goodman-Lavey (Eds.), *The occupational therapy manager.* Rockville, MD: American Occupational Therapy Association.

Philips, John L. Jr. (1969). *The origins of intellect: Piaget's theory* (2nd ed.). San Francisco: W. H. Freeman and Company.

Purtilo, R. B. (2005). *Ethical dimensions in the health professions* (4th ed.). Philadelphia: Elsevier.

Rest, J. R. (1979). *Development in judging moral issues.* Minneapolis: University of Minnesota Press.

Rest, J. R. (1983). Morality. In J. H. Flavell, E. M. Markman & P. H. (Eds.), *Cognitive development* (4th ed.). New York: Wiley & Sons.

Rest, J. R. (1986). *Moral development: Advances in research and theory.* New York: Praeger.

Rest, J. R. (1988). Why does college promote development in moral judgment? *Journal of Moral Education,* 17(3), 183–194.

Rest, J. R. (1994). Background: Theory and research. In *Moral development in the professions.* Hillsdale, NJ: Lawrence Erlbaum Associates.

Rest, J. R. & Narvaez, D. (Eds.) (1994). *Moral development in the professions.* Hillsdale, NJ: Lawrence Erlbaum Associates.

Roosevelt, Eleanor (August 7, 1941). My day. Newspaper column.

Slater, D. Y. (September 6, 2004). Legal and ethical practice: A professional responsibility. *OT Practice,* 1–4.

Talmud. First to Fifth Centuries C.E.

Veatch, R. M. & Flack, H. E. (1997). *Case studies in allied health ethics.* Upper Saddle River, NJ: Prentice Hall.

Wittman, P. P. (1990). Cognitive developmental level and clinical behaviors in occupational therapy students: An exploratory investigation. (Doctoral Dissertation, North Carolina State University, 1990).

Wood, W., Nielson, C., Humphry, R., Coppola, S., Baranek, G. & Rourk, J. (2000). A curricular renaissance: Graduate education centered on occupation. *American Journal of Occupational Therapy,* 54, 586–597.

Interactive and Conditional Reasoning: A Process of Synthesis

Barbara A. Boyt Schell

OBJECTIVES

After reading this chapter, the learner will be able to:

1 Explain the reasoning that therapists use to guide interactions with clients.
2 Recognize the effect that both verbal and nonverbal behavior may have on the therapist-client relationship.
3 Explore the links among personal development, theoretical perspectives, power and practice culture as they relate to interactive reasoning.
4 Describe the concept of conditional reasoning and explain its role in both short- and long-term intervention planning.

KEY TERMS

Interactive reasoning
Intrapersonal intelligence

Interpersonal intelligence
Conditional reasoning

I t should be clear by now that clinical or professional reasoning is a complex process, which involves attention to a variety of factors. Fleming (1991) stated this well when she summarized findings from her work with Mattingly: "Eventually, we realized that the therapist-subjects attend to the patient on three levels: (a) the physical ailment, (b) the patient as a person, and (c) the person as a social being in the context of family, environment, and culture" (Fleming, p.1007).

Fleming went on to identify this phenomenon as the "therapist with the three-track mind" (1991, p. 1008). Earlier chapters in this unit build on the idea of multiple tracks of thinking, each of which serves to help therapists attend to different ways of thinking about therapy. Therapists reason about their clients' health problems, the impact of these problems in clients' lives, and the practical and ethical factors that guide therapy decisions. Therapists take a logical or objective stance when seeking to understand a person's health condition and potential to benefit from intervention. They move to narrative modes of thinking when attempting to understand the subjective experience of the health condition to the person and those who are important to the client. On top of all this, therapists have to negotiate on behalf of clients to obtain needed resources and to select among possible therapy options those that fit the practice setting as well as their own skill set. Finally, therapists must use ethical judgment when faced with therapy situations in which there are competing issues to address and when it is not clear which will promote the most good or minimize harm most effectively. This chapter focuses on how therapists integrate and use these varying ways of thinking about practice.

Thinking About Thinking 9-1

The difference between listening and pretending to listen, I discovered, is enormous. . . Real listening is a willingness to let the other person change you. When I'm willing to let them change me, something happens between us that's more interesting than dueling monologues. Like so much of what I learned in the theater, this turned out to be how life works, too.

—Alan Alda, 2005, p. 160

The first part of this chapter addresses the interpersonal processes that are required to move therapists' reasoning to effective action in each therapy encounter. In Chapter 6, Narrative Reasoning, Hamilton provided extensive examples on the importance of understanding each therapy situation as part of an unfolding story. Here, we look at **interactive reasoning,** which is used to make and sustain the human connections that are the lynchpin of the therapy process. Interactive reasoning is necessary for obtaining narratives and information on the person's health condition, as well as for encouraging clients as their lives shift in light of the therapy process. Skilled therapists are very mindful of what and how they are communicating, even though it is in many ways a very automatic process. Interactive reasoning requires a synthesis in the "here and now" of scientific, narrative, pragmatic, and ethical knowledge, which is then transformed into skillful communication acts. Obviously, there are both verbal and nonverbal aspects to this process. Readers are encouraged to reflect back on the information provided in Chapter 4 about the embodied nature of practice as we explore the use of both words and gestures as therapy acts.

As more expert therapists communicate with their clients, they may do so in light of how the clients' health and performance might unfold over their lives. This requires the construction of trajectories to guide the overall therapy process as well as to predict different possible occupational performance outcomes. These mental roadmaps are based on therapists' combined understanding of the client's health condition, anticipated developmental changes, and life story, along with practical supports and constraints. As discussed in Chapter 2, this sort of expertise typically requires extensive experience and reflection. **Conditional reasoning** is the term used to describe the process of imagining the longer trajectories needed to anticipate the future. The latter part of this chapter discusses examples of conditional reasoning. In both current interactions and longer term predictions, therapists weave together and shift among their various "tracks" of thinking to respond to the demands of each therapy situation.

REASONING AS AN INTERPERSONAL PROCESS

There is a long history in occupational therapy literature dealing with the interpersonal aspects of the therapeutic process. In the founding years, Meyer commented that "It takes rare gifts and talents and rare personalities to be real pathfinders in this work" (1922, 1977, p. 641). Decades later, Yerxa (1967) emphasized the importance of personal and professional authenticity in entering into "*mutual* relation with the client" (1967, p. 8). This aspect of reasoning seems to rely on personal intelligences such as those described by Howard Gardner (2004) (discussed in Chapter 4). Two of those types of intelligence are specifically related to aspects of personal aptitudes. The first is **intrapersonal intelligence,** which relates to a person's capacity to "access one's own feeling life" and to ultimately draw upon these feelings as a "means of understanding and guiding one's behavior" (p. 239). In contrast to the inward focus of *intra*personal intelligence is **interpersonal intelligence,** which is directed outward to other individuals. Interpersonal intelligence is the "ability to notice and make distinctions among other individuals, and in particular, among their moods, temperaments, motivations, and intentions" (p. 239).

The ability to build and maintain effective therapy relationships is especially critical in occupational therapy because occupational therapy involves "doing with" as opposed to "doing to" clients (Mattingly & Fleming, 1994, p. 178) Mattingly and Fleming labeled the thinking associated with building client collaboration "interactive reasoning" (1994, p. 196). Practitioners must gain the trust of their clients and of those persons important in their world. Peloquin (1990, 1993a, 1993b) convincingly argues the importance of the relationship as a critical component of the therapy process, noting that:

> The therapist brings to each exchange some understanding, or vision, of what a therapeutic relationship (and perhaps what a "good patient") should be, and the patient brings needs, memories of past experiences, and expectations of how a helpful caregiver should behave. The exchange of needs, visions, and expectations helps to shape the image that each person will hold of the other (Peloquin, 1990, p. 13).

Interactive reasoning represents a potent mix of intra- and interpersonal skills. Research to date shows some recurring communicative acts that reflect attention to client interaction. In the next section are examples of how communicative acts or strategies are observed as therapists appear to exercise their interactive reasoning abilities.

ACTS OF COMMUNICATION TO PROMOTE INTERACTION

A number of studies of clinical reasoning surface on the ways in which occupational therapists build rapport with their clients using both verbal and nonverbal communicative strategies (Alnervik & Svidén, 1996; Mattingly & Fleming, 1994; Kautzman, 1993; Peloquin,1990; Schwartzberg, 2002) . There are likewise many examples of successful and unsuccessful attempts to build relationships with clients. For example, in Burke's (1997) study of therapists evaluating young children, she records the thoughts of a therapist who was grappling with the communicative aspects of the therapy session (see Case Study 9-1 below).

CASE STUDY 9 - 1

Stabbing in the Dark

I kept stabbing the dark. I felt ineffective. I felt really lost. I couldn't read this mom's cues. I don't know if I didn't explain what therapy was. I usually find people. I don't know what I didn't do for her.

What can I do to engage her? What is her affect—is something else going on? Where is the husband in all this? Can I get her down on the floor?

Should I go up to her eye level? She kept the other baby in her arms and didn't make eye contact. She kept the other baby on her lap, like she was protected by her. I felt there was a fence between us and I couldn't tear it down. Usually, I can find a way. She didn't lay out anything for me. (Burke, 1997, p.101)

Although the therapist is being very self-critical, notice all the strategies she considers in trying to build a better connection with the mother: reading cues, explaining therapy, changing her body position, getting the mother to change her body position, acknowledging the mother's behaviors and how they impacted building a relationship.

Langthaler, a graduate student of Fleming's found hundreds of "subtle and obvious behaviors" when she examined short video segments from a therapy session with a physically disabled client; Bradburn, another graduate student, was able to surface multiple strategies used by two therapists working with psychiatric patients (both cited in Mattingly & Fleming, 1994, p.194-196) . *Table 9-1* summarizes strategies that have surfaced in various clinical reasoning studies as examples of therapist's therapy actions used to communicate with clients and build rapport.

Some of these therapy behaviors related to interaction are likely subjected to explicit reasoning. An example of explicit reasoning is provided in Case Study 9-1. Other behaviors may be quite automatic and a function of embodied practices such as those described in Chapter 4. Often, they are a mix of both. I often find that it is easiest to detect the importance of these practices when I make a mistake or get an unexpected reaction, as described in Case Study 9-2 below.

TABLE 9-1

Therapist Strategies for Communicating with Clients

Questioning	Asking about client experience of health problems, concerns, and desires
Listening	Taking time to allow client to respond to questions fully, initiate conversation, or expand on earlier discussions
Creating choices	Providing a range of options for client to choose from; number of choices often limited to how much therapist believes client can attend to
Individualizing treatment	Creating or providing therapy activities that meet therapy goals and that also relate to client interests or preferences
Structuring success	Selecting activities that the client can successfully perform
Providing special services or "gifts"	Doing something personal or extra for a client that goes beyond the therapy process
Exchanging personal stories	Creating an alliance by sharing stories about topics of common interest
Joint problem solving	Asking client to define problems and work with therapist to come up with possible solutions
Using different therapy personas	Assuming different ways of speaking and acting, such as levels of formality, degree of authority, use of professional jargon to match client needs and expectations
Teaching about health condition	Explaining to clients about their health condition for client to understand own experiences and frame future expectations
Using humor	Use of jokes or humorous comments to relieve tension, provide diversion, or encourage participation
Negotiating	Use of bargaining about therapy tasks, length of session, level of assistance to elicit participation and reward desired action
Encouraging	Communicating hopeful outcome possibilities either directly or through use of stories and arranging interactions with role models with similar conditions
Social chat	General discussions about current events used to relieve tension, ease client into therapy session or divert client during rest
Shifting conversation	Moving discussions between therapy work and other communicative activities such as social chat, humor or stories as way of providing relief from tension, frustration, discomfort
Positioning of self relative to client's eye level	Use of nonverbal strategies, such as being at eye level, sitting closer or farther from client, gesturing to convey empathy and understanding or to minimize power differentials
Positioning body in relation to client	Sitting closer to client to convey empathy and understanding, or farther away to promote independent action
Eye gaze	Use of eye contact to invite interaction
Gesturing	Use of arms, hands, head position, or other bodily actions to communicate positive regard, provide direction, or provide feedback

Summarized from Burke (1997), Crepeau (1991), Lyons & Crepeau (2001), Mattingly & Fleming (1994), Schwartzberg (2002), and Weinstein (1998).

CASE STUDY 9-2

Hallway Therapy

Occasionally, I get involved in what I have come to call "hallway therapy," which is my term for short interventions that I do in the course of my daily rounds. These usually occur because friends or colleagues are dealing with some sort of injury or health problem either themselves or with a family member. Technically, these are not therapy in the full sense of the word, since it is not a formal relationship (and there is certainly no intent to bill!), but these little interactions I find are very telling as to whether I am using my interactive reasoning skills effectively.

One example is when I listened to our minister talking about her problems with her preschool son who had gotten "kicked out of nursery school" for biting. As we sat over a potluck dinner and she told her story, I wondered if he might have sensory processing issues. I told her about how we all have different nervous systems and went on to tell her about our experiences of how therapy helped one of our grandchildren. She was fascinated to hear this possible explanation of her son's behavior and followed up by having him assessed and subsequently treated by an occupational therapist specializing in dealing with children who have sensory processing challenges. In this example, I demonstrated effective interactive reasoning (along with diagnostic reasoning). In reflecting on this, I remember *sitting near her, attentively facing her, providing eye contact* and keeping my *voice calm* as I gave practical *advice on where she might go for assistance. I questioned, provided answers,* and *offered choices of action.*

In contrast, I recently had a "hallway therapy" encounter with a person with whom I share some committee responsibilities. He had just barely been able to make the meeting because he had some shoulder surgery the week before and was currently in a positioning sling. I observed him during our meeting, and while talking to him after the meeting attempted to provide some help for him to be more comfortable in his sling. I noticed that the pad that came with the sling was not over his neck area where it should be, but it had slipped down over his chest. While asking him how he was doing, I automatically started to adjust the pad. He exclaimed "whoa" and immediately moved back about 2 feet. I knew right away I had made several errors (that was my interactive reasoning clicking in). First of all, I had not obtained his permission to touch him, nor had I spent the time to be sure that he even wanted my help. By moving too quickly to touch him, I frightened him. I suddenly realized that he really didn't know me that well and may not even realize that I was an occupational therapist. I could say more, but the point should be clear . . . here is what happens when interactive reasoning misfires! I quickly reflected on what was going on and realized what I had done. I switched gears by first of all apologizing for scaring him and then explained in words (while maintaining a significant space between us) that I was an occupational therapist and had seen lots of folks be uncomfortable in slings. I told him that I had just meant to help him since I was concerned that he would have neck pain. After a bit more discussion, it was apparent he was willing to receive some help. I asked him how he would like me to help him, and he replied that I should just tell him what needed to happen and he would make the adjustments himself. In this example, I initially demonstrate a number of errors: I didn't *question,* didn't initially *regulate the distance between my body and his,* and *didn't engage in joint problem solving.* In short, I was so focused on the biomechanical concern, that I didn't take the time to build rapport. Once I realized my mistake, I was very careful *not to touch* him, to *apologize,* and to *use his preferred approach* by *talking* him through some options, rather than to attempt a physical adjustment.

I want to emphasize that neither of these incidents is really "therapy" in the sense that we use the word in the profession, but rather just examples of informed care giving that we often provide to friends and colleagues outside of formal therapy relationship. With that disclaimer, I do think they illustrate well the importance of effective interactive reasoning and what can go wrong when we don't attend to this aspect of therapy.

With a better understanding of what is meant by interactive reasoning and related therapy behaviors, we turn next to considering some of the apparent influences on interactive reasoning.

INFLUENCES ON INTERACTIVE REASONING

Interactive reasoning is in many ways an extension of both our personal and professional personas. This is one reason why evidence of strong interpersonal skills is considered to be critical in the admissions processes of many occupational therapy programs. Development of these "people skills" is one part of the picture, but another part appears to be the ways in which therapists frame the nature of the therapy process itself and their theoretical stance. A third factor is a recognition and management of power relations inherent in any human encounter.

Development of Interactive Reasoning

Interactive reasoning requires nuanced development of therapists' skills in communications. In part, this is framed by the therapist's values and worldview, as described in Chapter 2. Ranka and Chapparo (2000) suggest that the development of interactive reasoning starts with basic skills for listening, observing, and "feeling at ease when entering purposive social interaction within the context of an interview" (p. 193). Therapists then build on these skills to accurately collect and interpret information from these purposeful interactions, as well as to develop appropriate management of power relations. The ability to take the perspective of the client requires a degree of reflective judgment, in which the therapist interprets both verbal and non-verbal cues in light of the different perspectives held by the client. The Thinking about Thinking quotation that opened this chapter, by the actor Alan Alda, illustrates the importance and challenges of being truly open to the perspectives of others and willing to change behaviors based on that feedback. Chapters 10 and 11 include more discussion about educational philosophy and theories that explain the development of reflective judgment.

Theoretical Stance and Interactive Reasoning

Therapists' theoretical perspectives appear (not surprisingly) to frame the degree and manner in which they engage in interactions with clients. One of Burke's major findings in her study of pediatric therapists was that the way in which therapists framed their therapy practice influenced the degree and manner in which they engaged the parent in the therapy process. Therapists with advanced training who had more of an occupational and client-centered perspective demonstrated more attention to inter-acting with the child and his or her mother than therapists who did not have advanced training and who practiced from a medical model perspective. These find-ings echo the results of a much earlier study of therapists who practiced within a hos-pital setting. Rogers and Masagatani (1982) qualitatively studied 10 therapists doing initial assessments of patients with physical problems being seen in a medical setting. Although therapists "stressed the importance of developing rapport" (p. 198), the researchers concluded that the overarching focus of these therapists was on the bio-logical body. Psychosocial data obtained did not appear to be integrated into therapy goals and plans for future assessment of occupational functioning in areas outside of self-care. These results raised the concern that the espoused philosophy of occupa-tional therapy in which humans are seen as unitary biopsychosocial beings was dichotomized in practice into the biological (physical body) and the psychosocial (psychiatric) areas (p. 216). These issues have continued to surface during the ensu-ing quarter of a century since this study, in spite of the arguments put forth that emphasize the importance of using theoretical frameworks more consistent with occupational therapy's core philosophies and values (Fisher, 1998; Gray, 1998; Peloquin, 1993a&b; Trombly, 1995) . For instance, a study by Trigillio (2003) demon-strated that participants specializing in mental health used significantly more interac-tive reasoning when presented with a familiar case than did therapists specializing in working with individuals with physical disabilities or those working with children. Other studies are needed to more fully examine the communicative aspects of occu-pational therapy and how they are influenced by theoretical stance of the therapist. It makes sense that the way that therapists frame the nature of therapy is likely to have an impact on how they relate to their clients. The core of this stance may be therapist awareness of power relations as they affect the therapy process.

Power and Interactive Reasoning

The communication techniques used by therapists help them gain information and build alliances. Equally important, these techniques help to level out the power rela-tionships that are inherent in most professional–client interactions (Crepeau, 1991). As is often stated, occupational therapy is a "doing with" profession, rather than a "doing to" profession (Mattingly & Fleming, 1994). For therapists to effectively develop a partnership with the client, it is important to manage power differentials. Whether it is by creating opportunities for choice (see, for example, Duncan-Meyers & Hubner, 2000), or adjusting your posture so that you are on the same eye level as the client (Crepeau, 1991), the way we interact as humans virtually always involves a negotiation of power relations. By effectively managing these relations, therapists can theoretically elicit better information about client values, interests, and concerns (Ersser & Atkins, 2000). This in turn sets the stage for understanding the client's health problem (requiring scientific reasoning) and the meaning of that problem (narrative reasoning) to the client.

It is not surprising that there appears to be a link between therapist use and skill in interactive reasoning and the practice culture in which the therapist is functioning. In other words, issues of power are not only negotiated between therapist and client, but they are also reflected by therapists' sense of freedom to engage in interactive reasoning within the dominant view of the therapy process found in the practice context. Unsworth found:

> . . . therapists' capacity to reason interactively seemed to hold the key to the degree to which they were client-centered in their practice, just as a departmental practice culture that engendered client-centered practice seemed to promote interactive reasoning in the therapists (2004, p. 15).

Thus, not only must therapists reason about power-based relationships with their clients, but they must also pragmatically reason about the degree to which their interactive reasoning is and will be supported by the practice culture of their setting. New practitioners who wish to develop skills to support interactive reasoning would be wise to examine the culture of prospective employers. Similarly, managers and supervisors interested in client-centered care can strive to create cultures in which therapists are rewarded for this aspect of clinical reasoning.

The elements described in the preceding section all blend in such a way as to enhance the therapists' use of theory to inform intra- and interpersonal aspects of interactive reasoning. This blend becomes more powerful when therapists are willing to develop higher levels of interactive reasoning to promote a client-centered program of therapy in which power is shared and used to achieve results that are in the best interest of the client.

Therapy as a Conditional Process

Practitioners blend different aspects of clinical reasoning to interact effectively with their clients, and they must flexibly modify interventions in response to changing conditions. Fleming (1994) calls this conditional reasoning. Conditional reasoning can be used to anticipate possible outcomes over short or long periods of time. For example, Creighton and her colleagues (Creighton, Dijkers, Bennett & Brown, 1995) noticed that occupational therapy practitioners pre-planned treatments in a hierarchical manner. They observed that practitioners typically brought several sets of supplies to a treatment session. One set would be directed to the expected level of performance, and the others to a stage higher and lower than expected performance. As an example, one practitioner, in preparation for a writing activity with a person who had a spinal cord injury, brought a short writing splint and unlined paper. This practitioner also brought a longer splint providing wrist support (in case the client's hand control was worse than expected) and lined paper requiring more precision (in case his hand control was better than expected). This practitioner blended scientific reasoning (knowing about central nervous system effects on hand use and adaptive strategies to promote performance) and pragmatic reasoning (not wanting to waste time in making several trips to get needed supplies) in such a way as to conditionally anticipate several possible situations that might occur.

This ability to see possible futures is found in research in other professions, such as nursing. Benner and her colleagues describe how nurses use "future think" or a "habit of thought which enables them to respond quickly to likely clinical eventualities" (Benner, Hooper-Kyriakidis & Stannard, 1999, pg. 62). Benner (1984) provided a great example of this from an interview with a pediatric nurse who was fairly far along in her expertise development:

> . . . OK, here's *this* baby, this is where *this* baby is at, and here's where I want *this* baby to be in 6 weeks. What can I do today to make this baby go along the road to end up being better? (p. 28).

Notice how the nurse in this situation takes a holistic perspective and views the baby over time. Rather than focusing on a particular clinical aspect, such as the baby's respiratory capacities or birth weight, the nurse views the client from the point of view of interactive systems that can improve over time. As discussed in Chapter 3, clinical reasoning at this level requires that practitioners cognitively synthesize many different kinds of knowledge, as well as experiences with many other clients, to help them form these future possibilities.

Similarly, physical therapy researchers suggest that therapists use "predictive reasoning" to "envisage and then inform the patient" about likely therapy outcomes, as well as possible future scenarios (Jones, Jensen & Edwards, 2000, p. 124). This later work from other professions echoes the Fleming's description of how skilled occupational therapy practitioners "form an image of future life possibilities for the person" (Fleming, 1994, p. 234).

Unique to occupational therapy practice, in contrast to the examples from nursing and physical therapy, is the way in which occupational therapists "enlist the person in the construction of the image and in the activities that will help make these possibilities come about" (Fleming, 1994, p. 234). A cooking activity becomes a step toward returning to the role of motherhood, using a splint to assist in computer use helps an accountant see return to work as an option, and flipping pages in a textbook becomes a link back to college for the injured student. Thus, therapy activities are not only selected for their impact on the client's current health status, but also for their symbolic value in helping clients develop visions of themselves as they return to their regular lives. Crabtree (1998) uses the metaphor of a camera to explain how conditional reasoning seems to work:

> **Therapists position themselves where they can gain a panoramic view. From this point, they zoom in on the details that will help them to understand what they see. The may zoom in at different points and see different things, such as problems, stories and people. In contrast, they can also grasp the immensity of the landscape. This is conditional reasoning. It is more than just using a wide-angle lens, it includes the details as well. Both kinds of view serve a purpose: the details to guide the daily practice and the wider picture to grasp the meaning of the endeavor (p. 122).**

By using conditional reasoning, therapists can shape their practice to simultaneously use a macro- and microview that includes a forecast for the future and concern for the details of the present.

SUMMARY

This chapter highlights the complexities inherent in forming and managing the therapy relationships critical to the occupational therapy process, as well as the need for therapists to envision future possibilities to orchestrate the therapy process over time. Interactive reasoning describes the thinking and related actions that therapists use for developing positive interpersonal relationships with clients. Conditional reasoning is a way of anticipating various therapy scenarios, and the therapy process over time. Conditional reasoning in particular seems to require significant therapy experiences to accumulate the range of possibilities needed to inform such thinking.

LEARNING ACTIVITY 9-1

Interacting with Clients and Caregivers
Mary Shotwell

Purpose

To help learners notice factors influencing their relationships with clients and client families and caregivers

Connections to Major Clinical Reasoning Constructs

This activity provides the learner with practice in observations, insights, and skills needed for interactive reasoning.

Directions for Learners

1 Choose some clinical interaction that took place on fieldwork.
2 Give some background as to the events that happened.
3 Break down the interaction into action steps, listing each step separately. Pay attention to shifts in thought and/or action.
4 Analyze your interactions with the client and the family or caregivers.

Background/summary of events

_____

_____

Action steps

_____

_____

_____

_____

Family/Caregiver Interaction Analysis

Describe participation of the caregiver:

• How did they contribute to the intervention session?

• What did they ask from the OT?

_____

_____

Describe how you included the caregiver:

• What verbal strategies did you use?

• What nonverbal strategies did you use?

• In what ways did you attend to cultural issues relevant to the caregiver?

• In what ways did you attend to the learning needs of the caregiver?

_____

_____

Identify any biases about the family/caregiver (good or bad) that impacted your thoughts about the client.

_____

_____

How did the treatment session impact or relate to the client's performance at home, school, or other setting after the session?

_____

_____

How has the client's health condition impacted the family?

_____

_____

LEARNING ACTIVITY 9-2

Self Analysis Survey: Interactive Reasoning with Children
Robin Underwood

Purpose

To help learners anticipate areas of comfort and areas of concern in relating to children at different ages

Connections To Major Clinical Reasoning Constructs

This activity provides the learner with an opportunity to anticipate interactive reasoning strategies with children.

Directions for Learners

1 Circle rankings for each item on survey.
2 For any rankings above 3, make notes about interactive strategies you find successful.
3 Share your findings and thoughts with a group of peers.
4 Note strategies to try for any age groups in which you identified discomfort, as well as any new ideas for age groups you are comfortable with.

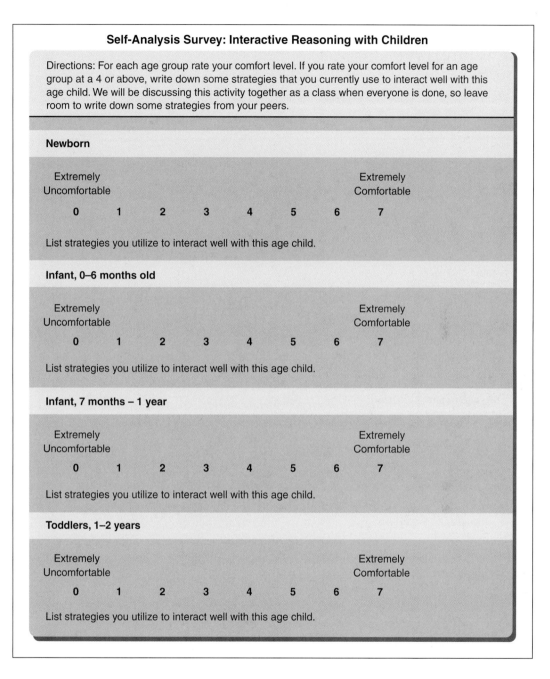

Self-Analysis Survey: Interactive Reasoning with Children

Directions: For each age group rate your comfort level. If you rate your comfort level for an age group at a 4 or above, write down some strategies that you currently use to interact well with this age child. We will be discussing this activity together as a class when everyone is done, so leave room to write down some strategies from your peers.

Newborn

Extremely Uncomfortable							Extremely Comfortable
0	1	2	3	4	5	6	7

List strategies you utilize to interact well with this age child.

Infant, 0–6 months old

Extremely Uncomfortable							Extremely Comfortable
0	1	2	3	4	5	6	7

List strategies you utilize to interact well with this age child.

Infant, 7 months – 1 year

Extremely Uncomfortable							Extremely Comfortable
0	1	2	3	4	5	6	7

List strategies you utilize to interact well with this age child.

Toddlers, 1–2 years

Extremely Uncomfortable							Extremely Comfortable
0	1	2	3	4	5	6	7

List strategies you utilize to interact well with this age child.

Child, 3–4 years

Extremely   Extremely
Uncomfortable   Comfortable

0   1   2   3   4   5   6   7

List strategies you utilize to interact well with this age child.

Child, 5–6 years

Extremely   Extremely
Uncomfortable   Comfortable

0   1   2   3   4   5   6   7

List strategies you utilize to interact well with this age child.

Child, 7–8 years

Extremely   Extremely
Uncomfortable   Comfortable

0   1   2   3   4   5   6   7

List strategies you utilize to interact well with this age child.

Preadolescent, 9–10 years

Extremely   Extremely
Uncomfortable   Comfortable

0   1   2   3   4   5   6   7

List strategies you utilize to interact well with this age child.

Adolescent, 11–13 years

Extremely   Extremely
Uncomfortable   Comfortable

0   1   2   3   4   5   6   7

List strategies you utilize to interact well with this age child.

Adolescent, 14–18 years

Extremely   Extremely
Uncomfortable   Comfortable

0   1   2   3   4   5   6   7

List strategies you utilize to interact well with this age child.

LEARNING ACTIVITY 9-3

Analysis of Self—Your Cultural Competence Challenge
Ellen Cohn and Diana Bailey

Purpose

To reflect on your own social identities and the meanings you and society attach to them

To help you understand how these factors influence your ability to engage in culturally relevant and meaningful occupations, and your therapeutic use of self

Connections to Major Clinical Reasoning Constructs

This activity supports learners in developing insights as to how their social identities impact their reasoning and interactive relationships with clients.

Directions for Learners

1 In each social identity category listed, describe your position and reflect on its implications. For example, if you are privileged in one of the categories, what, most likely, have you taken for granted? Where you may be subordinate or disadvantaged, how do you cope, and what have you learned about yourself and your response to oppression?

2 In each case, what are the challenges you are likely to encounter when developing your awareness, knowledge, and skills to become an occupational therapist? What do you need to learn?

From Bailey, D. & Cohn, E.S. (2001). Understanding others: A course to learn interactive clinical reasoning. *Occupational Therapy in Health Care* 15, 31–46.

Social Identity Categories

This information is for your personal use only, and you will not be asked to show it to peers or instructors. You have control over what and how much information you choose to disclose and with whom you wish to share.

Age _____

Race _____

Nationality/ethnicity _____

Language facility _____

Socioeconomic class _____

Gender _____

Religion _____

Sexual orientation _____

Disabilities _____

_____

Health _____

_____

Physical size and appearance _____

_____

_____

Education level _____

_____

Occupation/occupational roles _____

_____

_____

Mannerisms and styles of presenting and interacting with others _____

_____

REFERENCES

Alda, A. (2005). *Never have your dog stuffed and other things I've learned.* New York: Random House.

Alvernik, A. & Svidén, G. (1996). On clinical reasoning: Patterns and reflections on practice. *Occupational Therapy Journal of Research,* 16, 98–110.

Benner, P. (1984). *From novice to expert: Excellence and power in clinical nursing practice.* Menlo Park, CA: Addison-Wesley Publishing Company.

Benner, P., Hooper-Kyriakidis, P. & Stannard, D. (1999). *Clinical wisdom and interventions in critical care: A thinking-in-action approach.* Philadelphia: W. B. Saunders.

Burke, J. P. (1997). Frames of meaning: An analysis of occupational therapy evaluations of young children. *Dissertation Abstracts International,* 58(03), 644.(UMI Number: 9727199).

Crabtree, M. (1998). Images of reasoning: A literature review. *Australian Occupational Therapy Journal,* 45, 113–123.

Creighton, C., Dijkers, M., Bennett, N. & Brown, K. (1995). Reasoning and the art of therapy for spinal cord injury. *American Journal of Occupational Therapy,* 49, 311–317.

Crepeau, E. B. (1991). Achieving intersubjective understanding: Examples from an occupational therapy treatment session. *American Journal of Occupational Therapy,* 44, 1016–1024.

Duncan-Meyers, A. M. & Hubner, R. A. (2000). Relationship between choice and quality of life among residents in long-term care facilities. *American Journal of Occupational Therapy,* 54, 509–521.

Ersser, S. J. & Atkins, S. Clinical reasoning and patient-centred care. In J. Higgs & M. Jones (Eds.), *Clinical reasoning in the health professions* (pp. 68–77). Oxford: Butterworth Heinemann.

Fisher, A. G. (1998). Eleanor Clarke Slagle Lecture—Uniting practice and theory in an occupational framework. *American Journal of Occupational Therapy,* 52, 509–521.

Fleming, M. H. (1991). The therapist with the three-track mind. *American Journal of Occupational Therapy,* 45, 1007–1014.

Fleming, M. H. (1994). Conditional reasoning: Creating meaningful experiences. In C. Mattingly & M. H. Fleming (Eds.), *Clinical reasoning—forms of inquiry in a therapeutic practice* (pp. 197–235). Philadelphia: F. A. Davis.

Gardner, H. (2004). *Frames of mind: The theory of multiple intelligences (Twentieth anniversary ed.).* New York: Basic Books.

Gray, J. M. (1998). Putting occupation in practice: Occupation as ends, occupation as means. *American Journal of Occupational Therapy,* 52, 354–364.

Jones, M., Jensen, G. & Edwards, I. (2000). Clinical reasoning in physiotherapy. In J. Higgs & M. Jones (Eds.), *Clinical reasoning in the health professions* (pp. 117–127). Oxford: Butterworth Heinemann.

Kautzman, L. N. (1993). Linking patient stories and family stories to caregiver's use of clinical reasoning. *American Journal of Occupational Therapy,* 47, 169–173.

Lyons, K. D. & Crepeau, E. B. (2001). Case report: The clinical reasoning of a certified occupational therapy assistant. *American Journal of Occupational Therapy,* 55, 577–581.

Mattingly, C. & Fleming, M. H. (1994). Interactive reasoning: Collaborating with the person. In C. Mattingly & M. H. Fleming (Eds.), *Clinical reasoning: Forms of inquiry in a therapeutic practice* (pp. 178–196). Philadelphia: F. A. Davis.

Meyer, A. (1922/1977). The philosophy of occupation therapy. *American Journal of Occupational Therapy,* 31, 639–642. (Original work published 1922).

Peloquin, S. (1990). The patient–therapist relationship in occupational therapy: understanding visions and images. *American Journal of Occupational Therapy,* 44(1), 13–21.

Peloquin, S. M. (1993a). The depersonalization of patients: A profile gleaned from narratives. *American Journal of Occupational Therapy,* 49, 830–837.

Peloquin, S. (1993b). The patient-therapist relationship: beliefs that shape care. *American Journal of Occupational Therapy,* 47(10), 935–942.

Ranka, J. & Chapparo, C. (2000). Teaching clinical reasoning to occupational therapists. In J. Higgs & M. Jones (Eds.), *Clinical reasoning in the health professions* (pp.191–197). Oxford: Butterworth Heinemann.

Rogers, J. & Masagatani, G. (1982). Clinical reasoning of occupational therapists during the initial assessment of physically disabled patients. *Occupational Therapy Journal of Research,* 2, 195–219.

Schwartzberg, S. (2002). *Interactive reasoning in the practice of occupational therapy.* Upper Saddle River, NJ: Prentice Hall.

Trigillo, J. T. (2003) *Variations in clinical reasoning among occupational therapy practitioners.* Dissertation Abstracts International-A 64/01, Publication Number AAT 3076538, Obtained from http://proquest.umi.com 1/13/2006

Trombly, C. A. (1995). Eleanor Clark Slagle Lecture—Occupation: Purposefulness and meaningfulness as therapeutic mechanisms. *American Journal of Occupational Therapy, 49,* 960–972.

Unsworth, C. A. (2004). Clinical reasoning: How do pragmatic reasoning, worldview and client-centredness fit? *British Journal of Occupational Therapy, 67*(1), 10–19.

Yerxa, E. J. (1967). 1966 Eleanor Clarke Slagle Lecture: Authentic Occupational Therapy. *American Journal of Occupational Therapy, 21,* 1–9.

Weinstein, E. (1998). Elements of the art of practice in mental health. *American Journal of Occupational Therapy, 52,* 579–585.

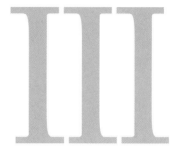

Teaching Professional Reasoning

Epistemology: Knowing How You Know

John W. Schell

CHAPTER OUTLINE

Elements of Western educational philosophy
  Epistemology
  Metaphysics
  Axiology
Common schools of Western educational thought
  Perennialism (idealism)
  Essentialism (realism)
  Behaviorism
  Progressivism (pragmatism)
  Reconstructionism
  Existentialism

Knowledge development and social constructivism
  Knowledge construction
  Types of constructivism
Expert knowledge
Ways of knowing
Reflective judgment and reflective practice
  Stages of reflection judgment
  Reflective Practice
Summary

OBJECTIVES

After reading this chapter, the learner will be able to:

1 Describe epistemology as an element of educational philosophy.
2 Articulate common schools of Western educational philosophy by teacher characteristics, curriculum emphasis, instructional assumptions, instructional methods, and goals of student assessment.
3 Explain elements of constructivism as a way of knowing.
4 Develop knowledge structures that are unique to experts in a professional field.
5 State elements of reflective judgment as a way of knowing.
6 Articulate elements of reflective practice as a way of using knowledge.

KEY TERMS

Epistemology	Realism	Progressivism
Metaphysics	Behaviorism	Reconstructionism
Idealism	Behavioral engineering	Existentialism
Perennialism (idealism)		

I n Unit III, our attention shifts from understanding clinical and professional reasoning to how we can best teach and support the ongoing development of reasoning in practice. In this and subsequent chapters, authors provide both theoretical and practical information designed to help readers become better teachers, researchers, and scholarly thinkers. Our questioning turns toward the philosophic and resulting epistemological perspectives of the nature of knowledge. In the beginning of the chapter, we scrutinize the most common elements of educational philosophy, followed by an epistemological discussion of the most common western schools of educational thought. Later in the chapter, we turn our attention to knowledge development in the contexts of social constructivism. Continuing with our discussion with regard to the nature of knowledge we will then examine how specific groups conceive, develop and use their knowledge. In this regard, we discuss Mary Field Belenky's epistemology of "Women's Ways of Knowing" (1997). Finally, we observe King and Kitchener's (1994) associated stages of reflective judgment and Schön's (1983) work on reflective practice. Now we begin our exploration of epistemological foundations commonly found in education programs for the therapeutic professions.

Thinking About Thinking 10-1

It is important that students bring a certain ragamuffin, barefoot irreverence to their studies; they are not here to worship what is known, but to question it.

—Jacob Chanowski

ELEMENTS OF WESTERN EDUCATIONAL PHILOSOPHY

The histories of education and philosophy are often intertwined. Several famous educators are also well known as philosophers (O'Hear, 1995). John Dewey may be the best example of a modern philosopher, educator, and social commentator. Dewey is often cited in educational circles as the father of pragmatism, which is known as the philosophic home of progressive education. As a social activist, Dewey was deeply immersed in matters of national and international politics in addition to reform of American education (Westbrook, 1991).

Western educational philosophy is often discussed in light of its role in perpetuating a liberal democratic society. However, the pendulum of educational purpose continues to swing. Since the early 1900s, many have believed that education should be focused on the development of independent individuals who, in an existential sense, take precedent over the preservation of societal institutions or cultural traditions (White, 1995). In the last decade of the 20th century and the beginning years of the new millennium, many educational policies and practices seem to have returned to a mode of promotion and conservation of traditional values and mastery of basic skills. This end of the continuum is characterized by an educational atmosphere of accountability and a curriculum of recall and standardized testing.

These contradictions of educational purpose nicely illustrate a tension common among today's educators. Today, preservation of traditional values seems to be a strong societal value. For example, recent public school curriculum reform is characterized as a "return to basics." In this era of conservatism, progressive education that promotes problem solving and innovative thought are not commonly included in today's curriculum of standardized testing (White, 2000). Among the questions we should be asking about the purpose of American education are the following: Should we promote individual autonomy over meeting the more generalized educational needs of our society? Is the purpose of education to socialize children and to indoctrinate them to our traditional way of life, or is it to maximize the intellectual potential of each individual? Can we indeed find truth through learning? Is a quest for truth a meaningful way to maximize human potential? No matter how we might answer these questions, consideration of educational context is a vital and important discussion. Every professional educator should examine questions such as these since they formulate a foundation of their professional practice.

Consistent with the writing of Carr and Shotwell in Chapter 3, professional educators approach questions like these within the context of their own experiences and the resulting mental frameworks. Thus, a scholar's quest for a greater understanding of the applications of educational philosophy must take them through an exploration of concepts like epistemology, metaphysics, and axiology.

So, let us take the first steps on our initial journey. As with any passage, it is important to know something about the various roads that lead to our eventual philosophic destination. In the next section, we briefly explore a conceptual roadmap that traverses the philosophic landscape. Our investigation should include a brief definition and discussion of three philosophic elements including epistemology, metaphysics, and axiology.

Epistemology

Kincheloe, Slattery, and Steinberg (2000) have defined **epistemology** as "the study of knowledge and knowing" (p. 27). In many ways epistemology is concerned with questions about the nature of truth. Kincheloe and others (2000) frame these philosophic questions: What is truth? Is truth the same in every context? How is truth ordained, by "God, or gods, or nature?" (p. 27). Is knowledge inert or is it constructed?

Epistemology is both a philosophic and a theoretical construct. So, in the first part of this chapter we are going to investigate several of the best-known Western schools of educational philosophy. Each philosophic position has its own version of "the ways of knowing." To understand how we know what we know, it is important to examine our assumptions of educational values, beliefs, and ethics.

Metaphysics

What is real? What does it mean to be a human being? **Metaphysics** is a branch of philosophy devoted to the examination of such questions. Of course, it is critically important. As a matter of course, teachers of any subject make philosophic decisions about what is real and what is true. This is a by-product of daily judgments about which content is included or excluded from our course materials. Do our curriculum decisions come from our best estimate of reality? Is that reality extracted from research and supporting evidence? Or, is there an absolute reality that exists just out of human sight that we take on faith that must be included?

Perhaps there is more than one version of reality. Allow me to share a brief personal story that may illustrate this point. Uncle Austin was my childhood hero—he remains a hero even now, many years after he has passed away. Austin was uneducated, rough-hewn, loving, delightfully homey, brilliant, and a deeply philosophic man. Living quietly in remote southern Missouri for most of their adult lives, Uncle Austin and Aunt Lizzy were a strong influence on my upbringing when I spent summers on their small farm in the 1950s. It was during these long summers when Uncle Austin educated me about many of life's mysteries. Many of his lessons came as we sat in the evenings on the front porch of their modest farm house listening to Harry Carey announce the St. Louis Cardinal Baseball games on a battery-powered radio. Large sections of rural America were still without electrical power well into the 1960s. Uncle Austin and Aunt Lizzy were among those who lived most of their adult life with their only heat and food made possible by wood fires and very hard physical work. A major "reality" for Lizzy and Austin was the hardwood trees to be chopped down, cut to length, aged, and split for next winter's fire wood. Because their daily existence depended on wood fires, Austin maintained the hand tools that enabled him to create much needed fuel. Cutting and splitting firewood was so important that 8-year-old nephews were often drafted for the summer because of their willing nature and the high quality of their spirited labor.

During a water break on a hot July log-splitting day, Uncle Austin showed me his axe with a hand-carved handle. "John," he said in his slow rural Missouri drawl, "see this axe? I've had this here axe for more than 60 years now. It came down the Ohio River on a flat-bottom boat with Grandpa Walter. It's had two new heads and I'd guess 12 new handles. Yes sir, this here's the same axe he used."

Now, more than 40 years later, I still do not know if the story is true; it is entirely possible that my metaphysical leg was being pulled. Regardless of its authenticity, the truths I have drawn from this story have stuck with me. I still recall it 50 years later when I discuss the nature of reality with doctoral students. Was it indeed the same axe Uncle Austin inherited even though it had been entirely reconstituted with replacement parts many times over? What was the nature of Austin's perceived reality when he regarded his axe? I think he believed that the reality of this important tool had never changed. For him, it was an article of fundamental faith; this axe was a tool for survival. But as a young boy I questioned his version of reality and allowed (silently, of course) that the present axe is now an entirely different tool evolved from its original state by the inclusion of new heads and new handles. In spite of our unspoken philosophic differences, we could easily agree on the necessity of a warm fire on cold Missouri winter evenings and those great apple pies that Aunt Lizzy baked in the wood-fired oven—all made possible because of the "multiple realities" of Austin's physical and metaphysical axe.

Axiology

"What is good?" (ethics) and "What is beautiful?" (aesthetics) (Kincheloe et al., 2001, p. 28). Axiologists are concerned with questions such as these. As I am writing this section, I am at a table in the library of a small liberal arts university that is known for its contributions to the visual and performing arts. All around me are artistic sculptures, drawings, prints, and ceramic renderings of extraordinary beauty. Some are exacting representations of a known reality while others are more suggestive of reality and are less focused representations of perceived beauty and truth. Each type of art is an expression of truth understood by the artist of what is real and beautiful in life. Some I find are reassuring and suggestive of the past; others even push me to confront aesthetic barriers by making the view slightly uncomfortable. Each approach is valuable. In art we confront life. It is the emotionality of art that makes it have meaning.

The other sides of axiology are the important questions of values. Even as I spend this very enjoyable day in the company of great beauty, I recognize that we also live in a world at war. Later this afternoon, will I turn on National Public Radio and hear of the latest atrocities of the current wars in the Middle East? Terrible times of war like these make most of us reflect deeply on our personal values and ethics. What is the value of human life? When should lives be sacrificed for the larger societal good? Which society and groups of individuals should benefit from war? Is God (or are the gods) on one side or the other?

How do these elements of philosophy lead us to think about education? To begin the next part of our conversation, we will examine a number of schools of educational thought. Of course, each of these positions is drawn from classical schools of Western philosophy.

COMMON SCHOOLS OF WESTERN EDUCATIONAL THOUGHT

Classical philosophy has emerged over centuries owing to reflective thought and scholarly debate about the meaning and purpose of life. Socrates, Aristotle, and Plato were students and teachers of philosophy who built on each others' thinking. Socrates (469–399 BC), considered by some as the father of modern philosophy, believed that ideas were the only true reality. Known as a teacher, Socrates engaged in question-based dialogue as a method for discussing and examining philosophic ideas. This type of questioning has become known as the Socratic method of instruction. From this and many other traditions, schools of educational thought have emerged. Each of these paradigms is concerned with the epistemological question of how do we know that our knowledge is true and therefore worthy of inclusion in the curriculum?

Perhaps another brief personal story will shed additional light. On a recent drive home from a Thanksgiving holiday spent with family, Barbara and I came across a program on National Public Radio as the 1988 book written by Joseph Campbell was being discussed: *The Power of Myth with Bill Moyers*. Of course, philosophy has been represented in one mythological form or another for many centuries. This radio discussion caught our attention because the commentators were describing the cultural nature of ritual dinners such as those served to the family on the Fourth of July, Thanksgiving, Hanukkah, Kwanzaa, or Christmas. The radio journalists and researchers pointed out that we often celebrate these holidays by preparing our favorite holiday foods. For example, in the United States hot dogs and hamburgers are grilled on the Fourth of July. These foods are frequently supplemented by regional favorites such as sweet iced tea served in our region of the southern United States. A dish peculiar to each extended family often accompanies the traditional meal that is prepared out of a sense of tradition. You know the famous (or infamous) dish that your aunt makes that perhaps has become known among members of your family as "Aunt Judy's Corn and Spinach Soufflé." In the case of my family, it was an unfortunate potato salad concoction.

My parents, as survivors of the depression of the 1930s and 1940s, were fiscally and politically conservative. This world view inevitably led to a lifestyle and diet that could only be characterized as "basic." Food dishes included simple ingredients often grown in our own garden. Potatoes were a dietary staple for a family of five living in rural Missouri on a Post Office salary. When combined with my mother's disagreeable culinary skills, this "depression era" approach to finances, menu planning, and cooking could only result in a basic and bland diet. Even bland food was preferred to the vulcanized dishes that resulted from my mother's probable attention deficit disorder. But she did have her culinary moments: "Aunt Mickey's Potato Salad" was her unfortunate concoction, which assumed mythological status among members of the extended family.

For years, summer family picnics featured this bland and mostly tasteless blend of boiled and cut potatoes, a stingy dash of French's mustard, several spoonfuls of bargain brand mayonnaise and perhaps a light sprinkling of salt. Each Fourth of July, this dish was carefully prepared and placed in the refrigerator several hours before company arrived. The Midwestern culture of politeness that permeated our family annually prevented a frank appraisal of that year's batch of "wall paper paste." However, as the Schell boys moved toward adulthood, our assorted girlfriends and wives began to anticipate and covertly avert the annual potato salad assault. Each in turn, one of the younger women distracted my mother while another began the process of adding exotic ingredients such as celery, more seasonings, spices, and more interesting mustards. Over the course of several family picnics, my mother ironically became famous for her zesty potato salad. In the years since her passing, "Mickey's Potato Salad" has assumed an epic role as a family myth and is lovingly discussed among the relatives even to this day.

By now, you are probably wondering how this story is connected with educational philosophy. To make that connection, I want to direct your attention back to Joseph Campbell and Bill Moyers (1988). In his writings, Mr. Moyers responded to a question about the nature of myth by stating: "These myths [stories] speak to me because they express what I know inside is true" (p. 37). It is in this spirit that I share the potato salad story. What are the meanings of this dish among members of the extended family? How do we know the true formulation of the potato salad and how is that position justified?

As we continue this discussion of educational thought I will present a brief summary of the most common educational philosophies followed by a discussion of Aunt Mickey's potato salad from that point of view. Finally, I briefly describe educational interventions and instructional strategies typical of each philosophy. Although there are other schools of educational thought these are the most commonly accepted positions:

- Perennialism
- Essentialism
- Behaviorism
- Progressivism
- Reconstructionism
- Existentialism

Table 10-1 represents a summary of the assumptions of learning, curriculum, instructional, and assessment practices for each of these epistemological positions.

TABLE 10-1

Common Western Educational Philosophies

Elements of Education	Perennialism	Essentialism (Realism)	Behavioral Engineering	Progressivism	Reconstructionism	Existentialism
Philosophic presuppositions	▪ (Wo)Men seek "ideal" universal order ▪ Faith & reason coexist & are mutually supporting ▪ Truth is represented by an ideal existence ▪ Past & present exist to achieve divine purpose *Superior intellectual development is limited to "philosopher kings"*	▪ (Wo)Men seek essential & universal reality ▪ Ultimate good exists—probably unattainable by mortals ▪ Truth is absolute even if unknown ▪ Education conserves basic principles & values	▪ (Wo)Men acknowledge supremacy of scientific method ▪ Truth is scientifically proven ▪ Behaviors are to be controlled ▪ Behavior is programmed from birth by culture ▪ Learner is conditioned via response to stimuli	▪ (Wo)Men progress toward better solutions to problems ▪ Truth is relative to context ▪ Ability to select among options is nurtured ▪ Skill in evaluating practical outcomes is critical ▪ Democratic society depends on informed participation	▪ (Wo)Men must participate in achievement of a better society ▪ Truth is relative to context ▪ Education is key to democratic perfection ▪ Isolate deterrents to human progress ▪ Education promotes & protects individual rights & equality ▪ Interested distribution of societal powers	▪ (Wo)Men must seek their own path ▪ Human existence has no universal purpose ▪ Humans are free agents to decide for themselves ▪ Truth is subjective; open for individual interpretation ▪ Education gives courage to seek meaning ▪ No promise of external reward
Teacher characteristics	Teachers who are: ▪ Master artisans with complete command of discipline content ▪ Living examples of best ethics & morals	Teachers who are: ▪ Proven masters of discipline content ▪ Capable teachers of content ▪ Fact oriented	Teachers who: ▪ Demonstrate appropriate content behaviors ▪ Are expert in performance-based instruction	Teachers who are: ▪ Master facilitators teaching to learner interests, abilities, curiosity & motivation	Teachers who are: ▪ Master facilitators teaching to learner interests, abilities, curiosity & motivation	Teachers who are: ▪ Master facilitator teaching to individual learner interests, abilities, & motivation

(continued)

TABLE 10-1

(continued)

Elements of Education	Perennialism	Essentialism (Realism)	Behavioral Engineering	Progressivism	Reconstructionism	Existentialism
	▪ Capable teachers of content	▪ Acquainted with latest science & technology within field	▪ Associate reward & punishment for proper performance	▪ Capable professional practitioners	▪ Capable practitioners ▪ Social activist in democratic workplace	▪ Capable & experienced practitioners
Curriculum emphasis	Emphasis on: ▪ High-quality scholarship ▪ Ideals extracted from "Great books" of Western society ▪ Ideals of the past which are essential for the future	Emphasis on: ▪ Transmission of essential (basic) skills ▪ Sequence arrayed from simple to complex ▪ Established practices well regarded in the field	Emphasis on: ▪ Mastery of sequenced & incremental tasks ▪ Achievement of minimum levels of performance ▪ Reward for correct performance ▪ Punishment for incorrect performance	Emphasis on: ▪ Core professional skills ▪ Overview of entire profession & relationship to healthcare systems ▪ Authentic contexts & experiences ▪ Problem solving ▪ Critical thinking	Emphasis on: ▪ Adaptable skills ▪ Critical thinking for political & social impact ▪ Achieving & maintaining social justice ▪ Strategies for intervention & change of injustice	Emphasis on: ▪ Critical thinking skills promoting self interpretation & meaning making ▪ Authentic context & individual experience ▪ Problem solving
Instructional assumptions	Teacher-oriented instruction assuming: ▪ A student who is a learner ▪ Learning is independent; not a social phenomenon	Teacher-oriented instruction assuming: ▪ A student who is a learner ▪ Learning is independent; not a social phenomenon	Teacher-oriented instruction assuming: ▪ A student who is a learner ▪ Learning is independent; not group oriented ▪ Student is guided by external learning objectives	Student-oriented instruction assuming: ▪ Learners who are also students ▪ Instruction within a community of practice	Student-oriented instruction assuming: ▪ Learners who are also students ▪ Instruction within a community of practice	Student-oriented instruction assuming: ▪ A learner who is a student ▪ Learner seeks unique intellectual pathways ▪ Instruction for individuals or groups

Associated methods	■ Lecture ■ Seminar ■ Demonstration ■ Coaching ■ Scaffolding & fading	■ Lecture ■ Demonstration ■ Coaching ■ Scaffolding & fading	■ Individualized programmed instruction ■ Demonstration ■ Coaching ■ Scaffolding & fading	■ Authentic experiences ■ Scaffolding & fading ■ Exploration ■ Articulation ■ Reflection	■ Authentic experiences ■ Scaffolding & fading ■ Exploration ■ Articulation ■ Reflection	■ Tutorial-based exchange ■ Scaffolding & fading ■ Exploration ■ Articulation ■ Reflection
Goals of assessment	Ascertain if: ■ Student skills are historically sound ■ Student skills reflect excellent scholarship	Ascertain if: ■ Students have mastered learning objectives ■ Essential or basic skills have been met ■ Student learning meets or exceeds standardized measures ■ Novice performance is acceptable in the workplace	Ascertain if: ■ Students have mastered basic competencies ■ Minimum entry-level skills for the workplace have been mastered	Ascertain if: ■ Learner can accommodate to technical & societal change Learner can solve ill-structured workplace problems	Ascertain if: ■ Learners are agents of social change ■ Learners are adaptable to changing social, economic and technological contexts Goals for a humane workplace and equal opportunities are met	Ascertain if: ■ Mutually negotiated subjective goals are met ■ Learners "know themselves"

These summaries can be used as a reference to provide a brief explanation of the positions of each educational philosophy.

Each of these philosophic positions are presented in light of the unique presuppositions, teacher characteristics, curriculum emphasis, instructional assumptions, instructional methods, and the goals of assessment. The first philosophy is Perennialism.

Perennialism (Idealism)

Plato (427–347 BC) was considered by historians as a devoted but questioning student of Aristotle. As his own reflections matured, Plato thought more specifically about the nature of human existence. He wrote about his goal of the "philosopher king" who was said to be an intellectual who could guide an entire society toward the highest ideals. The origin of the word perennialism is taken from the Latin term *philosophia perennis*, which was a reference to the "perennial wisdom of God" (Lerwick, 1979, p. iv).

A central concept of Plato's emerging thinking was the ponderous question of reality. What is real? What makes it real? For him, reality was based on the existence of an "ideal" world that exists in the ideas of the mind (Kincheloe et al., 2000). This world of ideas of the mind has become known philosophically as **idealism.** In educational terms, the philosophy of **perennialism** is the application of idealism in education (Kincheloe et al.) (Box 10-1).

BOX 10-1

Perennial Potato Salad

The perennial potato salad is the real thing and is based on ideal ingredients according to the beliefs of the intellectual aristocracy (in this case, my mother) who divines the perfect potato salad (i.e., this is how God would make it). However, bad potato salad made by mortals will always be with us; "drought, famine, sickness, war and suffering are by nature part of the order of the universe" (Lerwick, p. 28). In the context of her privileged standing, Mickey as philosopher-queen understood that the perfect potato salad existed within an "unfolding unity of spiritual and divine purpose" (p. 28). She left it to mere mortal women and men of this earth to use faith and reason to seek perfection within the "rationale of the complete and eternal ideal [potato salad]" (p. 28).

Perennialist teachers are most often content experts with complete command of their discipline. Although most are capable teachers, their best qualification is a complete mastery of professional content. Perennialists come from a tradition of artisans where the focus is on expert performance of an ideal way to practice their profession. In many cases, instructional expertise is secondary to their knowledge of the content.

A perennialist curriculum often consists of ideas extracted from the classic works of great artists, writers, and researchers in a search for truth that is foundational to the creation of an ideal and enduring professional practice. From this perspective past "best practices" often represent the ideal way to conserve the

same time as the pragmatist movement (circa 1900), behaviorists in education began to focus on "observable behaviors . . . that could be isolated, measured, compared, categorized and empirically defined" (Lerwick, 1979, p. 63). Many early psychologists and behaviorists believed that learning was the result of a stimulus external to the learner, their response to that cue, and a systematic program of reinforcement. "Motivation to learn was assumed to be driven primarily by drives, such as hunger, and the availability of external forces, such as rewards and punishments" (Bransford, Brown & Cocking, 2000, p. 6). Lerwick (1979) describes behaviorists as anxious to improve society by "engineering" behavioral changes in the culture (Box 10-3).

BOX 10-3
Behavioral Potato Salad

The behaviorally engineered potato salad is a product of a recipe that has been carefully derived from scientific study conducted specifically for the "improvement of the human environment" (Lerwick, 1979, p. 64). Even though each Schell daughter-in-law made individual contributions to the dish, they did so because of their prior conditioning. In this situation, they were responding to stimuli inherent in this current culinary situation. In other words, behaviorists hold that the helpful sous-chefs added special ingredients because they have been rewarded for avoiding the "bad behavior" of serving or eating pitiable food. Or, perhaps they have been rewarded in the past for their "good behaviors" when preparing interesting and zesty-tasting potato salad.

Behaviorist teachers, like their perennialist and essentialist brothers and sisters, also operate in a teacher-oriented learning environment. They assume a directing position in relationship to the student. This position of dominance affords the teacher the right to shape behaviors through application of operant and classical conditioning strategies. Effective behaviorist teachers are experts at associating a systematic program of rewards with proper student performances. Many behaviorist teachers operate "competency-based" instructional schemes which are based on measurable goals and objectives.

The behavioral curriculum is thought to engineer the mastery of appropriate skills and abilities among students that are based on de-constructed series of tasks that comprise a larger skill set (Lerwick, 1979). "Once the proper sequence of behaviors has been learned, the student should be encouraged toward increased quality and speed of performance" (p. 68).

A curriculum developed from a behaviorist perspective consists of linear and incremental concepts and tasks, arrayed in an instructional sequence with appropriate rewards and punishments, that eventually leads to a desired performance. As an example, an occupational therapist learns to transfer a patient from a wheeled chair to a bed. Based on a systematic task analysis, this activity is deconstructed into a series of smaller steps and taught individually (i.e., body mechanics, methods for coaching patients, how to lock wheelchair brakes). Behaviorist instructors would subsequently reward appropriate behaviors while withholding praise or punishing inappropriate student responses (i.e., by low grades on competency checklists). This instructional approach is a form of operant-reinforcement (Bigge & Shermis, 2004).

Behaviorist assumptions of instruction are, once again, teacher oriented in nature. Instruction is designed to promote the acquisition of skill sets among individual students learning independently from others. A further assumption is the need to direct and shape student performance as measured by highly structured behavioral objectives.

Behaviorist instructional methods are often "individualized programmed instruction." Such programs of instruction are linear in nature and rely on many traditional methods that generate lower-order cognitive, affective, and psychomotor skills. Traditional methods include programmed instructional materials supplemented by demonstration, coaching, and systematic programs of rewards and punishments to determine grades.

Assessment within a behaviorist paradigm of instruction is based on the student's level of achievement when compared with measurable instructional objectives. Standards for successful completion are most often based on the lowest acceptable level of performance.

Behaviorist approaches are easy to recognize as elements of behaviorism common in today's pre-schools, elementary, middle, high schools and postsecondary institutions. The principle of **behavioral engineering** is foundational to standardized testing, now so common in schools under state initiatives and the current No Child Left Behind Act of the U.S. Department of Education (2005).

Progressivism (Pragmatism)

William James and John Dewey were fathers of the progressive movement during the first part of the 20th century. Philosophically, progressivists "test hypotheses to see what works" from a lifetime of experiences (Kincheloe et al., 2000, p. 29). Truth is based on experience, morality is left to society to determine, and beauty is changeable according to current public tastes (Kincheloe et al.). Progressive educators are dedicated to preparing students who can solve problems encountered in life. This requires a curriculum that is "student centered" and based on skills of critical thinking and solution of challenging problems. This approach is thought by progressives to be critical to the preservation of a liberal democracy. Therefore, principles of democracy are foremost as foundational to progressive educational beliefs. Lerwick (1979) writes that the preservation of human liberty takes precedent over the conservation of institutions, property, or social mores (p. 45). Educationally, progressivists are committed to education as a tool for preserving a democratic way of life. "Education can serve the needs of democracy by providing the individual citizen with the knowledge, competencies and skills necessary for participation in a free society" (Lerwick, 1979, p. 45) (Box 10-4).

Progressive teachers are expert teachers with a mastery of child and adult development. In addition, progressive teachers are capable practitioners of their professional discipline. Teaching from this perspective requires strong facilitation

---

BOX 10-4
Progressive Potato Salad

The progressive potato salad evolved because of the individual efforts of each Schell daughter-in-law as she sought her own solution to an easy problem within a potentially difficult social context. The true essence of the progressive dish is based on a "reality" that is relative to each chef. The annual reinvention of Aunt Mickey's Potato Salad was inherently democratic in that each contributor was free to add ingredients according to her beliefs and tastes. Education and learning are important in the creation of progressive potato salad because it is the source of "appropriate knowledge, competencies and skills necessary for participation" (p. 45) in a society characterized by freedom to create an infinite number of progressive potato salad concoctions. Therefore, Aunt Mickey has been indirectly made (in)famous for her culinary powers.

---

skills in which student's interests, abilities, curiosity, and motivation are matched with the content to be learned.

A progressive curriculum has at least two foci: problem-solving and learning through experience. Under this paradigm, the purpose of education is to learn to solve difficult problems (Lerwick, 1979). It is assumed that this level of problem solving and associated critical thinking will transfer to the workplace and more generally to the creation of a better society through democratic processes. Progressivists assume that experience is the greatest teacher. The progressive curriculum will most likely feature realistic learning experiences that are directly linked to classroom content. For example, an occupational therapy professor might ask a student therapist to analyze a case study about a teenager with a head injury and suggest how to teach him to use the computer again. In this case, students are encouraged to use their own knowledge and ability to generate approaches or find needed information. Level I fieldwork experiences in occupational therapy curricula are also good examples of a progressive curriculum.

Progressive assumptions of instruction start with a learner-centered approach designed to enhance practical and logical applications of progressive ideas to the solution of practical problems. Progressive instruction is essentially a social activity in which learners are assumed to be social equals with teachers. This is why **progressivism** is often associated with socialization theories of learning such as situated cognition (Lave & Wenger, 1991) and communities of practice (Wenger, 1989).

Progressive instructional methods often focus on the acquisition of higher-order thinking and problem-solving skills. When possible, authentic learning experiences can be used to illustrate an overall or global picture of the materials to be mastered. Once such a global perspective has been achieved, the learner can reference an intellectual framework within which smaller details fit like pieces of a puzzle. Other methods common to this approach are exploration, articulation, and reflection. Exploration is an opportunity for the learner to walk around the landscape of an area of interest using his or her own interest and curiosity. Articulation is the opportunity for learners to express their knowledge. Of course, this does not need to be limited to oral expression. Written work, videotape, and PowerPoint presentations or a portfolio are just a few ways that acquired knowledge can be articulated by learners. Reflection is a closely associated instructional method with articulation. Stated in simple terms, reflection is an opportunity for the learner to attach meaning and value to the knowledge that they have acquired. Reflection is not a new idea. John Dewey wrote about the importance of reflection in his famous book, *How We Think* (1910; 1933).

> **In every case of reflective activity, a person finds himself confronted with a given, present situation from which he has to arrive at . . . what is present carries or bears the mind over to the idea and ultimately the acceptance of something else. (p. 190)**

This tradition has been carried forward by modern theorists such as Donald Schön and Kathleen Blake Yancey. Much more is shared on the topic of reflection as an educational strategy in subsequent chapters in this unit. In fact, the effective use of reflection as a foundation for professional practice is a central point of this book. Progressive assessment is designed to ascertain whether students can accommodate to social and technological change. In addition, progressive teachers are concerned with their students' abilities to demonstrate their knowledge through the solution of complex problems that are common in a democratic society.

Reconstructionism

Reconstructionism is a brand of philosophy that acquired its name from socially active advocates who wish to reconstruct society in light of more radical but still pragmatic conclusions. Many educational philosophers consider the reconstructionist position as a drastic form of progressivism (Lerwick, 1979). Reconstructivists believe that "in a democracy, all people ought to plan, prepare for and participate in achieving a more desirable society" (Lerwick, p. 52). From this viewpoint of social concern, education becomes a central actor as a "facilitator of change" (p. 51). Reconstructionist teachers are social activists who seek change and betterment through the actions of their students. Philosopher and writer, Paulo Freire (1997), wrote of the "pedagogy of the oppressed." From his perspective, education was a critical tool in encouraging economically and socially disadvantaged populations to gain sufficient power to overcome oppression imposed by those holding social and economic control (Box 10-5).

Reconstructivist teachers are social activists committed to equitable distribution of social justice, economic resources, and preservation of democratic principles. In many ways, reconstructivist and progressive teachers share similar interests in critical thinking and problem solving because these are thought to be important elements in keeping and maintaining a democratic society. Teachers who practice from this perspective are often master teachers who may be only competent (as opposed to expert) practitioners.

A reconstructivist curriculum places an emphasis on creating adaptable skills in a changing society. Emphasis is place on critical thinking skills used for social, economic, and social impact. The reconstructivist curriculum is likely to be a platform for social intervention and redress of injustice.

BOX 10-5
Reconstructivist Potato Salad

The existence of the reconstructivist potato salad is a natural by-product of the hegemonic power structure that sometimes resides within a mother-in-law and daughter-in-law family constellation. Daughters-in-law have been known to feel somewhat disempowered and marginalized by their extended family of marriage. Under these circumstances, it can be difficult to create an entrée of mythological proportions. As a result, social and culinary upheavals have occurred. The true reality of reconstructed potato salad is assumed to be relative to each chef and therefore open to interpretation and negotiation among reasonable cooks. Of course, the chief mother-in-law chef has been known to aggressively retain her traditional supremacy. In this case, education can play a crucial role in the planning, preparation and participation in the creation of a more democratic potato salad. Reconstructivist educators often play a critical role in these acts of social Darwinism. In this way, potato salad and "society can be rebuilt to be more humanly and personally fulfilling" (Lerwick, p. 52).

Reconstructivist assumptions of instruction are learner-centered in approximately the same way that progressive teachers put their students in the forefront of the learning process. Often it is assumed that learning is most effective when conducted in authentic political, economic, or social contexts.

Reconstructivist instructional methods in this paradigm are often contextualized and oriented toward the real world. Methods are likely to be rooted in social exploration with an emphasis on achieving social justice for under-represented groups. Again, similar to a progressive approach, reconstructionist teachers provide appropriate scaffolding and fading as needed. However, an important instructional method is the twin concepts of articulation of knowledge and subsequent reflection on meaning to the democratic life of the learner and for social justice within the larger society.

Assessment within a reconstructive paradigm is designed to ascertain the extent to which learners have become agents of social change. Are they adaptable change agents for greater social, economic, moral, and technological equality? Reconstructionists are often concerned with the establishment and maintenance of a humane workplace where the goal of equality among workers is met.

Existentialism

Existentialism, for many, is a difficult philosophy to understand and appreciate because it often defies systematic definition (Lerwick, 1979). The most common existential point of view comes from the nihilists who consider the world tragic and absurd (Kincheloe et al., 2000). "In other words, we find truth when we examine our present existence rather than some preconceived notion of the essential characteristics of the world and human beings" (p. 30). Lerwick (1979) identified three characteristics of existentialism. The first characteristic is a preoccupation with "philosophic paradoxes." Humans often attempt to make order of a disorderly world. One example is the strong human need to resolve cognitive dissonance such as the need to understand the mind of teenaged therapy patients. The second existential characteristic is the subjective nature of truth. "Each person exercises his or her freedom of choice to discover the truth" (Kincheloe et al., p. 30). Finally, many existentialists believe existence is a tragic consequence of being alone in an "arbitrary and random universe" that ends in personal anxiety (Lerwick, 1979, p. 58). Existentially speaking, it is up to each individual to promote human freedom while creating goodness and beauty in the world according to his or her own individual and subjective standards (Box 10-6).

B O X   1 0 - 6

Existential Potato Salad

The existential potato salad is created by individuals who seek to suit their own unique tastes—they can add ingredients as they wish. In fact, existential potato salad does not really have to have potatoes. In our family, each daughter-in-law exercised her existential right by adding the ingredients present at this "existential moment." As a free agent each avoided the anxiety of consuming potato salad that was absurd and not a part of her personal existence. For each, it was an attempt to identify the relative existence and nature of existential potato salad and to create a dish of goodness and beauty appropriate for their life's unique culinary journey.

Existentialist teachers are focused on assisting the learner to find his or her own understanding of the content. The emergence of the learner as his or her "authentic self" is an important goal. Teachers from this point of view recognize that they are free to "set goals for their own lives and destinies" (Lerwick, 1979, p. 60). Of course, this idea impacts on their practice as a teacher. It is critical to facilitate others as they set their own goals and seek their personal destiny.

The existentialist curriculum features content, methods, and sequence that are devoted to educational experiences that become a personal life project for the learner. Individualism and choice making constitute a constant curricular theme along with the inevitable consequences and accountability for decisions made.

Existentialist assumptions of instruction include an individual-oriented approach in which the learner is seeing a unique intellectual pathway that will guide his or her own personal and professional life. Although there may be both individual and group instruction, the emphasis is always on the development of the person.

Existentialist instructional methods are in many ways similar to those used by progressive and reconstructionist teachers. A difference might emerge around the use of individual tutorial-based exchanges between the teacher and the learner. A strong instructional emphasis is placed on articulation of knowledge as it is interpreted by the individual accompanied by an emphasis on meaning-making activities.

Assessment within an existentialist paradigm seeks to ensure that goals and objectives mutually negotiated between the teacher and the learner have been met. An existential teacher is also concerned that learners are prepared to seek their own destiny and that they know themselves as a person and a practitioner.

In summation, I contend that an understanding of the values, ethics, and views of truth and reality that inform practice are of critical importance to anyone who assumes an instructional role. Without some philosophic guidance, curriculum and instruction can appear to be without direction. In my early days of pre-service teacher preparation, I was warned not to become a "triple-threat teacher" who gives lectures on one subject, readings on another, and tests on a third. Without philosophic guidance, it is easy to become a learning threat to our students, and it is more difficult to keep the instructional train on the track and heading in a desirable and predictable direction.

In the next section, we explore an epistemological area that many educational experts reflect on through the lenses of philosophy, psychology and sociology.

KNOWLEDGE DEVELOPMENT AND SOCIAL CONSTRUCTIVISM

Here, our conversation turns to how we have come to believe that humans construct and use their knowledge. We will examine an emerging view of constructivism that can be thought of from the perspectives of philosophy, psychology, and sociology. This section concludes with a brief review of expertise and the epistemology of experts in a given field.

Knowledge Construction

The scholarly debate about constructivism as epistemology versus pedagogy has always been a highly charged discussion. Von Glasersfeld believes, however, that many of the debates are frivolous and distracting. He states, "constructivism does not claim to have made earth-shaking inventions in the area of education; it merely claims to provide a solid conceptual basis for some of the things that, until now, inspired teachers had to do without theoretical foundation" (1995, p. 35). It is in that spirit that we consider constructivism as an educator's "way of knowing" and teaching.

Many researchers of cognitive science have stated that learners create cognitive or mental structures. This premise has been extensively covered in Chapter 3. These mental models provide meaning and organization to the learners' experiences. It is in this way that individuals construct new ideas or concepts and learners become active participants in building new knowledge based on what they have already learned. This construction of knowledge has become known as "constructivism." An operational and generalized definition of constructivism is "the learner's contribution to meaning and learning through individual and/or social activity" (Biggs, 1996, p. 348).

Types of Constructivism

The most common three types of constructivism are connected via a unifying theme: The assumed cognitive orientation of the learner. One might ask: How is the learner cognitively oriented to his or her world? Does the learner's worldview take precedent in the construction of mental frameworks or schema? Another constructivist from a competing point-of-view might ask: Does the learner's prior knowledge (or schema) strongly influence his or her interpretation of the world? Or, does it happen both ways as a blended interaction between environmental influences and existing cognitive structures? These competing forms of constructivism are known in the literature as *exogenous* (oriented to environmental influences), *endogenous* (existing mental frameworks interpret environment), and *dialectical* constructivism (a blend of the two above types of constructivism). These educational perspectives are discussed in much greater detail in Chapter 11 as we begin to think about how learning theories such as these influence teaching practices.

From an epistemology point of view, exogenous constructivism represents knowledge as a true reality that corresponds with the learner's accepted environment. This is consistent with the assumed truth in both essentialist and perennialist philosophic positions; there is little room for truth with shades of gray. Many early constructivist learning theorists have viewed humans as possessing machine-like mental qualities. Information is taken in, stored in mental frameworks, and then recalled when needed in much the same way that a computer might store and recall bits of data on magnetic media. It is the conception of mental frameworks that gives this perspective the characteristics of constructivism. This metaphor of frameworks and cognitive associations remains common among today's educators and policy-makers, who place a high premium on information retention and recall on standardized tests to measure student achievement. The historical and theoretical traditions supporting this exogenous perspective come from the early research in the area of cognitive science. "This general orientation to psychology . . . goes under a variety of names most commonly the 'information processing approach' and the 'cognitive science' approach" (Phillips & Soltis, 1998, p. 75). The information processing or "mind as machine" concept remains a strong influence in our metaphorical understanding of the mind.

Endogenous constructivism represents knowledge acquisition that begins with the learner's internal cognition and shapes an understanding of the external environment through that mental lens. This second view of constructivist learning has many implications for instructional design, methods of delivery, and assessment of student accomplishment. The instructional emphasis is on the learner as an individual.

Epistemologically speaking, knowledge acquired is abstract and is constructed through intense cognitive activity. This is in contrast to the exogenous assumption that knowledge creation is primarily passive in nature. Another perspective is that knowledge is invented, not discovered, as would be asserted by other constructivists. The invention of knowledge suggests that the nature of what is true is likely to be different for each learner. To the extent that knowledge is constructed, learning is then a matter of understanding the meaning of information and how it fits with other bits of knowledge.

The third type of constructivism is dialectical, a blend of both internal and external constructivism. The cognitive orientation moves from the individual to how groups of individuals construct knowledge in social settings. This perspective assumes an interaction between learners and their physical and social environments. Dialectical knowledge development is often associated with "contextualism," in which *"thought and experience are inextricably intertwined with the contexts or settings where learning occurs"* (Bruning, Schraw & Ronning, 1999, p. 217, italics added).

Within blended constructivism, the epistemological nature of knowledge is relative to the interpretation of the individual learner and those who might have social influence in the learner's environment. Truth from this perspective is submerged in cultural beliefs, tools, and artifacts. Although some might believe that truth can be known absolutely, here it is as if understanding of what is true is negotiated through internal and external mental interactions.

Knowledge gained from this social form of constructivism places great value on the experiences of the learner and his or her ability to extract meaning from experiences. The work of Lev Vygotsky (1978) has contributed to the construction of a theoretical framework that embraces physical and more abstract social-psychological tools. Many theorists now believe that learners use physical tools when engaged with the external world. Conversely, sociopsychological tools are symbol systems employed by individuals when engaged in thinking (John-Steiner, 1997). The use of both physical and sociopsychological tools enables change over time as learners internalize and transform interactions into mental frameworks. Using Vygotsky's zone of proximal development (ZPD) as a way to think about learning and teaching, teachers and learners can engage in mutual work in what might be called the "construction zone" (Newman, Griffin & Cole, 1989). The ZPD is thought to be the difference between the level of difficulty that a child can demonstrate with independence and a level that can be achieved with the help of a facilitating adult teacher (Vygotsky, 1978). This interaction between learner and teacher is similar to the scaffolding/fading strategies described by internal constructivism, but now the emphasis turns to social interactions and mutual interpretations of knowledge and subsequent understandings.

How does one gain and apply knowledge that is exemplary? What are the epistemological characteristics of experts? Is their knowledge construction and use different from a novice or a mid-level practitioner? The research suggests that such differences do exist.

EXPERT KNOWLEDGE

From the perspective of theory and research on expertise, outstanding performance must be considered to occur within a given domain of knowledge and as a result of domain-specific training and practice (Ericsson & Smith, 1991). The assumption underlying this approach is that intelligent, flexible thinking emerges as the individual develops a rich understanding of a domain and the ability to use this knowledge in multiple contexts. For example, an expert occupational therapist not only has years of education but has extensively practiced the use of learned knowledge and skills.

Expertise is more than book learning; it is the ability to use knowledge to solve problems within a domain. Outstanding performance within a domain is the outcome of years of study and training in a given field. A novice therapist may have a more difficult time with an unusual set of performance problems. Conversely, a more experienced therapist will have had sufficient experience to deal with the novelty of unusual situations. Many educational programs in therapeutic healthcare fields cite the work of Patricia Benner (1984) as a way to think about expertise and its meaning to the development of helping professionals. Benner's work, popularly known as the Novice to Expert Continuum, is drawn from the Dreyfus Model of Skill Acquisition (Dreyfus & Dreyfus, 1980) and applied to the field of nursing. In their review of occupational therapy clinical reasoning development, Schell, Crepeau, and Cohn (2003) proposed a model of expertise development in different strands of reasoning (*Table 10-2*).

TABLE 10-2

Clinical Reasoning Developmental Stages and Characteristics in Occupational Therapy Practice

Stage	Years of Reflective Practice	Characteristics
Novice	0	No experience in situation of practice and therefore dependent on theory to guide practice. Uses rule-based procedural reasoning to guide actions, but doesn't recognize contextual cues and therefore not skillful in adapting rules to fit situation. Narrative reasoning used to establish social relationships, but does not significantly inform practice. Pragmatic reasoning stressed in terms of job survival skills. Recognizes overt ethical issues.
Advanced beginner	<1	Begins to incorporate contextual information into rule-based thinking. Recognizes differences between theoretical expectations and presenting problems. Limited experience impedes recognition of patterns, difficulty identifying salient cues, consequently doesn't prioritize well. Gaining skill in pragmatic and narrative reasoning. Begins to recognize more subtle ethical issues.
Competent	3	Automatically performs more therapeutic skills, and attends to more issues. Able to develop communal horizon with persons receiving service. Sorts relevant data, and able to prioritize intervention goals related to desired outcomes. Planning is deliberate, efficient and responsive to contextual issues. Uses conditional reasoning to modify intervention but lacks flexibility of more advanced practitioners. Recognizes ethical dilemmas posed by practice setting, but may be less sensitive to justifiably different ethical responses.
Proficient	5	Perceives situations as wholes. Reflects on expanded range of experiences, which permits more focused evaluation, more flexibility in intervention. Creatively combines different diagnostic and procedural approaches. More attentive to occupational stories and relevance for intervention. More skillful in negotiating resources to meet patient/client needs. Increased sophistication in recognizing situational nature of ethical reasoning.

(continued)

TABLE 10-2

(continued)

Stage	Years of Reflective Practice	Characteristics
Expert	10	Clinical reasoning becomes a quick intuitive process, which is deeply internalized and embedded, in an extensive range of case experiences. This permits practice with less routine analysis, except when confronted with situations where approach is not working. Highly skillful use of occupational story making during intervention to promote long-term occupational performance satisfaction.

From Schell, Crepeau & Cohn. (2003). Professional development. In: Crepeau, Cohn & Schell (Eds.). *Willard and Spackman's occupational therapy,* 10th ed. (p. 143). Philadelphia: Lippincott Williams & Wilkins. Used with permission.

From an epistemological point of view, research on expertise is important because it allows insight into how individuals at differing levels of experience conceptualize problem states and how they use their knowledge to engage in problem solving. This concept is also important because it affords a view of the nature of truth as seen by individuals at differing stages of professional development.

WAYS OF KNOWING

Other researchers and writers have explored ways in which members of individual groups have come to know what it is that they know. Probably the most famous and most often-cited work in this area is the work of Belenky, Clinchy, Goldberger, and Tarulet in *Women's Ways of Knowing* (1997). Their work consisted of 135 case studies of women in which respondents were interviewed with regard to their knowledge of gender, relationships, the epistemological nature of their knowledge, and applications within assorted moral dilemmas. The qualitative research data of Belenky et al. provided evidence that women's perspectives on knowledge development and use could be summarized in five intermittent categories. These divisions included (a) silence, (b) received knowledge, (c) subjective knowledge, (d) procedural knowledge, and (e) constructed knowledge. The category of *silence* gave evidence that many women experience themselves as an entity without a socially valued voice and are frequently marginalized by external sources of auditory authority. Other women cited themselves as receptacles of *received knowledge* that is reproduced by relying on evidence drawn from external authorities. At this stage, women infrequently speak for themselves and see words as concrete, specific, and dualistic opposites. *Subjective knowledge* is a conviction that right or correct answers exist within themselves. These women often believe that truth is localized to the person and external sources of evidence are unnecessary. Fortunately, many women at this stage are developing a sense of self, appreciation for life experiences, and are becoming more vocal, but evidence for opinions is often underdeveloped and incomplete. In later stages of epistemological development, many women develop *procedural knowledge* in which a sense of knowing is based on more careful observation and the nature of problems are increasingly viewed as more complex or ill-structured. Belenky et al. report that this can be a difficult stage of development for many women as the world becomes less certain and their inner voices become more critical. *Constructed knowledge* is a higher-order stage in which women engage in integration of complex concepts. Here, a high tolerance for ambiguity and uncertainty is developed and appreciated. Now knowledge is not easily placed into gift-wrapped boxes, but is represented by contradictive evidence and relative representations of truth and reality.

The importance of Belenky's work is that it gives evidence of hope for the development of higher-order thinking among practicing professionals. Teachers and professors should take heart that experience and strategic education can lead to higher levels of thoughtfulness and problem solving at relatively earlier stages of career development.

To achieve greater levels of problem solving, it is important to be able to sort useful information from that which has more limited applicability. For example, practitioners need to be able to make judgments based on valid evidence and reflections on practice.

REFLECTIVE JUDGMENT AND REFLECTIVE PRACTICE

Here, we examine two main bodies of literature that can be woven together to shed light on learning and practice: King and Kitchener's theory of reflective judgment (1994) and Schön's (1983) work with the everyday actions of a professional's practice.

Stages of Reflective Judgment

The work of King and Kitchener (1994) describes stages of growth in terms of how individual judgment is drawn. The model stages judgment is based on the level and quality of evidence used by individuals to support a particular position. Epistemologically, this theory is also based on the nature of the problem to be studied and the nature of truth. King and Kitchener make a distinction between problems that are structured and those that are ill-structured. They argue that as a learner advances through these stages of reflective judgment, the nature of acceptable evidence becomes more stringent while what is known to be true becomes more relative to specific situations. Structured problems are those that lend themselves to logical and direct solutions. For example, administration of the *Motor-Free Visual Perception Test* could be an example of a highly structured standardized test that is accompanied by standardized scoring procedures. Here, solutions can be described with confidence, completeness, and certainty. Experts have agreed with these solutions when the standardized instrument was validated and tested for reliability before being commercially published. However, OTs often face problems that are much more difficult to solve. These are known by King and Kitchener as ill-structured problems in which the nature of the problem cannot be described with completeness and is often not completely solved. Even when some ill-structured problems are partially resolved, experts often disagree on the effectiveness of the solution. An example of an ill-structured problem for an occupational therapist is helping a young parent learn to care for an infant who has cerebral palsy while also caring for other typically developing children and maintaining his or her role as marriage partner. A middle position between structured and ill-structured problems could be illustrated by the administration of the Canadian Occupation Performance Measure (COPM). This assessment procedure consists of standardized guidelines and format, but also requires expert interviewing skills on the part of the administering therapist.

King and Kitchener (1994) cluster these stages into *prereflective, quasi-reflective*, and *reflective* groups.

Prereflective Stages

Stages 1, 2, and 3 represent prereflective thinking. In Stage 1, knowledge is assumed to exist absolutely; there are no abstractions and truth is obtained with certainty by simple observation. There is no need for justification at this first stage, as knowledge is absolute and alternate perspectives are not permitted.

At Stage 2, knowledge is still certain or has the potential to be certain when it becomes available. Knowledge becomes known and justified through direct observation or from another authoritative human source. Truth is thought to be absolute and often little thought is given to the solution of highly ill-structured problems. An example might be a robust patriotic belief that one's country is always on the side of God in any international conflict or dispute.

Stage 3 knowledge is again certain or, if unknown, to be considered so only on a temporary basis. Only personal opinions are known absolutely, but other knowledge can be swayed by an authoritative person with evidence to prove his or her point. Justification of this level of knowledge is based on the word of a person assumed to be an expert. For example, urban legends such as alligators in an urban sewer system are often perpetuated by authorities who report having seen such a reptile in a toilet bowl.

Quasi-reflective Stages

At the quasi-reflective thinking stages (4 and 5), knowledge and its nature become slightly more complex and situated. Stage 4 thinking involves increasing levels of ambiguity and the acceptance of knowledge as uncertain. Justification for an individual's knowledge is based on reasons given and the use of evidence. The evidence, however, is unique to the point being made by the individual. An example of Stage 4 quasi-reflective thinking revolves around the mystery of Egyptian pyramids. No one alive today can give an exact answer to how these marvels were constructed. Consequently, many theories and varying levels of proof of those theories are offered to explain their existence.

Knowledge at Stage 5 is subjective and contextualized. It is often based on personal perceptions and an individual's selected criteria for making such a judgment. Justification for such beliefs is extracted and interpreted from rules of inquiry unique to that context. However, different individuals might interpret data differently owing to a variety of cognitive and emotional predispositions. A timely example might be how different and well-meaning groups propose to solve the persistent problem of teenaged pregnancies outside marriage. One group might examine the problem from a moral perspective, citing evidence of scripture and biblical teaching while prescribing a solution of sexual abstinence among teenaged partners. Other groups might choose to consider the same problem from the perspective of personal development and strongly advocate for a curriculum that promotes maturity and good decision-making skills among teens as a solution. Still others may look at unwanted pregnancy as a much larger social problem.

Reflective Stages

Stages 6 and 7 are described by King and Kitchener (1994) as reflective thinking. Individuals practicing at these levels are often independent and inclined toward reasoned arguments and valuable analysis. In Stage 6, knowledge is also constructed. Conclusions are drawn about difficult and ill-structured problems on the bases of high-quality data extracted from a variety of sources. In this stage, problem solvers are concerned with solutions to complex (ill-structured) problems and make supporting judgments based on (a) the quality of the evidence collected, (b) the practicality of a given solution, and (c) the importance of the problem. An example might be how a well-informed person might construct their position on right-to-life issues such as abortion, sustaining life in a persistent vegetative state, applications of the death penalty, and appropriate conventions when prosecuting a war.

At Stage 7, knowledge as an outcome of inquiry is constructed on the basis of evidence that is the most reasonable and probable. All such solutions are re-evaluated when new or better evidence is made available. Often Stage 7 solutions are justified based on probability and consideration as to the weight of the evidence, adequacy and consistency of the explanation drawn from the evidence, and the calculated risk of making a mistake. An example of Stage 7 reflective judgments might be those of astrophysicists who develop their arguments based on photographic, radiographic, and digital data downloaded from satellite technology such as the Hubble Telescope. From these data, and other collaborating sources, hypotheses about the origins and true nature of the universe are often constructed.

Developing and using reflective judgment constitutes only the first step toward becoming a reflective practitioner. In the next section, we discuss reflective practice and make associations with concepts such as the above-mentioned reflective judgment that might assist readers as they strive to become reflective practitioners.

Reflective Practice

Reflective practice can be considered foundational when building professional expertise. Lessons learned about most psychosocial learning theories strongly suggest that specific learning contexts are important when taken alone (insufficient). Contextualized learning experiences should be "examined" in light of how reflective judgments can be made and meaning extracted. Such reflective educational practices bring about opportunities to explore newly acquired knowledge that results in more meaningfulness and an emerging identity for the learner. It is one thing to have command of facts and figures, but quite another to be able to use those facts in a practical way to solve ill-structured problems in the clinic, workplace, or home.

The promotion of reflective practice is one instructional strategy that exposes learners to the "next step of learning." Learners often want to know, "What does this information mean to me?" "How will this help me solve problems that I encounter at work or in my learning community?" These are natural questions and come from the famous question we all asked our algebra teachers: When will I ever use this stuff?

Both endogenous and dialectical constructivists, along with learning theorists who write from a socialization perspective, speak to the importance of concepts such as reflective practice as a way for learners to make topics relevant and meaningful. A model that is often adopted when reflecting on importance of reflection is the work of Donald Schön (1983). His work *reflection in action* and *reflection on action* is widely accepted and does appear to have application to the education of teachers in higher education settings who are concerned with bridging the gap between theory and practice.

Reflection-in-action is a slight pause during practice to mentally connect current actions with a conceptual framework of theory that gives authority and legitimacy to what the professional is doing at the moment (Schön). Bruning, Schraw & Ronning, (1999) describe this practice as an "on-the spot thought experiment" (p. 222). A teacher of occupational therapy might make a quick, but value-free, judgment to test some type of alternative instructional strategy—a type of working hypothesis about their instructional practice. Reflection-on-action is a look behind to connect with reflections-in-action previously taken and evaluate their effectiveness or efficiency. Both are metacognitive strategies that can help students understand how information might be applied and have meaning in real life (Bruning et al.).

Of course, there are many ways to reflect and many metacognitive processes supported by instructive activities. When students are asked to verbally articulate their knowledge and their thought processes when solving a problem, the result can be a powerful opportunity for students to compare their thinking with that of others. Students and teachers, as members of learning communities, can readily observe theoretical and practical constructs from many perspectives. This can be especially powerful when both learners and teachers are held accountable for the quality of their judgments and the evidence that they select to justify their position. When this happens, it is learning at its best.

SUMMARY

We have touched on the surface of epistemology or the nature of knowledge. Our philosophic examination has taken us through common elements of educational philosophy and the most common Western schools of educational thought. Later, we turned our attention to knowledge development in the contexts of social constructivism and then continued with insights into how specific groups conceive, develop, and use their knowledge. Finally, we discussed stages of reflective judgment and how it is related to reflective practice. In the next chapter, we refocus our attention to the intentional act of teaching for expert practice.

LEARNING ACTIVITY 10-1

Draw Your Philosophy

Purpose

To represent your educational beliefs on paper without having to write the standard, two-page "My Philosophy" assignment

Connections to Major Clinical Reasoning Constructs

This activity will connect with various schools of educational philosophy and begin to allow learners to see themselves in a philosophic home.

Directions for Learners

Working alone for 10 to 15 minutes, use the provided marking pens, construction paper, glue, glitter, puppet eyes, etc., to do the following:

1 Create a representation of what you now believe to be your educational philosophy. (It is okay to represent yourself in more than one philosophic position; in fact, it is quite common.)
2 Present your artwork to your colleagues and explain why you have represented your educational philosophy as you have.

A variation on this activity is to make a philosophy tee-shirt. Collect the artwork, scan it as a .jpg file, and print it out using an InkJet printer and iron-on transfer materials. Be sure that your reverse the image before you print it out. Iron the transfer material onto a plain white cotton tee-shirt and give it to the artist as a way to commemorate his or her initial educational philosophy.

LEARNING ACTIVITY 10-2

Where is Billy?

Purpose

To illustrate how King and Kitchener's States of Reflective Judgment can be used to understand more about a stated position

Connections to Major Clinical Reasoning Constructs

This activity will connect with the use of evidence and the construction of the problem.

Directions for Learners

Allowing approximately 20 minutes, in groups of four or five people:

1 Read the attached article in which Dr. Billy Graham is reflecting on his life-long ministry.
2 Reflect on his comments and then place him at one or more of King and Kitchener's Stages of Reflective Judgment. Arrive at a consensus among members of your group.
3 Prepare to defend your choices on the basis of the type of problem that Dr. Graham is addressing, and the quality of the evidence that he has chosen to cite.

The article can be obtained from the *USA Today* website. Search for "Billy Graham Humble Before God, Clinton. February 4th, 1998." Note that the use of this article should not be construed as condoning or criticizing a particular religious conviction. The attached article was selected because it illustrates one person's thoughtful reflection on a lifetime of practice.

REFERENCES

Benner, P. (1984). *From novice to expert*. Menlo Park, CA: Addison-Wesley.

Belenky, M.F., Clinchy, B.M., Goldberger, N.R. & Tarule, J.M. (1997). *Women's ways of knowing: The development of self, voice and mind. Tenth Anniversary Edition*. New York: Basic Books.

Bigge, M.L. & Shermis, S.S. (2004). *Learning theories for teachers* (6th ed.). Boston: Allyn & Bacon.

Bransford, J., Brown, A. & Cocking, R. (Eds.) (1999, 2000). How People Learn: Brain, Mind, Experience, and School. Washington, D.C.: National Academy Press. Online at: http://www.nap.edu/html/howpeople1/

Bruning, R. H., Schraw, G. J. & Ronning, R. R. (1999). *Cognitive psychology and instruction*. Upper Saddle River, NJ: Prentice-Hall.

Campbell, J. & Moyers, B. (1988). *The power of myth*. New York: Doubleday.

Biggs, J. (1996). Enhancing teaching through constructive alignment. *Higher Education*, 32, 347–364.

Dreyfus, S. & Dreyfus, H. (February, 1980). *A five-stage model of the mental activities involved in directed skill acquisition*. Unpublished report supported by the Air Force Office of Scientific Research (AFSC), USAF (Contract F49620-79-C-0063), University of California at Berkeley.

Dewey, J. (1910: 1933). *How we think. A restatement of the relation of reflective thinking to the educative process* (rev. ed.), Boston: D. C. Heath.

Dewey, J. (1948). *Reconstruction in philosophy*. Boston: Beacon Press.

Ericsson, K. A. & Smith, J. (1991). Prospects and limits in the empirical study of expertise: An introduction. In K. A. Ericsson & J. Smith (Eds.), Toward a general theory of expertise: Prospects and limits (pp. 1–38). Cambridge: Cambridge University Press.

Freire, P. (1997). *Pedagogy of the oppressed* (20th Anniversary Edition). New York: Continuum.

John-Steiner, V. (1997). *Notebooks of the mind: Explorations of thinking* (rev. ed.). New York: Oxford University Press.

Kincheloe, J.L., Slattery, P. & Steinberg, S.R., (2000). *Contextualized teaching: Introduction to education and educational foundations*. Boston: Addison Wesley Longman.

King, P.M. & Kitchener, K.S (1994). *Developing reflective judgment: Understanding and promoting intellectual growth and critical thinking in adolescents and adults*. San Francisco: Jossey-Bass.

Lave, J. & Wenger, E. (1991). *Situated learning. Legitimate peripheral participation*, Cambridge: University of Cambridge Press.

Lerwick, L. (1979). *Alternative concepts of vocational education*. ERIC Document Retrieval Service (ED: 169 285).

Newman, D., Griffin P. & Cole M. (1989). *The construction zone: working for cognitive change in school*. Cambridge: Cambridge University Press.

O'Hear, A. (1995). History of the philosophy of education. In T. Hondrich (Ed.), *The Oxford companion to philosophy*. New York: Oxford University Press.

Phillips, D. C. & Soltis, J. F. (1998). *Perspectives on learning* (3rd ed.). New York: Teachers College Press.

Rojewski, J.W. & Schell, J.W. (1994). Instructional considerations for college students with disabilities. In K.W. Prichard & R. McLaren Sawyer (Eds.), *Handbook of college teaching*. Westport, CT: Greenwood Press.

Schell, B.A.B. Crepeau, E.B. & Cohn, E.S. (2003). Professional development. In E.B Crepeau, E.S. Cohn & B.A.B. Schell (Eds.), *Willard and Spackman's occupational therapy* (10th ed., p. 143). Philadelphia: Lippincott Williams & Wilkins.

Schön, D. A. (1983). *The reflective practitioner: How professionals think in action*. New York: Basic Books.

von Glasersfeld, E. (1995). *Radical constructivism: A way of knowing and learning*. London & Washington: The Falmer Press.

Vygotsky, L. S. (1978). *Mind in society*. Cambridge, MA: Harvard University Press.

Wenger, E. (1989). *Communities of practice*. Cambridge, U.K.: Cambridge University Press.

Westbrook, R.B. (1991). *John Dewey and American democracy*. Ithaca, NY: Cornell University Press.

White, J. (1995). *Problems of the philosophy of education*. In T. Hondrich (Ed.), *The Oxford companion to philosophy*. New York: Oxford University Press.

Teaching for Expert Practice

John W. Schell and Barbara A. Boyt Schell

OBJECTIVES

After reading this chapter, the learner will be able to:

1 Articulate theories and frameworks that constitute contextual learning and teaching concepts.
2 Strategically utilize elements of context and matching learning perspectives to maximize the effectiveness of contextualized instruction.
3 Strategically utilize interactive elements of curriculum to contextualize and energize their teaching.
4 Apply concepts of contextual learning and teaching (CLT) in management and supervisory contexts.
5 Facilitate the development of expertise among novice therapists.

KEY TERMS

Context	Expertise	Dialectical constructivism
Transfer	Exogenous constructivism	Instructional content
Learning transfer	Endogenous constructivism	Instructional sequence
Settings	Instructional methods	

I n this chapter, we focus on teaching for expert practice. We use selected learning theories associated with teaching practices that promote earlier expertise and reflective practice. Recent research on teaching clearly suggests the important role of context. The form of teaching discussed here promotes higher-order thinking and the use of information to solve problems in the context of professional practice. Next, we examine supportive teaching and curricula that use the aforementioned learning theories to promote expert behaviors among our students. Last, we discuss how these practices can be used to transcend the higher education classroom to real practice settings where student and practitioner learning is supported by field supervisors and program managers.

Thinking About Thinking 11-1

Thought flows in terms of stories—stories about events, stories about people, and stories about intentions and achievements. The best teachers are the best story tellers.

—Frank Smith

I (John) would like to begin with three brief but important caveats about learning and teaching. There are many ways to successfully approach the job of teaching. Many successful teachers effectively use direct teaching techniques such as abstract lecture in isolated contexts. Other teachers are equally effective by using indirect forms of teaching such as facilitation. In my nearly 40 years of teaching experience, I have found that there is a time and a place for almost all instructional strategies. However, for the purposes of this book and this chapter our focus is on a form of learning and teaching used for the purpose of promoting and enhancing professional reasoning. For that reason, I have selected a specific body of educational literature with regard to teaching, which can guide learners toward the goal of meaning-making and reflective practice.

Second, Barbara and I have been collaborating in this area of learning and teaching for professional reasoning for several years. I have learned a great deal about occupational therapy during that time, but my day job still remains in the area of the education of teachers. Our collaboration, however, has pointed out to me how integral teaching is to effective occupational therapy and to the education of expert therapists. Because of a recent knee replacement surgery, I have experientially relearned this lesson from both sides of the clinic. This important role of OT as teacher is equally true for OT educators and for OTs themselves as they engage in daily practice. So, it is important that OTs learn about how learning theories support good teaching.

The third caveat is a language convention that I have adopted in recent years. In my writing, I always use the term "learning and teaching" as opposed to the more common expression of "teaching and learning." To me, this is a small but important difference. After many years of research, writing, and learning about learning, I have come to appreciate the many diffcrences between learning and teaching. For example, college teachers cannot simply teach harder or differently and then expect learners to magically learn and retain more information. The dynamic between learning and teaching is far too complex to assume a direct relationship. Students still must accept responsibility and engage deeply in learning. These efforts can be facilitated by effective teaching but learning may not be the result. Teaching can only facilitate learning and possibly motivate the learner, but it cannot directly cause the neurological changes required for learning to occur. So, learning always precedes teaching, especially when the educator is engaged in curriculum or instructional planning. My admittedly unconventional point is that teaching can be more effective when it is based directly on specific assumptions of learning. When this is done, targeted teaching strategies can address students' needs. If teachers would routinely match their teaching practices to their perceptions of how individuals learn, our mutual profession of teaching professionals and subsequent instruction for clients would be more effective. Now, I would like to begin the exploration of the meaning of contextualized learning and teaching.

CONTEXTUAL LEARNING AND TEACHING

Now let us look at contextualized learning and the scholarly arguments that suggest that learning in realistic situations can be more effective when the expectation is to enhance levels of expert professional practice. In the following text, I provide operational definitions for key terminology, discuss the nature of contextual learning in classrooms and in real-life settings, and then turn to a brief examination of social and psychological learning theories that support contextual learning and teaching.

Definitions of Key Terms

The term **context** is defined as social and psychological constructs including (a) the level of conceptual knowledge, (b) learners' interpretation of instructional goals, and (c) participant roles that the learner brings to bear in the setting. **Transfer** across settings depends on the ability of the individual to interpret the social setting in such a way that enables them to apply and use the knowledge within that setting (Schell, 1999). Other key terms here are "settings" and "transfer." **Settings** are defined as physical places or tasks in which learning occurs. Unfortunately, instruction within formal or informal settings does not guarantee transfer unless the learner recognizes similarities across contexts (Detterman & Sternberg, 1993; Schell, 1999). Transfer is defined as learners' independent use of knowledge and skills across settings (Detterman & Sternberg, 1993). **Learning transfer** is thought to be dependent on how the learner interprets the setting and the nature of the learning context.

Another key aspect of this chapter is what we mean when we use the term **expertise**. From the perspective of theory and research on the term, expertise is outstanding performance within a domain of knowledge and is the result of domain-specific training and practice (Ericsson & Smith, 1991). The assumption underlying this approach is that intelligent, flexible thinking emerges as the individual develops a rich understanding of a domain and the ability to use this knowledge in multiple contexts. For example, an expert physician not only has years of education but has practiced the use of learned knowledge and skills.

Expertise is more than "book learning"; it is the ability to use that knowledge to adroitly solve problems within that domain. Outstanding performance within a domain is the outcome of years of study and training in a given field. The theory that supports contextual learning and teaching assumes that learning is tied to a specific context; an expertise approach assumes that learning is tied to a domain of knowledge. As the student acquires more expertise within a domain, that knowledge becomes more flexible, and the student is more able to deal with novel and complex problems. A new doctor may not be able to deal with an unusual set of symptoms or may be fooled by a common illness that presents an uncommon set of symptoms. Conversely, a more experienced and expert doctor has a greater repertoire to successfully deal with the novelty of unusual situations.

Expertise is assumed to gradually emerge with experience within the context of a specific domain. When students are novices, they are unlikely to have a deep understanding of a domain but will focus on surface features of usually complex problems. Their problem solving will be more hit-or-miss rather than planned. As their skills and knowledge emerge with experience, they begin to have a deeper understanding of a domain and, as a result, are able to create more effective plans of action. This ability comes from both a rich knowledge of a field and from experience using that knowledge. Thus, the main purpose of this chapter is to illustrate a form of teaching that is thought to promote earlier expertise among new professionals.

Continuum of Contexts and Settings

Let's begin with this question: What does it mean to contextualize instruction? I argue that all learning is contextual in one fashion or another. But qualitative differences do seem to exist, depending on the context in which learners are expected to eventually apply their knowledge. As a foundational part of an extensive research grant from the U.S. Department of Education on contextual learning and teaching (CLT), researchers at The University of Georgia, College of Education created a graphic depiction of the relationship of contexts and settings (*Figure 11-1*). This graphic is an array along a continuum that ranges from "abstract" to "authentic contexts and settings" (Schell, 1999). As we continue in this chapter, this continuum is used to help you locate the theories relative to their use of natural contexts. Note that this discussion in many ways parallels the discussions that the occupational therapy profession has been having about occupation, and the importance of the context in performance (AOTA-COP, 2002; Fisher, 1998; Schell, 2003).

CLT rests on the assumption that learning should be to the extent possible situated in authentic contexts and settings. This element is drawn from the extensive literature on situated cognition (Lave, 1988) and communities of practice (Wenger, 1998) and other forms of socialization within a variety of professions (Brown, Collins & Duguid, 1989).

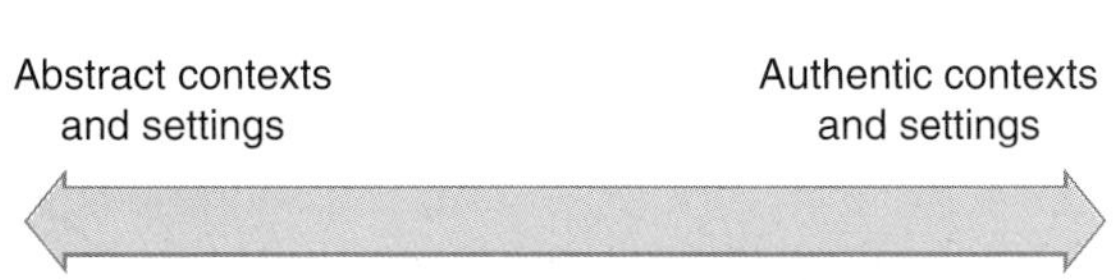

Abstract contexts
and settings   Authentic contexts
and settings

Figure 11-1   Continuum of contexts and settings.

Assumptions of Contextual Learning and Teaching

What does instruction look like when contextual learning and teaching (CLT) is practiced? Box 11-2 is a list of key attributes of CLT practice. Here, I refer to these principles in the boxed examples and relate them to associated learning theories.

> **BOX 11-1**
>
> ## Attributes and Instructional Practices of CLT
>
> 1. *Authentic learning contexts* promote actively *engaged learners* using *higher-order thinking and problem-solving skills.*
> 2. Learners increase *levels of expertise* using knowledge *relevant* to their professional life.
> 3. Learning in *multiple contexts* allows learners to *identify and solve problems* in unique contexts (transfer).
> 4. Learners learn through community of practice framework, which can enhance *cooperation, discourse, teamwork,* resulting in *self-reflection.*
> 5. Learners take *metacognitive* responsibility for *reflecting on practice* resulting in *meaning making* and *application* (learning to learn reflectively is as important as the content that is learned).
> 6. Learners' *mental frameworks* and *prior experiences* are used to guide instruction.
> 7. Teachers act as facilitators of learning using a *repertoire of contextualized instructional methods.*

The key to this teaching approach is the use of authentic contexts to promote relevance to the learners and to extend that recognition to the creation of instructional opportunities that promote reflection and meaning making. Crist, Wilcox, and McCarron (1998) provide a wonderful example of such reflective professional development using transitional portfolios. These professors of occupational therapy assume that professional competence is an outcome of self-directed reflective activities. Their model is based on the assumption that reflection on clinical reasoning is at the intersection of the modes of (a) practice, (b) information, and (c) knowledge. The transitional portfolio emphasizes practice as experience and associated problem solving. The information mode is based on evaluation, whereas knowledge assumes the creation of pertinent information via research, writing, and presentation. In addition, these researchers illustrate the use of a transitional portfolio at differing stages of professional development, beginning with the novice practitioner and concluding with the advanced reflective practitioner. This approach is clearly consistent with the reflective elements of CLT, especially when the transitional portfolio documentation can be described using adjectives such as relevant, problem oriented, social, metacognitive, diverse, and reflective.

More about the attributes of CLT is presented in the following sections. However, if I were asked to justify contextual learning and teaching, I would have to say that the greatest benefit comes from moving students into higher levels of reflection and expertise at earlier phases of their career. This is accomplished mostly because the instructional emphasis is on relevant learning requiring higher-order thinking and problem solving and extensive reflection on authentic and relevant practice.

Elements of Constructivism

Contextual learning and teaching is consistent with many of the constructivist learning theories that were briefly introduced in Chapter 10. Although it is true that these theories have application to reflective practice and learning in context, it is also true that there are many ways to be a constructivist. A generalized definition of constructivism is ". . . the learner's contribution to meaning and learning through individual and/or social activity" (Biggs, 1996, p.98). However, not all of the constructivist theories are oriented to the social nexus that most people commonly associate with constructivism.

Constructivist Theories

Constructivism is an important learning theory in today's technological society. The rapid economic, social, and cultural changes seem to promote a society in which knowledge has a very short shelf life. A high degree of thinking and problem solving is required to live well in today's society. Constructivist pedagogy (as well as andragogy) appears to have a good deal of face validity when thought of as a potential educational solution to the preparation of occupational therapists to meet the demands of a highly volatile technology-enhanced lifelong-learning society. Constructivist pedagogy appears to have the potential to promote self-directed and intentional learning. It is expected that teachers and students trained from this learning perspective may become more self-motivated and mature as life-long learners.

The scholarly debate about constructivism as a way to think about epistemology and pedagogy is highly charged. Von Glasersfeld believes that many of the debates are frivolous and distracting. He states, "Constructivism does not claim to have made earth-shaking inventions in the area of education; it merely claims to provide a solid conceptual basis for some of the things that, until now, inspired teachers had to do without theoretical foundation" (1995, p. 26). In that spirit, this framework embraces a range of constructivist theories and celebrates the attempts of all faculties to construct learning opportunities that result in meaningful education for all students.

Types of Constructivism

The teacher who wishes to practice as a constructivist has to make many decisions with regard to the type of constructivist he or she wish to be. To simplify the topic somewhat, we are going to examine three types of constructivism: exogenous, endogenous, and dialectical. Choosing among these models depends on the assumptions one makes about the nature of learning and the context in which knowledge will be used. In this chapter, we are limiting our discussion to a brief introduction to exogenous constructivism in favor of a more detailed discussion of endogenous and dialectical constructivism. This decision is also consistent with the work of Hooper and Wood (2002), in which the philosophic elements of pragmatism and structuralism were compared and contrasted. Although certainly not rejecting a structuralist (objectification) approach to education as illegitimate, a pragmatism approach appears to be more consistent with the goal of educating reflective practitioners in the current culture of occupation-based, holistic OT practice (Hooper & Wood). As we proceed, text boxes highlight instructional elements and strategies that are appropriate for those who want to teach or become reflective practitioners.

EXOGENOUS CONSTRUCTIVISM

Exogenous constructivism was articulated by early cognitive scientists. Learning was portrayed by them as "a rather passive or mechanical process—the acquisition of a new behavior, was more or less something that happened to a learner rather than being something that a learner did or achieved" (Phillips & Soltis, 1998, p. 33). Exogenous constructivism represented a movement away from such passive views of learning, focusing on the development of mental structures as a reaction to the external world (*Figure 11-2*).

The *cognitive orientation* for external constructivism is based on the assumption that learners rely on external sources to help them interpret their world. For these learners, the world is understood in light of cause-and-effect relationships, received information that is presented by authoritative figures, or observed behaviors. These interactions between the individual and his or her environment are believed to be incorporated into mental schemata, network models, or production systems (Bruning, Schraw & Ronning, 1999). This latter perspective is consistent with the work of Carr and Shotwell presented in Chapter 3.

Because of the exogenous emphasis on teacher-centeredness, instructional practice under this paradigm is almost always decontextualized and is therefore almost always abstract in the mind of the learner. Some learning theorists have come to the conclusion that, from the exogenous constructivist camp, knowledge is seen as more absolute and is often transmitted from the teacher to the learner with a hope that the student will be able to activate (transfer or generalize) the knowledge when it is required. In most cases, this type of direct instruction is delivered in the oral tradition in a traditional classroom using lecture as a favored medium. The teacher is a primary source of knowledge and an expert on the course content.

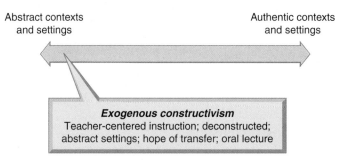

Figure 11-2 Continuum of contexts and settings: exogenous constructivism.

ENDOGENOUS CONSTRUCTIVISM

Endogenous constructivism represents a learning paradigm that begins with the learner's internal cognition and shapes an understanding of the external environment through that mental lens. This view of constructivist learning has many implications for instructional design, methods of delivery, and assessment of student accomplishment. At this point, the emphasis is still on the learner as an individual. In more radical forms of constructivism, our focus shifts from individuals to construction and interpretation of knowledge among social groups. This more radical view is discussed as dialectical constructivism later in this chapter.

Learning theorists believe that, from the internal constructivist paradigm the *cognitive orientation* of learners determines how they view and interpret their world.

This is accomplished according to their existing mental frameworks constructed and modified over time. There is a strong biological organism assumption associated with this perspective. "Piaget's stagewise view of cognitive development, for example, is a prominent representative of endogenous [internal] constructivism" (Bruning, Schraw & Ronning, 1999, p. 216). This view of the learner's mental frameworks gives many clues for instruction. Here, instruction is more learner-centered and requires an engagement between the facilitating teacher and the student that surfaces and then builds on the learner's prior knowledge as shown in the following Case Study:

CASE STUDY

Teaching for Reflective Practice: Principle 6

Learners' mental frameworks and prior experiences are used to guide instruction. Practitioners can enable critical reflection when learners' prior experience and life contexts are used for instructional purposes.
For example:

> **Bill, an OTR, is interested in taking the AOTA-sponsored advanced certification examination in neurorehabilitation. He has worked for 6 years in the neurorehabilitation unit of a major hospital . . . he knew that he met the qualifications to take the examination, but the [AOTA] brochure provided little information about the knowledge to be tested.**
>
> **"With his reflective journal at his side, Bill used a double-entry procedure to identify potential content that might be on the examination and one to identify and review resources he already had to prepare for the examination . . . A [previous] journal entry reminded him of a panel he heard at the Annual Conference that outlined state-of-the-art approaches related to occupational therapy in neurorehabiliation (Crist et al., 1998, p. 732).**

Bill reflected on and then used his prior knowledge and mental frameworks to formulate a plan to develop a study group to prepare for the examination.

Epistemologically speaking, knowledge is more abstract when viewed from this endogenous perspective, and it is constructed through intense cognitive activity. This is in contrast to the exogenous [external] assumption that knowledge is passively gathered in from external sources. Another perspective is that knowledge is invented, not discovered, as would be asserted by other sister and brother constructivists. The invention of knowledge would suggest that the nature of what is true is likely to be different or relative to each learner. "We always perceive and know the world from some socio-cultural, and historically situated, point of view. Hence human knowledge is always to be seen as a 'construct,' a product of the human mind" (Fox, 2001, p. 25). To the extent that knowledge is constructed, learning is then a matter of understanding the meaning of information and how it fits with other bits of knowledge.

In endogenous constructivism, the *assumption of learning* is the creation of new mental frameworks, based on the learner's engagement with the exterior world. Learning is about understanding and making meaning. This type of learning demands more than rote learning and recall (Fox, 2001). It implies a deeper examination of relationships between and among ideas and concepts.

Creating new mental frameworks occurs naturally as the learner is challenged to dig deeper. For example, OT students can be encouraged to explore reasons why sensory integration therapy techniques are effective with some hyperactive children. These students exploring SI theory can build new mental frameworks while "field testing" their assumptions in appropriate field work settings. This learning opportunity encourages the learners to add to their existing mental frameworks on the topic, but also encourages the meaning of making appropriate choices for varying conditions in real or simulated contexts and settings. In this way, learners can make meaning of their lessons while increasing the likelihood of making appropriate and socially responsible choices.

Instructional practices of endogenous constructivism can be envisioned as learner-first systems. Learners use knowledge and skills that have been previously converted into mental structures to understand and interpret this new knowledge. In many cases, the teacher may choose to follow the lead of the student in that she or he determines the context and settings for learning. For this reason, instruction may or may not be deeply immersed in an authentic context or physical settings. Learning and teaching rely on the learners' cognitive understandings of those realistic, imagined, or simulated contexts from their own mental frameworks, in which combinations of more abstract settings are interspersed with real life applications.

A key component of endogenous teaching is to use learning activities and resources that are appropriate to the learner's current stage of development. Using Piaget as an example, strategies and instructional activities are tied to the anticipated stage of development for the chronological age of the learner (Driscoll, 1994). See how demands are increased over time in the Case Study below.

The learner's own initiative, barriers, and expectations for what they want to learn can determine instructional content. Under the guidance of a skilled

CASE STUDY

Teaching for Reflective Practice: Principle 1

Authentic learning contexts promote actively engaged learners using higher-order thinking and problem-solving skills.

For example, a novice OT at preprofessional levels could be assumed to be capable of higher-order matching of theoretical constructs from the Model of Human Occupation (MOHO) (Kielhofner, 2002) to a client seen in her Level I Fieldwork setting. She would likely attend to motivational issues particularly, as she would have prior experience in her life with her own motivation and that of others, seeing MOHO as an elaboration of motivational factors. By the time she was on her Level II Fieldwork, she could be expected to understand the complexities of MOHO and further notice the similarities and differences between MOHO and other models, such as Occupational Adaptation, (Schkade & Schultz, 1992). Furthermore, she would be expected to synthesize these occupational theories with specific diagnostically oriented theories, such as the expected neurological recovery of a person after a stroke. In this way, she would build larger and larger constructs as her experience and expertise grew, learning to give client-centered interventions, using her knowledge of occupation and of various health conditions.

facilitating teacher, content to be learned would certainly vary, depending on the knowledge and level of expertise of the learner. Under the guidance of an expert teacher, therapists demonstrate understanding of how data are connected and then move to higher levels as they demonstrate newly acquired control of their knowledge. For example, beginning therapists at this stage would have the ability to use their knowledge to help school teachers solve a problem presented by a student with an attention deficit disorder. This earlier stage is often characterized by the learner's use of specific information to solve an unstructured problem, such as knowing the importance of minimizing distractions in the environment for the child with an attention deficit disorder. The highest level of content is when learners have achieved command of information and use it to create learning strategies to solve never before encountered problems (Case Study 11-3).

CASE STUDY

Teaching for Reflective Practice: Principle 2

Learners increase levels of expertise using knowledge relevant to their professional life.

For example, expert therapists demonstrate both interactive and conditional reasoning (see Chapter 9) by blending their deep understanding of human occupation with an equally deep appreciation of the various potential medical "futures" to find a way for clients to participate in desired activities. Instructional content is largely determined by the level of knowledge control demonstrated by the practitioner.

Instructional methods used by endogenous constructivist teachers are varied but are best described as strategies that "facilitate" the construction of increasingly more advanced mental frameworks. To begin an instructional sequence, an OT professor might engage in a conversation with a student or novice practitioner who has already partially explored an intellectual pathway of his or her own choosing. Probing questions might reveal some estimate of the learner's level of knowledge. This initial practice might also reveal any misconceptions that may have been incorporated into the schema of the learner. Other methods such as "scaffolding" and "fading" might be used to assist learners while they expand their cognitive abilities. Skillful teachers often provide the learner with a scaffold or bridge to other related information by performing some of the more difficult tasks for the student. At a later time, students will be able to perform this part of the task for themselves as the teacher fades from the direct instructional role.

CASE STUDY

Teaching for Reflective Practice: Principle 5

Learners take metacognitive responsibility for reflecting on practice resulting in meaning making and application.

Exploration is an important endogenous instructional strategy. A learner can be encouraged to identify or select among a range of topics that they find personally interesting. Teachers and learners can negotiate a project that will require the student to probe the topic. As that project is in process, the teacher works with the learner by acting as a guide and mentor. The teacher asks probing questions of students and encourages learners to think about their mental processes (metacognition) when engaged with practice topics that are important to them. This opens the instructional door to asking the student to articulate the meaning and applications of their newly acquired knowledge. At the beginning this approach requires the practitioner to probe deeply with the learner asking them to think genuinely about how this information is applied in practice. Later, learners are encouraged to become more independent in the way that they use their own thinking to extract meaning from their learning experiences.

For example, I ask students to find meaning from contextualized activities that I arrange for them. After one round of reflection, I ask them to consider their reflection in light of how their insights might impact on their own practice. In my whale course on communities of practice, I ask students to reflect on the importance of environmental stewardship; then I ask them about how their insights might change their own instruction in this area.

The most important role for the endogenous teacher is to provide educational opportunities for students to articulate their combined old and new knowledge (mental frameworks) and then to arrange for them to systematically reflect on the meaning of these ideas for their professional lives. This is the instructional foundation for prompting and promoting professional reasoning among occupational therapy educators, students and practitioners. Skillful endogenous teachers push their learners to see beyond their perceived barriers to learning as they engage with the world of professional practice. The educator is then able to physically or virtually enter that context and setting to aid the learners as they extract information and knowledge. Asking learners to articulate their knowledge and then to reflect on its meaning is often the curricular rationale for clinical reasoning courses that now exists in many professional therapy programs (*Figure 11-3*).

Endogenous constructivism is located on the context continuum as "moderately contextualized" when compared with our operational definition of context and settings. You will notice that the area of endogenous constructivism is marked along a gray arrow on the graphic. This would mean that students are mostly asked to use their imaginations to contextualize lessons as they are encountered and taught in

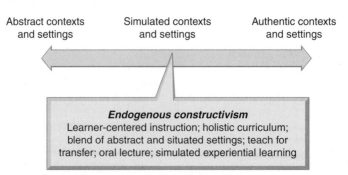

Figure 11-3 Continuum of contexts and settings: endogenous constructivism.

classroom-type environments. However, it is not entirely uncommon for endogenous instructors to use simulations or even authentic workplace settings as a context for teaching. Wolff summarizes endogenous constructivism by emphasizing the individuality of learning and the importance of different forms for each learner. "The outcome of any particular learning process varies from learner to learner, because knowledge is always subjective and takes different forms for each particular learner" (1994, p. 2).

Dialectical constructivism is a blend of both exogenous and endogenous constructivism. The cognitive orientation moves from the individual to how individuals organize and construct knowledge within social settings.

Dialectical Constructivism

Dialectical constructivism is an interaction between learners and their environments and is often associated with "contextualism," where ". . . thought and experience are inextricably intertwined with the contexts or settings where learning occurs" (Bruning, Schraw & Ronning, 1999, p. 217). Dialectical, or blended constructivism, is linked with the movement among psychologists and sociologists to jointly understand learning from the perspective of "contextualism" (Bruning, Schraw & Ronning, 1999).

The cognitive orientation is a focus on interaction of the external and internal origins of cognition. Learning theorists researching from this viewpoint are interested in the interaction between existing mental frameworks and how they are affected by the environment and how environmental influences affect the way that individuals think and formulate their mental frameworks. The dialectical belief is that traditional views of cognition are insufficient, and sociology and societal influences are also inadequate explanations of how humans learn (Bruning et al., 1999). In this blended way of thinking, it takes both psychology and sociology to begin to understand how individuals orient and learn from their environment and how those interactive influences shape their processes.

Within dialectical constructivism, the epistemology or nature of knowledge is relative to the interpretation of the individual learner and those who might have social influence within the learner's social environment. Truth drawn from this perspective is submerged in the learners' engagement with their cultural beliefs, tools, and artifacts. Although some might believe that truth can be known absolutely, dialectical constructivists often believe that understanding of what is true is negotiated through the interaction of cognitive and social influences.

As a central assumption of learning the dialectical constructivist places great value on experiences of the learner and his or her ability to socially extract meaning from these experiential encounters. The work of Lev Vygotsky (1978) has contributed to the construction of a theoretical framework that embraces both physical and abstract social-psychological tools. Many theorists believe that learners use physical tools when engaged with the external world, in the way that a carpenter might use a level to make a stud wall square. Conversely, sociopsychological tools are symbolic systems used by individuals when engaged in thinking (John-Steiner, 1997). The use of both physical and sociopsychological tools enables change over time as learners internalize and transform these mental and social interactions into mental frameworks or schemas.

In the same way that learning is an interaction between environment and mental engagement, so is the dialectical learning and teaching dynamic. Using Vygotsky's zone of proximal development (ZPD) as a way to think about learning and teaching, teachers and learners can engage in mutual work in what might be called the "construction zone" (Newman, Griffin & Cole, 1989). The ZPD is thought to be the difference between the level of difficulty that a learner can demonstrate with independence and a level that can be achieved with the help of a facilitating practitioner (Vygotsky, 1978). This interaction between learner and facilitator is similar to the scaffolding/fading strategies previously described in the discussion of endogenous constructivism. However, the emphasis turns to social interactions and mutual interpretations of knowledge and subsequent negotiation of understandings between the practitioner and the client.

Instructional content rests to the extent possible within authentically contextualized settings—in the real world. A learning goal in dialectical constructivism is to understand cultural relationships between and among knowledge elements. The educational goal is to promote understanding and command over information through social relationships between learners, their peers, and the practitioner. This is not to say that learners and educators are always close friends, but dialectical constructivists do believe a melody and rhythm make up the musical ensemble of social learning and teaching.

The characteristics of content are rooted in unstructured problems, complexities, and nuanced information. Practitioners of blended constructivism are concerned with how learners use information to solve complex problems encountered in authentic settings.

Instructional methods are widely varied but for the most part are designed to serve the needs of the learner. The role of teacher might be conceptualized as a safari guide for a mutual learning journey. The explorers are teacher and student, both as reciprocal learners. Instruction begins with the teacher as a learner and not the traditional authoritative fountain of absolute truth. Rogoff's work on "apprentices in thinking" is a natural fit with blended constructivism (1991). She argues that cognitive development is inherently social and requires mutual engagement with partners of greater skill. Context, according to Rogoff (1991), consists of the social relationships that children and adults encounter as they learn. The instructional side of the social relationship is with one who is more knowledgeable on a given topic. That instructional guide is likely to use an instructional method known as guided participation where the learner uses interpersonal communication and stage setting to build mental bridges between that which they already know and new information. She argues for enriched (reflective) mental processing because learning occurs in the context of the learner trying to accomplish something of personal relevance (Bruning, Schraw & Ronning, 1999).

CASE STUDY

Teaching for Reflective Practice: Principle 7

Teachers act as facilitators of learning using a repertoire of contextualized instructional methods.

This principle strongly suggests the importance of accomplishing something real as a contribution toward motivating learners to learn. For example, a student might be asked to do a review of the evidence relative to an intervention approach, which is commonly used in the fieldwork setting to which the student has been assigned. The faculty member, student, and the fieldwork supervisor could all participate in setting the question, seeking good resources, interpreting the findings, and deciding how to use this information with the targeted client population during the student's time at the setting. At various times, this might include scaffolding to help the student find resources, fading as they gained skill, mapping out the various concepts to develop relevant mental frameworks built on the research, reflecting on the findings in light of practice experiences.

Instructional sequences can vary depending on the journey that is taken jointly by the teacher and the learner. Taking trips is often conducive to finding alternate routes to a destination. During the trip, the learner often sets the sequence of instruction. The teacher and student engage in interpersonal communication along the way. In these interactions, information surfaces that the teacher can combine with his or her expertise and subsequently use to set the stage for later learning activities. As the journey continues to these new stages, the learner has opportunities to make new connections. It is during these events that Rogoff suggests new cognitive growth takes place. The skillful teacher can make the journey seem informal but meaningful for their fellow but novice scholars; formal, standup, direct teaching is not always necessary to realize extraordinary gains in learning (*Figure 11-4*).

Dialectical constructivism intersects with the continuum of context both right and left of center, signifying a strong inclination to contexts and settings that might be considered more authentic. This approach is learner centered and situated in real life. The often informal relationship between the learner and the teacher approximates more natural relationships as they are found in everyday society and culture. Blended constructivism is also more contextualized because it relies on cultural tools and symbols to promote interaction between the environment and the learner's cognitive processes.

The next learning perspective continues toward a more complete orientation toward learning occurring in social settings. In the next few pages, we explore situated cognition and communities of practice theories.

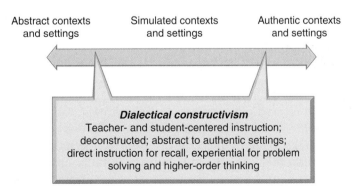

Figure 11-4 Continuum of contexts and settings: dialectical constructivism.

Situated Cognition and Communities of Practice

In recent years, Jean Lave and Etienne Wenger have written about learning in interesting and refreshingly different terms. From an ethnographic point of view, they have used critical elements of sociology while emphasizing the importance of context and participation in communities of practice as a foundation for learning (Lave, 1988; Wenger, 1998). Another distinction is that the authors consider situated cognition as a "socialization" theory; it is about how individuals become members of communities. They might ask how a novice OT becomes a member of the professional community of therapists within a given organization. These concepts and ideas are potentially important to the design, delivery, and assessment of contextual teaching and learning especially applicable to the training of new practitioners for the profession of occupational therapy.

Jean Lave, an educational anthropologist, has spent recent years studying learning as it occurs in natural settings. Her research often examines elements of partial and full membership in some type of community. This body of literature has come to be popularly known as *situated cognition*, or legitimate peripheral participation. Lave's collaborator, Etienne Wenger, has extended this body of research in his most recent publication, *Communities of Practice* (1998). Like the research on constructivism, this research also has important possibilities as a framework for authentic instruction and assessment.

Situated Cognition

From her naturalistic studies, Lave coined the term "situated cognition" to describe the cognitive process as a "nexus of relations between the mind at work and the world in which it works" (Lave, 1988, p. 1). She further proposed that cognition is not merely a psychological phenomenon, but rather it is "stretched across mind, body, activity and setting" (Lave, 1988, p. 18). This view of cognition is not new; it is similar to the work of other educational theorists and philosophers such as John Dewey (1938) and constructivist Lev Vygotsky (1978).

Lave and others have researched learning in everyday life contexts rather than abstract classroom or laboratory conditions (Lave, 1988; Lave & Wenger, 1991, Resnick, 1987). They have found that when individuals address problems requiring the same knowledge, the context in which the person was engaged greatly influenced how he or she used information to solve a problem. Lave gives an example of individuals attempting to follow weight reduction diets (1991). In their own kitchens, dieters relied on estimation techniques, often physically dividing food into appropriate portions. However, in a classroom setting, the same dieters attempted to use paper-and-pencil approaches to dividing fractions. This and other research strongly suggests the importance of learning context on how problems are thought about as well as how solutions are generated.

In reporting their research, Lave & Wenger (1991) used the term "legitimate peripheral participation" to describe how individuals gain opportunities to use learning as members of a community. In this community role, individuals must make a legitimate contribution to a situation that they value and consider "authentic." These contributions initially are likely to be at edges or the "periphery" of the socially constructed community. As new members progressively demonstrate competence, other members of the community gradually allow novices to engage in more complex activity. In this way, learners are eventually affirmed as full-fledged members. Through participation, learners also construct their identity relative to the community. As a result, learners achieve a mental "meaningfulness" that comes from participation as members of a valued community.

Communities of Practice

Wenger has extended this work in situated cognition into a more formalized construct that he now calls *Communities of Practice* (1998). Wenger's definition of communities of practice incorporates a learning viewpoint. To him, learning is a central element that connects at the intersection of *meaning, practice, community,* and *identity.*

Meaning is a way that we use our increasing abilities to create meaning from our lives and our work.

Practice (or collective participation) is a way in which our community constructs a mutual history, collective social resources, and common ways of looking at the world. These commonly held values guide our actions and promote continued engagement in the business of the community.

Community consists of the social networks that define our enterprises as worth pursuing and recognizes the work of an individual as competent.

Identity is a way of talking about how learners change as they learn. In this way, the learner creates a personal history of how he/she has become a member of a community of practice.

Based on the principles of community of practice, it is the "meaningfulness" that a learner attaches to the content that makes multiple uses of information possible. Social learning theorists such as Wenger (1998) and Westheimer and Kahne (1993) do not easily acknowledge learning transfer as a construct. They believe that learning is a new event in each new social setting. Wenger believes that community members ultimately achieve meaning through the interaction of their "participation" and the "reification" of imaginary and real objects that represent the tools and values of the community. For example, occupational therapists have a number of imaginary symbols that represent, in their own mind, elements that constitute tools available for learning within the context of a community of practice. These tools might be intangibles such as the common beliefs about the "best way" to do an initial evaluation with a person who had a stroke. Or, these beliefs could be actualized in a physical form such as the initial evaluation form or written therapy protocols. It is participation as therapists within a valued therapeutic enterprise along with the use of real and imaginary symbols and tools that gives meaningfulness to members of the professional community. It is also this sense of meaningfulness that helps to shape our professional identities (Wenger, 1989) and helps to explain research into clinical reasoning which surfaced the degree to which therapists tended to do things in similar ways within certain settings (Rogers & Masagatani, 1982; Barris, 1987).

Researchers who practice from a cognitive/social orientation believe that individuals learn in ways different from what traditional cognitive psychologists believe. When looking at situated cognition as a foundation for contextual teaching and learning, it is important to understand that the theory is moving away from traditional psychological views of learning. This is similar in many ways to dialectical constructivism, but situated cognition theorists strongly argue that learning is primarily a social phenomenon. Yet, there is an underlying recognition of the role of cognition. It is this recognition that brings this social view of learning and constructivism together and makes it possible to see philosophic and theoretical consistencies between the theories (St. Julien, 1997).

From this socialization learning perspective, the epistemology, or the nature of social knowledge, is deeply embedded in the practices chosen by members of the community. The practices and conventions of a community are determined as the group proceeds toward the accomplishment of its valued enterprise. Obviously, in this context truth is relative to what is perceived to work in a given context or setting. Acquiring mastery of the practices (knowledge) of the community is the journey toward full membership and increased expertise. Wenger also warns educators who would develop such a community of practice as a foundation for learning: "Learning cannot be designed. It can only be designed for—that is, facilitated or frustrated" (1998, p. 229).

Instructional practices within a community of practice viewpoint requires a thoughtful and learner-oriented approach. Wenger (1998) gives attributes of learning that have important implications for teaching within the context of communities of practice. Additional instructional practices within this paradigm are discussed further in a later section of this chapter and referenced in relation to *Table 11-1*.

All applications of situated cognition theory are based in authentic contexts and settings. This places applications of this theory at the far right end of our continuum of context. Learning allowances are made in the real world. It is in this way that learners are provided opportunities to learn practices and procedures that are actually used in businesses or other types of institutions (*Figure 11-5*).

TABLE 11-1

Joining a Community of Practice

Being Socialized as an Occupational Therapist within a Community of Practice Means:

2-1 The ability to negotiate new meanings, which	—involve the whole person in an interplay of participation and reification to find meaning & application.
2-2 The creation of new mental structures, which	—encourage a blend of old and new knowledge.
2-3 Both experiential and social learning activities performed	—in authentic social settings that require learners to engage deeply with the community.
2-4 A matter of engagement, which	—requires learners to engage with interesting & relevant material.
2-5 Opportunities for change that	—encourage self-reflection (reflective practice encourages individual and group change).
2-6 A matter of imagination that	—promotes reflection and exploration so that identities and practices can grow.

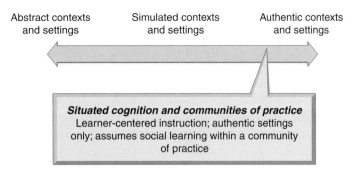

Figure 11-5   Continuum of contexts and settings: situated cognition and communities of practice.

This is appropriate because of the tradition of this theory for providing explanations of how peripheral members of a community become socialized as full-fledged members of a group. An underlying principle of contextualized contextual learning and teaching is this: The more learners perceive that the learning environment is authentic, the more likely they are able to use their learned information to solve problems in a similar practice setting.

CASE STUDY

Teaching for Reflective Practice: Principle 1

Authentic learning contexts promote actively engaged learners using higher-order thinking and problem-solving skills.

For example, Stern (2005) reported on the use of simulated real-life activities in the context of an OT education course on evidence-based practice. Her research results were highly encouraging with regard to the use of a simulated context as a way to "respond to the challenges of doing research" (p. 158). Are simulated contexts the same as authentic? No. But are they a realistic step towards using real-world contexts? Yes. This is also further evidence that use of contextualized settings can add to learning effectiveness.

Contextual Learning and Teaching for Reflective Practice

Reflective practice is an important step toward building expertise (Crist et al., 1998). All of our research with regard to the application of contextualized learning theories strongly suggests that experiential learning alone is insufficient (Schell, 1999). Contextualized experiences should be "examined" experiences. Such reflective examinations are examples of instructional practices that bring about opportunities for increased meaningfulness. It is one thing for the learner to have command of facts and figures, but it is quite another for him or her to be able to use those facts in a practical way in an authentic setting. Yet, application of knowledge is our goal as teachers of practitioners. Teaching for reflective practice represents a variety of instructional strategies that can expose learners to the "next step of learning." Learners should be asked to reflect on questions such as, What does this new information mean to me? How will this help me solve problems that I encounter at work or in my community? and many more questions.

Endogenous, exogenous, and dialectical constructivists along with their situated cognition colleagues all address the importance of reflection as an educational artifact. A model that is often adopted when thinking of reflection is the work of Donald Schön (1983). His work on reflection in action and reflection on action is quite famous and does appear to have application to the training of therapists. Reflection-in-action is a slight pause during practice to mentally connect current actions with a conceptual framework of theory that gives authority and legitimacy to what the therapist is doing at the moment. Bruning, Schraw & Ronning (1999) describe this practice as "an on-the spot thought experiment" (p. 222). An OT educator or practitioner might make a quick, but value-free, judgment to test some type of alternative instructional strategy—a type of working hypothesis testing. Reflection-on-action is a "look behind" to connect with reflections-in-action previously taken and evaluate their effectiveness or efficiency. Both are metacognitive strategies that apply to both professional practice and instructional strategies that help students understand how information might be applied and valued in real life (Bruning, Schraw & Ronning, 1999).

Of course, there are many ways to reflect and many metacognitive processes. For example, when students are asked to verbally articulate their knowledge and their thought processes when solving a problem, the result can be a powerful opportunity for other students and their teachers to compare their thinking with that of others. When reflection is viewed in this light, it becomes obvious that there is almost always more than one way to solve a complex clinical problem. This alone is a valuable learning outcome.

TEACHING FOR EFFECTIVE PROFESSIONAL REASONING

The use of reflection as an instructional strategy is only one tool that teachers have at their command to promote professional reasoning. There are many well-documented "instructional systems" that are appropriate for situated or context-based learning. Example instructional systems are Bransford's Anchored Instruction (1990) or Elaboration theory posited by Reigeluth and Stern (1983). For the purpose of this chapter, I have chosen to illustrate contextual teaching using the cognitive apprenticeship approach as described by Brown, Collins, and Duguid (1989). These researchers suggest that apprenticeships are a traditional and appropriate foundation because it is a good fit with a socialization theory such as situated cognition or legitimate peripheral participation in which novices become experts through experiences in authentic contexts. Brown et al. have written about the use of cognitive apprenticeship as a way to think about the design of instruction.

Cognitive apprenticeship is based on four interacting elements: (1) instructional content, (2) instructional methods, (3) instructional sequence, and (4) the sociology of the learning community. It is most helpful to think of these elements as a "system of instruction" in which decisions made in one arena are very likely to impact on the other three. *Figure 11-6* is an illustration of the interactive relationship among these instructional elements. Each of these elements is discussed in more detail in the next few paragraphs, along with how they are interrelated.

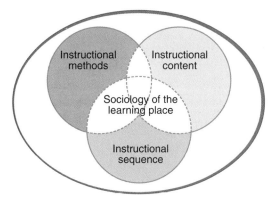

Figure 11-6   Elements of cognitive apprenticeship.

Instructional Content

This element refers to the types and levels of knowledge required by experts to solve complex problems in the real world. Content can be seen to range from basic knowledge to information that experts use to reflectively compose strategies for learning new things (Brown et al., 1989).

These researchers conceptualize instructional content as a hierarchy beginning with domain knowledge. This type of knowledge reflects basic subject matter. We often think of this as foundational knowledge that is prerequisite to the mastery of more advanced information. Heuristic knowledge can be thought of as tricks of the trade that competent professionals might use after significant experience with their work. At the next level are control strategies used by experts as they are solving problems. The last level of content is learning strategies, which are represented by knowledge of how to learn how to learn.

CASE STUDY

Teaching for Reflective Practice: Principle 2

Learners increase levels of expertise using knowledge relevant to their professional life.

Learning how to use and control knowledge is a key element of expertise. The implication here is that too often professional education programs such as those for therapists rely heavily on domain knowledge. In fact, students often feel this way: "Just give me the facts—and I can recall them on a test." Of course, over-reliance on this level of content knowledge within an abstract classroom context strongly suggests future difficulties with application of these isolated facts within an authentic practice setting. To meet the learning objective of expert application of knowledge to practice, teachers are encouraged to move beyond didactic views of knowledge by illustrating how professionals apply knowledge within the field; how they gain control of their practice strategies; and how they eventually became expert problem solvers who "know how to learn" when confronted with new and challenging circumstances.

Instructional Methods

Teaching strategies for contextualized learning include a variety of instructional strategies that can be used by a facilitating teacher. They range from traditional demonstration to higher-order methods of exploration, articulation, and reflection (Brown et al., 1989).

Basic instructional methods can be grouped and described as strategies for guided practice (Brown et al.). These lower-order methods such as modeling are effective when you as teacher might want to illustrate a skill set. A teacher using a modeling technique might begin a session saying, "watch me closely as I demonstrate because you will be doing it next." In the next instructional phase, you might utilize a coaching instructional strategy in which you are giving advice and encouragement from the sideline as the learners are attempting to apply the skills for themselves. As learners are becoming more independent, a teacher might apply scaffolding and fading methods. As a learner approaches an element of content that might require a safety procedure or a higher level of difficulty, the teacher might intervene by providing a scaffold or bridge for the student. As the student becomes more competent, the teacher can fade out and allow the student to be more independent and capable of accomplishing the complete task.

Guided practice methods give way to methods that promote knowledge control (Brown et al., 1989). Note the similarity in language that was used when we discussed higher levels of instructional content such as "control strategies" and "learning strategies." Knowledge control strategies are composed of instructional methods that promote higher-order thinking and administration of thinking and learning. This set of instructional methods is intended to go beyond direct teaching that is common to guided practice. Knowledge control strategies allow learners to develop skills to manage their knowledge and to draw meaning from their educational experiences.

Exploration as a learning strategy allows learners to "follow their own noses." By this, I do not advocate blanket exploration as unstructured exploration can inadvertently give permission to the learner to venture too far off the curricular target. Just as too much instructional structure often stifles learning, too little structure can be confusing and misguiding. However, allowing students to explore while choosing from a targeted range of topics can be an exhilarating way to learn. Often, exploration learning can be somewhat structured but in such a way that the organization of the topic is transparent to the learner but very useful to the practitioner.

Like scaffolding and fading, articulation and reflection are also twin instructional strategies used to encourage learners to articulate their knowledge, reasoning, or an approach to problem solving while reflecting on the meanings that they have extracted from a learning experience.

CASE STUDY

Teaching for Reflective Practice: Principle 1

Authentic learning contexts promote actively engaged learners using higher-order thinking and problem-solving skills

Articulation and reflection can promote expression of new learning and critical analysis of emerging mental frameworks. Articulation of knowledge can be in almost any form, using a variety of educational media. This is not simply an oral recitation of knowledge; it can be one of a variety of representations of understandings. Perhaps a videotape can be prepared by a learner to demonstrate his or her mastery of group therapy. Or, it could be in the form of a play, a puppet show, a song, a dance, a scrapbook, a formal paper, a reflective journal, or hundreds of other possible ways to express acquired knowledge. Creativity and innovation are always important elements in the design of instruction. I certainly encourage my students to be experimental with their teaching, especially when it comes to providing learners with opportunities to express their knowledge in a way that is a fit with their preferred style of learning (Spoon & Schell, 1997) or their preferred area of intelligence (Gardner, 2004). When students are encouraged to be creative, their work can provide surprising benefits for others within the learning community. For example, when a student OT describes his or her approach to a given therapy technique, it allows other students to compare their thinking and can result in even greater instructional opportunities.

As a mirror image of articulation, instructional methods that promote reflection can enable learners to draw meaning from their experiences (Nelson, 1988). Again, reflection strategies should not be limited to asking students, "how did you feel when you provided therapy to Ms. Brown?" Reflection is where learning is "unpacked" and students are asked to articulate the meaningfulness of that information. For example, students might be asked to choose a critical incident from their fieldwork experiences. This can be a therapeutic moment, or it could even be a time when an aspect of professional ethics is drawn into consideration. Once the incident is documented, it can be further diagramed using a mind-mapping technique in which students are asked to make connections between elements of the situation. For each connection that is made, learners are asked to describe the nature of the association and how it is related to other parts of the chosen learning experience.

This reflection technique makes the thinking of the learner more explicit. When their thinking is shared within a social learning situation, each member of the learning community is allowed to compare his or her own thinking, which can either be validating or lead to a re-consideration of that approach. This is also a good action example of dialectical constructivism in the classroom setting.

Instructional Sequence

The order of instruction is important. What to teach to whom and when? In many cases, teachers feel that they must begin any curriculum sequence at the beginning and move through a topic to the end in a logical sequence of steps. Most experienced teachers realize that they have more options than first meets the eye when they are thinking of how to progress. There are at least three basic sequencing strategies, including (1) linear progression through materials, (2) increasing capacity, and (3) global before local (Brown et al., 1989).

CASE STUDY

Teaching for Reflective Practice: Principle 5

Learners take metacognitive responsibility for reflecting on practice resulting in meaning making and application.

There are several options when considering the sequence of instructional content. Obviously, choice of sequence is related to level of instructional content and vice versa. When a given skill set to be taught is fairly low-order, logical sequence does make sense. Start teaching with basic content and progress to more difficult content in stepwise fashion; begin at the beginning and move progressively to the end. An example of this might be teaching students how to fabricate hand splints. Many instructors start with the fabrication of a simple wrist cock-up splint. Once the student has mastered this, the student might progress to making a full hand splint. More complicated splints such as antispasticity splints or dynamic splints would be taught later in the sequence. This approach assumes that information can be deconstructed for teaching in smaller increments. It also assumes that when these smaller increments are reconstructed, the greater whole will be recognized. That is, the teacher is relying on the learner to "transfer" or generalize the knowledge. For a lot of reasons, this supposition of transfer is not always a good bet (Detterman, 1993). We discuss the issue of transfer in greater detail in a later section of this chapter.

As a way to promote multiple uses of information a second sequencing strategy could be used: increasing capacities. This is where a concept is taught in a curriculum in several different times and locations. For example, a novice OT is expected to be able to analyze occupational activities in a variety of settings. Beginning students may first be challenged to identify the physical requirements of a simple task such as making coffee. Later, the same skills can be adapted to make more sophisticated judgments such as determining a client's safety risks when returning home. Both of these professional judgments require the use of activity analysis, but each requires a different level of skill on the part of the therapist. So, as a teacher of OTs, one could use increasing capacities to teach activity analysis at an early juncture of the curriculum with the caveat that "we will use this skill over and over during the next few years—but each time it will require more sophisticated judgment on your part." When those future junctures are encountered, the college instructor can say something like ". . . do you remember when we first learned about activity analysis? We are going to call on those skills again, but in a slightly different way." Now, prior knowledge can be used to build to a greater level of expertise.

Global before local details is a sequencing strategy in which the students are given the "big picture" about why they are learning a given topic. This strategy is designed to help instructors answer the second most common question that students ask: "When will I ever use this stuff?" By the way, the most frequent question asked by students is "What do I have to do to get an A?" Although asking about grades may have varying levels of legitimacy, asking about the application of a skill set is very appropriate.

When instruction resides within the context in which information is going to be used, the more likely students are to value that knowledge because it now has utility and relevance. It is valued information that gets future use or gets transferred to other contexts (Detterman, 1993). In this way, teachers can give the global context of a topic before they begin to explore the details of the topic, and this gives a natural framework that can organize the learning for the community. It is even more effective when such a global perspective can be drawn from an actual context and setting where good OT is practiced (Lave & Wenger, 1991).

Sociology of the Learning Place

The final and overarching elements of the cognitive apprenticeship model are the beliefs, values, and social settings in which real-world learning takes place. Three aspects of social contexts are crucial for situated learning:

1. Developing and maintaining a community of practice
2. Encouraging intrinsic motivation
3. Maximizing cooperation within the community

CASE STUDY

Teaching for Reflective Practice: Principle 7

Teachers act as facilitators of learning using a repertoire of contextualized instructional methods.

Communities of Practice can be a powerful way to organize learning for both good and bad results—use them with care. Wenger (1998) writes of the power of a community of practice. These are naturally forming groups that pursue a common enterprise. This is a good description of a class of OT students. However, because they are a community of practice does not mean that sweetness and light will be a constant element of the learning environment. Communities of learners can be and frequently are misguided and are subject to the many foibles faced by any group. What makes a community of practice a powerful and positive learning environment is the skill of the facilitator (teacher). When the social structure of learning community is positively used to build a learning environment of mutual trust and respect, the chances of meaningful reflection are greatly enhanced (Schell & Black, 1994).

Skillful use of community can also be inherently motivating to students. When instructional direction is known, members of the community do not have to guess at instructional intentions. This gives a fundamental soundness to the instructional program and future directions. It also provides an instructional stability and an aura of trust among members of the learning community, and this includes the professor. It takes such an environment to maximize learning through reflection. This type of approach should also emphasize higher-order thinking and problem solving. But once again, I must warn that setting expectations for higher levels of academic performance can be threatening to students and can contribute to unrest among those not used to such expectations. Once again, achieving scholarly performance often requires a gifted teacher who can blend learning theory, instructional content, and methods, and can positively influence the sociology of the learning place.

In summation, the interactive instructional elements of content, methods, sequence, and sociology of the learning place in the hands of an expert instructor can greatly enhance the power of education through reflection. The interested reader will also note that in Chapter 16, I have included a new model for contextualized instruction that encapsulates these principles into a comprehensive system.

LEARNING PERSPECTIVES FOR MANAGERS AND SUPERVISORS

One of the best arguments for the use of contextualized learning or communities of practice is the *probability* that learners will become competent earlier when taught by a skillful facilitator (Schell, 1999; Neistadt & Smith, 1996) or learn to use their powers of reflection (Crist et al., 1998). However, no matter how well prepared a new practitioner is for that first job, it is clear that supervisors and managers can play a critical role in supporting the ongoing development of that person's reasoning skills. It is also clear that practitioners themselves must take responsibility for upholding their professional obligations to maintain competency and ideally acquire greater expertise as they gain experience. The nature of the strategies to help professionals develop are likely to change over time, as practitioners become more experienced, although there is little empirical evidence within occupational therapy that explains exactly how these processes best occur. Extensive work by both AOTA (Hinojosa & Blount, 1998) and NBCOT on maintaining continuing competency, as well as the move toward evidence-based practice (Tickle-Degnen, 1999) suggests some strategies that are useful for helping individuals develop throughout their careers.

Helping Novices Become Competent

Because most research on expertise suggests that it takes several years to become competent (Dreyfus & Dreyfus, 1986; Benner, 1984), helping novices develop often involves a continuation of the strategies used in fieldwork situations. These can include the use of clinical reasoning guides (such as well-explained evaluation protocols), frequent meetings with more experienced colleagues for mentoring, skill-building continuing education opportunities (workshops, etc.), followed by supervised practice opportunities back at the work site. The common practice of having a therapist go to a workshop and report back on what they learned is probably less useful than having that therapist attempt to use the new learning with one or more clients, keeping careful records of the results and then sharing these case studies for discussion with other colleagues. The goal for these practitioners is to learn ever more complex mental frameworks related to their populations and to understand the usual cycle of events, so that they can become more confident in predicting (i.e., goal setting, client education about the future).

A challenge for novices in today's healthcare delivery system is finding the professional support that is needed. When one practices in a setting where there is little professional interaction with colleagues in the same discipline (e.g., in school-based practice or in medical settings where interdisciplinary teams are also organizational units), the likelihood that he or she will have regular access to mentors within the profession is diminished. Supervisors and managers in these settings must acknowledge and facilitate access to appropriate mentors if the practitioner's experience is to be maximally used to advance professional reasoning. In addition, practitioners themselves can seek necessary support in the form of informal or contracted mentors, as well as through engaging in local and internet-based special interest sections and groups that can provide guidance and support reflection and development. This is why leaders in the profession emphasize active membership in professional organizations and interest groups.

An important strategy for all levels of practice can be started in the early stages of professional practice, and that is the development of "ready access to current evidence" resources on clinical issues important to the practice setting (Tickle-Degnen, 2000, p. 103). Tickle-Degnen's tutorials in her Evidence-Based Forums (see Tickle-Degnen 1999, 2000 for examples) provide strategies for all practitioners to use. Strategies to support learning and using an evidence-based approach are discussed in more detail in Chapter 13.

Helping Competent Practitioners Become Experts

Increased competency means that the person has formed effective chunking of information and has learned to prioritize the care process because he or she has enough experience to effectively predict what routinely occurs. At this juncture, practitioners in fact may need to learn new skills or need to evaluate their routine skills in light of new empirical evidence and practices emerging in the field. It can be especially challenging for practitioners at this level to be open to critically reflecting on their practices, primarily because of the impact that it has on their efficiency. Competent practitioners are less reliant on theory than they are on their own experiences, and the routine of their therapy approaches make for efficient practice. Changing or updating practice patterns may necessarily result in decreased efficiency while new routines are being learned. There is also the need to deal with the fear that prior knowledge and skills in which the practitioner was enjoying the sense of competence will be replaced by the struggles of learning something new. This is all counterbalanced, of course, by the intrinsic motivation of the therapist to provide the best care possible for the client, and the human desire to avoid boredom by increasing mastery.

A good strategy for pushing increased expertise at this level is to engage the person in teaching, as the teaching process naturally requires explanation, which in turn creates a press for reflection. Teaching can be in the form of fieldwork supervision, providing continuing education opportunities to others, and guest lecturing in academic programs.

At this stage, the pursuit of more systematic educational programs can also effectively challenge competent therapists to push themselves. Examples would be to pursue a post–entry-level graduate degree or to seek specialty certification (Crist et al., 1998). By engaging in more formalized educational opportunities, practitioners expose themselves to teachers who are likely to engage them in reflective learning activities that promote higher-order thinking and problem-solving.

Helping Experts Become More Expert

Promoting higher levels of expertise is often best done by having field supervisors teach or mentor higher-level competent folks, which requires them to "codify" their clinical reasoning in the form of treatment protocols, guidelines, and the like. Another effective method is to have experts engage in clinical research, so that they can look at empirical support for their highly developed assumptions in their area of expertise (Benner, 1984). At this level of expertise, learners become teachers and contributors to the professional practice through presentations, publications, and provision of consultation.

SUMMARY

In this chapter, assumptions underlying the teaching process included a look at the roles of both the teacher and the learner. Teachers are proposed as facilitators of learning, whereas learners must be active participants. In addition, the role of the learning context, both physical and social, is critical in helping learners gain and use knowledge for practice. Learning theories can be characterized in part by the degree to which they attend to the learning context. A community of practice perspective was recommended, and the implications of this perspective for instructional content, methods, sequencing, and the sociology of the learning place were all examined. Finally, the implication of this information for increasing expertise throughout professional development was suggested.

LEARNING ACTIVITY 11-1

Teaching to Make Mental Connections

Purpose

To demonstrate how authentic experiences can be used to facilitate the creation of mental frameworks within a community of practice in a Fieldwork II setting

Connections to Major Clinical Reasoning Constructs

This activity is associated with endogenous and dialectical constructivism.

Directions for Learners

1 Read the scenario (see below) and answer the Questions for Reflection.
2 In a small group of three to five novice OT practitioners, choose a constructivist perspective (endogenous or dialectical) around which a contextualized therapy session can be designed for Mrs. Brown. Ask yourself: How do you think Mrs. Brown best learns? Does she want to set the learning agenda for herself? Does she want me to do it for her? Or, are we going to learn together? (Of course, the answers to these questions are a matter of speculation, but draw from any hints you might find in the above biography).
3 As a member of a community of learners, utilize your Fieldwork II setting to find artifacts, ideas, symbols, systems, etc., which can be used to provide occupational therapy based on a theory such as occupational science, sensory integration, or Model of Human Occupation (MOHO). Feel free to investigate other theories and concepts that others may not have thought about.
4 Document the objects that you found. This may be done with a digital or video camera, a sketchbook, discussing with a classmate, making mental or physical notes, or other method(s).

5 Return to the classroom and construct a group mind map to demonstrate the various ways that the documented ideas and evidence relate to the main concept and to each other (see *Figure 11-7* for an example of a mind map).

6 Document at least two possible therapy approaches that could be constructed by members of your learning community by blending (a) your selected view of constructivism, (b) a theory of occupational therapy, and (c) the ideas, objects, symbols, etc., you have identified from an authentic therapeutic setting. Using a mind map, illustrate the relationships among the ideas, objects, symbols, and theories of occupational therapy treatment.

Scenario

Mrs. Brown is a retired 65-year-old elementary school teacher who had a stroke six months ago. You are a member of a team of occupational therapists who will be working with Mrs. Brown. She is very well known for the artistic and colorful quilts she has created for many years. Mrs. Brown has six grandchildren, and she has made a customized quilt for five of the six children in her family. Each of these quilts illustrates that child's branch of the Brown family tree. She considers herself an artist and is very anxious to return to her hobbies in needlework and fabric crafts. In her career

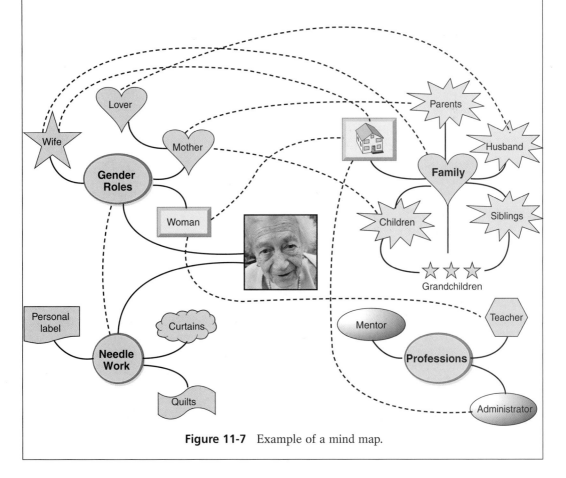

Figure 11-7   Example of a mind map.

as an early childhood teacher, Mrs. Brown was known for her open smiles and her willingness to let children explore and learn for themselves. However, she always made sure that children had mastered basic competencies and could apply them when solving problems.

Questions for Reflection

Use these questions to guide reflection on this activity:

1 How does Mrs. Brown best learn? Does she prefer to set her own learning agenda? Does she expect you to do it for her? Or, did you team up with her to set the expectations for learning?

2 What mental frameworks do you think that Mrs. Brown has formulated: With regard to her needlework? About her family? With regard to her maternal role within the extended family? Why are these mental frameworks so important?

3 Why do you think fabric arts are so important in Mrs. Brown's life? Why do they have meaning for her? What meaning does Mrs. Brown's hobby have to you as her therapist?

4 What is the importance of therapists who are working within a learning community when engaging in this learning activity?

5 How do you think individuals learn and change when they are acting as members of a learning community? Did you observe any practices that were used by your group when designing a learning-based therapy session for Mrs. Brown?

6 In what ways are your mental frameworks the same or different from those of Mrs. Brown?

7 How can you use this activity in your future as an occupational therapist?

Note: Mind mapping is a common instructional strategy that can be used when it is important to metaphorically illustrate the connections made among ideas that are generated within groups of learners.

REFERENCES

AOTA-COP (2002). Occupational therapy practice framework: Domain and process. *American Journal of Occupational Therapy, 56,* 609–639.

Barris, R. (1987). Clinical reasoning in psychosocial occupational therapy: The evaluation process. *Occupational Therapy Journal of Research, 7,* 147–162.

Benner, P. (1984). *From novice to expert.* Menlo Park, CA: Addison-Wesley.

Biggs, J. (1996) Enhancing teaching through constructive alignment. *Higher Education, 32,* 347–364.

Bransford, J .D. (1990). Anchored instruction: Why we need it and how technology can help. In D. Nix & R. Sprio (Eds.), *Cognition, education and multimedia.* Hillsdale, NJ: Erlbaum Associates.

Brown, J. S., Collins, A. & Duguid, P. (1989). Situated cognition and the culture of learning. *Educational Researcher, 18*(1), 32–42.

Bruning, R. H., Schraw, G. H. & Ronning, R. R. (1999). *Cognitive psychology and instruction* (3rd ed.). Columbus, OH: Merrill.

Crist, P., Wilcox, B. L. & McCarron, K. (1998). Transitional portfolios: Orchestrating our professional competence. *American Journal of Occupational Therapy, 52,* 729–736.

Detterman, D. K. (1993). Case against transfer. In D. K. Detterman & R. J. Sternberg (Eds.), *Transfer on trial.* Norwood, NJ: Ablex.

Dewey, J. (1938). *Experience and education.* New York: Kappa Delta Phi.

Driscoll, Marcy Perkins (1994). *Psychology of learning for instruction.* Needham Heights, MA: Allyn & Bacon.

Dryfus, H. L. & Dryfus, S. E. (1986). *Mind over machine: The power of human intuition and expertise in the era of the computer.* New York: Free Press.

Ericsson, K. A. & Smith, J. (1991). Prospects and limits in the empirical study of expertise: An introduction. In K. A. Ericsson & J. Smith (Eds.), *Toward a general theory of expertise: Prospects and limits* (pp. 1–38). Cambridge: Cambridge University Press.

Fisher, A. G. (1998). Uniting practice and theory in an occupational framework. *American Journal of Occupational Therapy, 52,* 509–521.

Fox, R. (2001). Constructivism examined. *Oxford Review of Education, 1*(27), 23–34.

Gardner, H. (2004). *Frames of mind: The theory of multiple intelligences* (twentieth anniversary ed.). New York: Basic Books.

Hinojosa, J. & Blount, M.-L. (1998). Nationally speaking: Professional competence. *American Journal of Occupational Therapy, 52,* 765–769.

Hooper, B. & Wood, W. (2002). Pragmatism and structuralism in occupational therapy: The long conversation. *Journal of Occupational Therapy, 56,* 40–50.

John-Steiner, V. (1997). *Notebooks of the mind: Explorations of thinking.* New York: Oxford University Press.

Kielhofner, G. (2002). *Model of human occupation* (3rd ed.). Baltimore: Lippincott Williams & Wilkins.

Lave, J. (1998). *Cognition in practice: Mind, mathematics and culture in everyday life.* Cambridge: Cambridge University Press.

Lave, J. & Wenger, E. (1991). *Situated learning: Legitimate peripheral participation.* Cambridge: Cambridge University Press.

Neistadt, M. E. & Smith, R. E. (1997). Teaching diagnostic reasoning: Using a classroom-as-clinic methodology with videotapes. *American Journal of Occupational Therapy, 51,* 360–368.

Nelson, D. (1988). Occupation: Form and performance. *American Journal of Occupational Therapy, 42,* 633–641.

Newman, D., Griffin, P. & Cole, M. (1989). *The construction zone: Working for cognitive change in school.* Cambridge, UK: Cambridge University Press.

Phillips, D. C. & Soltis, J. C. (1998). *Perspectives on learning* (3rd ed.). New York: Teachers College Press.

Reigeluth, C. & Stein, F. (1983). The elaboration theory of instruction. In C. Reigeluth (Ed.), *Instructional design theories and models.* Hillsdale, NJ: Erlbaum Associates.

Resnick, L. B. (1987). Learning in school and out. *Educational Researcher, 16,* 13–20.

Rogoff, B. (1991). *Apprenticeship in thinking: Cognitive development in social context.* New York: Oxford University Press.

Rogers, J. C. & Masagatani, G. (1982). Clinical reasoning of occupational therapists during initial assessment of physically disabled patients. *Occupational Therapy Journal of Research, 2,* 195–219.

Schell, B. A. B (Oct 6, 2003). Clinical reasoning and occupation-based practice: Changing habits. Continuing Education Article for *Occupational Therapy Practice.*

Schell, J. W. (1999). *Contextual teaching and learning in pre-service teacher education.* Accessed July 31, 2006 from: http://www.coe.uga.edu/ctl/theory.html

Schell, J. W. & Black, R. S. (1997). Situated learning: An inductive case study of a collaborative learning experience. *Journal of Industrial Teacher Education, 34*(4), 5–27.

Schkade, J. K. & Schultz, S. (1992). Occupational adaptation: Toward a holistic approach to contemporary practice, Part I. *American Journal of Occupational Therapy, 46,* 829–837.

Schön, D. (1983). *Educating the reflective practitioner: Toward a new design for teaching and learning in the professions.* San Francisco: Jossey-Bass.

Spoon, J. & Schell, J. W. (1997). Aligning student learning styles with instructor teaching styles. *Journal of Industrial-Technical Teacher Education, 35*(2), 38.

St. Julien, J. (1997). Explaining learning: The research trajectory of situated cognition and the implications of connectionism. In D. Kirshner & J. A. Whitson (Eds.), *Situated cognition: Social semiotic and psychological perspectives* (pp. 261–279). Mahwah, NJ: Lawrence Earlbaum Associates.

Stern, P. (2005). Holistic approach to teaching evidence-based practice. *American Journal of Occupational Therapy, 59,* 157–165.

Tickle-Degnen, L. (1999). Organizing, evaluating, and using evidence in occupational therapy practice. *American Journal of Occupational Therapy, 53,* 537–539.

Tickle-Degnen, L. (2000). Gathering current research evidence to enhance clinical reasoning. *American Journal of Occupational Therapy,* 54, 102–105.

von Glasserfeld, E. (1995*). Radical constructivism: A way of knowing and learning.* London: Falmer Press.

Vygotsky, L. S. (1978). *Mind in society*. Edited and Translated by M. Cole, V. John-Steiner, S. Scribner & E. Souberman. Cambridge, MA: Harvard University Press.

Wenger, E. (1998). *Communities of practice*. Cambridge, UK: Cambridge University Press.

Westheimer, J. & Kahne, J. (1993). Building school communities: An experience-based model. *Phi Delta Kappan,* 75(4), 324–329.

White, N., Blythe, T. & Gardner, H. (1992). Multiple intelligences theory: Creating the thoughtful classroom. In A. Costa, J. Bellanca & R. Fogarty (Eds.), *If minds matter: A foreword to the future*. Palatine, IL: Skylight.

Wolff, D. (1994). *New approaches to language teaching: an overview CLCS* Occasional Paper No.39. Dublin: Trinity College.

12

Communities of Practice
A Curricular Model That Promotes Professional Reasoning

John W. Schell and Barbara A. Boyt Schell

OBJECTIVES

After reading this chapter, the learner will be able to:

1 Articulate a compelling argument for the need for educational approaches that promote professional reasoning among members of a learning community.
2 Use principles of a learning community as a foundation for learning and teaching in higher education settings.
3 Facilitate the adoption of a practice of reasoning among learners within a communal learning context.
4 Facilitate the extraction of meaning among learners within a communal learning context.
5 Facilitate the development of self-identity among learners within a communal learning context.
6 Anticipate challenges inherent in a communal learning approach.

Community of practice	Identities
Practices	Meaning

Previous chapters in Unit III discussed epistemology, then turned to principles of learning and teaching appropriate for the education of occupational therapists. In this and the next chapters, discussions focus on practical approaches about how these concepts and ideas can be used in higher education programs, particularly entry-level programs. We believe these approaches advance professional reasoning skills among students, such that graduates enter the field with higher level (or "advanced beginner") practice skills.

Thinking About Thinking 12-1

It is the tension between creativity and skepticism that has produced the stunning and unexpected findings of science.

—Carl Sagan

First, we make an argument citing research that suggests the advantages of communities of practice in promoting professional reasoning. In the body of the chapter, we give practical suggestions that promote the practice of reasoning, draw meaning from that reasoned thinking, and eventually impact on the personal and group identity of the individual learner. Throughout, we illustrate the points made using a case study of the curriculum in place at Brenau University in Gainesville, Georgia (see Addenda A and B). This curriculum was developed and implemented based on legitimate peripheral participation and communities of practice as the educational philosophies guiding the program. We conclude by examining the challenges of implementing and maintaining a curriculum based on a communities of practice model.

COMMUNITIES OF PRACTICE

Communities are all around us. We are often engaged in overlapping communities. For us, these include our professional occupational therapy and educational communities, our family membership at the university golf course, the choir we both sing in at our fellowship, John's friends in our local remote control model airplane club and Barbara's friends in the local art community. Each of these communities is a community because they pursue common interests and enterprises (Wenger, 1998). As a married couple, we enjoy a shared life that weaves through our work, our play, and our commitment to a healthy lifestyle. This means that our separate and shared communities often overlap. For example, John serves on a number of college committees. Sometimes colleagues on those committees also sing in the choir in which we both sing. Others play golf at the university golf course with us. In some of these organizations, we assume leadership roles, such as when Barbara was department chair or John was a program chair and research team leader. Other times we are at the periphery of the community, such as when John stands on the sidelines at the model airplane club watching the planes flown by more expert pilots. Regardless of the role, in a **community of practice** we each interact with other members in the pursuit of the group's enterprise. At the air-plane club, when she goes along with John, Barbara sits on the sidelines reading a book and usually doesn't talk to anyone besides John. No one in that group considers her as a member of that community of practice—rather, just as John's wife.

Interaction among members of a community of practice shapes a network of relationships and the capabilities of our community, including our commonly shared **practices** (expertise) and our individual and collective **identities.** Participation in communities also enables us to draw **meaning** from that experience. In short, we are learning, just as we learn through living our lives. Most of us are socialized through what we learn from our participation in communities of one sort or another.

Theoretical Traditions

The insights shared in this chapter come from our own work, both empirical and experiential, as well as from social learning theories. Barbara extended her current area of research on clinical reasoning from the framework of social learning theory (Schell, 1996). In addition, Lindsay, a student of John's, conducted qualitative dissertation research on the community of practice within the Brenau University OT program (1999). Other practical and theoretical information used in this chapter is drawn from the results of a 5-year study funded by the U.S. Department of Education conducted at the UGA College of Education and other research universities, including The Universities of Wisconsin and Washington, the Ohio State University, and Johns Hopkins University. This project resulted in a national contextual teaching and learning (CTL) theoretical framework for teacher education. Finally, self-studies in association with re-accreditation by the Accreditation Council for Occupational Therapy Education (ACOTE) have provided data drawn from faculty, alumni, and those who employ Brenau graduates. Throughout, this chapter is supplemented by lessons drawn from our own experiences as collaborating researchers and teachers who strive for reflective practice among our own graduates.

To us the most important outcome of this research is a language of contextualized teaching and learning by which Barbara and John have guided their own instructional practices for several years. For example, John is a professionally trained career and technical education teacher. Yet, he now rejects most of the behaviorism that he learned in his teacher education program. For years, he practiced using a "gut feeling" or instinct to guide his teaching. John's impulses have always led him to be student-oriented and contextualized, but until about 20 years ago, he never knew exactly why he practiced in this manner.

He was a young assistant professor at the University of Pittsburgh when he first realized that there was substantial and meaningful research that gave definition and direction to his intuitive teaching. Over the years, many of his doctoral students have also commented on the importance of acquiring an instructional language for situated learning that enabled more focused teaching in their educational practice. Of course, learning the language of learning is an important step toward becoming a legitimate member of a teaching community. Even intuitive teachers can move toward fuller and more meaningful practice as they learn the language and apply elements of situated learning.

Before we move into the body of this chapter we would like to re-emphasize the primary reasons for choosing a social learning framework. It is because we believe that it can result in therapists educated to be reflective practitioners. In her practice, Barbara strives to accomplish this by immersion of the novice learner in authentic OT practice contexts from the very first days of the learner's professional OT education.

PHILOSOPHICAL BASE AND GUIDING ASSUMPTIONS

All accredited occupational therapy programs are required to explicate the fundamental organizing concepts guiding the learning process. For instance, ACOTE requires that the curriculum design:

> . . . reflect the mission and philosophy of both the occupational therapy program and the institution and shall provide the basis for program planning, implementation, and evaluation. The design shall identify educational goals and describe the selection of the content, scope and sequencing of coursework (ACOTE, 1998, standard 5.3).

We believe the educational theories and implied practices reflected in the terms "community of practice" are an excellent basis for occupational therapy education. The educational theories we refer to were primarily extrapolated from research conducted by Jean Lave and Etienne Wenger on situated cognition (Lave, 1988), legitimate peripheral participation (Lave & Wenger, 1991), and communities of practice (Wenger, 1998). As discussed in Chapter 11, these learning perspectives are rooted in sociology and vary from traditional psychological assumptions that learning occurs within an individual. Along with Wenger, we also do not believe in the common assumptions that learning "has a beginning and an end"; that it is best separated from the rest of our activities; and that it is the result of teaching" (Wenger 1998, p. 3). In contrast, like Wenger, we assume that learning is a function of living. In many instances, knowledge is drawn from participation in everyday life within a variety of communities that have adopted specific practices (Box 12-1).

B O X 1 2 - 1
Operator's Guide to Communities of Practice

A number of operational principles guide the development and support of a community of practice curriculum which uses context based teaching and learning approaches. Keys principles are:

- Support and maintain the learning community.
- Recognize and attend to issues of power and trust.
- Build on life experiences of the learner.
- Have learners use knowledge in authentic practice situations.
- Expect behaviors consistent with the professional community's standards.
- Coordinate learning opportunities to maximize knowledge acquisition, knowledge use and reflection on practice.
- Build in reflection and articulation time at the curricular level, as well as within course design.
- Provide opportunity for multiple perspectives in order to appreciate key concepts.

There is a synergy among these educational theories and many occupational therapy theories in that they emphasize the importance of participation in meaningful activity, whether the goal is to restore healthy or maximize learning. In Addendum A that follows, we show how these ideas, along with those related to the nature of professional reasoning described in Units I and II, are woven into a statement about educational philosophy.

ASSUMPTIONS OF CONTEXT-BASED TEACHING AND LEARNING

To guide faculty and other instructors in the development and implementation of teaching activities that were consistent with social learning theory and professional practice, assumptions of teaching and learning must be articulated for both faculty and students. *Table 12-1* provides an example of how this is done in a student handbook used as part of program orientation.

Addendum B (Brenau University OT Program: A Working Community of Practice) continues the description of the curriculum at Brenau and provides commentary on the thinking behind some of the decisions made as the curriculum was designed and implemented. Refer to this Case Study as you read through the next few paragraphs, in which we highlight elements critical to implementing a community of practice approach to teaching.

Building on Life Experience

Most psychologists and sociologists would agree that learners attempt to acquire new knowledge in light of what they already know. Although this is not an earth-shaking insight into learning, it is an important assumption that teachers who wish to strategically use authentic contexts as a foundation for their teaching must consider. Therefore, students are encouraged to share their personal, work, and volunteer experiences and to relate these to their new learning.

Using Knowledge for Authentic Practice

In Chapter 11, we discussed the importance of authenticity with regard to teaching that is intended to guide learners into professional practice. Our practice has always been to immerse learners into the real world of professional practice at the earliest point possible. For example, at Brenau, students are considered to be novice practitioners from their first moments in the program. Key to this is the extensive use of Level I Fieldwork as described earlier. For example, students are taught to do the Role Checklist (Oakley, Kielfhofner, Barris & Reichler, 1986) and Canadian Occupational Performance Measure (Law, Baptiste, Carswell, McColl, Polatjko & Pollock, 1998) during their first semester. After practicing use in labs, they then use these assessments with individuals in hospital or community settings. When truly authentic contexts are not practical, a simulated approach may be in order. For example, pediatric courses make liberal use of the on-site daycare children for learning developmental assessments and interventions such as splinting.

TABLE 12-1

Student and Faculty Responsibilities

As an occupational therapy student here at Brenau University, you have joined a community of learners that includes you, other students, faculty, staff, and occupational therapy practitioners. Each member of the community has a responsibility to promote development and learning for themselves and every other member of the community. Because you are entering a profession, you will have experiences and expectations that go beyond a typical student role to that of a developing therapist. In addition, because we believe that you have to use knowledge in meaningful ways to really gain control of it, you will be in many learning situations that involve or parallel the real demands of clinical practice. For many students, this is a shift in expectations of the student-teacher relationship. The table below summarizes some important expectations of faculty and of students as developing therapists.

Developing Therapist Responsibilities	Faculty Member Responsibilities
Use and share life experiences as a basis for gaining new knowledge for self and others.	Recognize the life experience of students, and use it to support new learning.
Shift from being a passive learner (i.e., note taker, listener, observer) to an active learner who contributes to discussions and solves problems.	Facilitate active discussion, problem solving, and student contributions. Avoid teacher-centered as opposed to student-centered approaches.
Shift from being an individual learner to becoming a member of the learning community.	Facilitate active discussion, problem solving, and student contributions. Avoid teacher-centered as opposed to student centered approaches.
View self as a developing therapist, not a student waiting to become a therapist.	Treat students as colleagues from whom one can expect professional behavior.
Actively seek, use, and give feedback to improve knowledge and professionalism.	Actively seek, use, and give feedback to improve knowledge and professionalism.
Accept responsibility for timely and dependable completion of assignments, attendance at class and informed participation and learning.	Communicate assignments in a timely manner and manage class meetings in a responsible manner that supports informed participation and learning.
Take risks and use learning opportunities to act like a therapist.	Develop learning opportunities in real or closely simulated practice situations.
Reflect on personal assumptions and be open to alternative understandings.	Provide opportunities for reflection. Model the reflective process.

Brenau University Occupational Therapy Student Handbook, 2005-2006. Used with permission.

Coordination of Learning Opportunities

It is important to maximize the potential synergy across and among learning experiences. Since, as discussed in Chapter 11, learning transfer does not reliably occur, faculty must point out to students the relationships designed into the learning opportunities. For instance, all courses under the control of the OT Department at Brenau focus at some level on the development of skills that have some practical application in professional practice. Each semester reflects a careful blending of lecture, laboratory, fieldwork, and reflection seminars, and assignments are coordinated to reinforce each other across courses. Aspects of supervision, accessing research related to practice, professional communications, and behavior are addressed in all courses. For example, students may learn about an assessment in lecture, practice it in lab with each other or on volunteer clients, administer it in "real life" on fieldwork, write it up for class, and then reflect on it during seminar. Later, students may be challenged to look more critically at the research supporting the assessment or intervention approach.

Building in Reflection Time

It is important to provide opportunities for reflection on underlying assumptions that shape both problem finding and problem solving in professional practice. The opportunities require instructional activities that promote reflection on newly acquired knowledge. Although there is commonly talk among educators about critical thinking and the use of reflective activities, there is often something missing in educational practice: the strategies that require students to use their metacognitive skills at a sufficient depth to promote meaning, professional identity, and some form of generalizability. Specifically, reflection activities should systematically require learners to:

- Articulate their authentic field experiences
- Afford opportunities to make comparisons of those experiences with appropriate theoretical assumptions
- Draw a purposive and meaningful lesson
- Illustrate at least one other practice circumstance in which this new knowledge might be applied (Schell, 2001)

For example, at Brenau during clinical reasoning seminars, students have weekly opportunities for open discussion with regard to any aspect of their developing knowledge and practice. This is combined with structured reflection activities in which each student, often with a student facilitator, discusses an in-depth analysis of their own reasoning of a particular therapy encounter during fieldwork practice. This formalization of reflection as a curriculum strategy in separate courses enhances the expected reflection that also occurs in other seminars, labs, and lectures.

Use of Multiple Perspectives

Students must have opportunities to appreciate key concepts from a variety of perspectives. This promotes a richer appreciation of the complexity of occupational therapy processes, and flexibility in finding approaches consistent with the client's unique situation. To make the greatest impact, different contexts and multiple experiences should be afforded in which the learner is required to view the same construct from multiple perspectives. This is a critical point. Often students gaining knowledge in abstract contexts such as classrooms or seminars do not learn to appreciate the complexities of activating this knowledge in practice. The application of reflection and principles of reflective practice can provide affordances for appreciating and exploring subtle but complex patterns of relationships between and among concepts. At Brenau, for example, students are given many opportunities to plan, implement and reflect on the use of meaning-ful therapeutic activities in a variety of different settings and with clients who have a range of physical, emotional, cognitive and developmental problems. Students are challenged to integrate more "impairment-oriented" intervention approaches, such as strengthening, range of motion, and cognitive activities with-in activities that are occupationally relevant to the client. Students also see how client performance is shaped by contextual factors such as physical setting and social norms. These challenges are revisited as students deal with clients in dif-ferent settings with different problems, requiring differing blends of therapy approaches.

CREATING AND MAINTAINING A COMMUNITY OF PRACTICE

Practically, the implementation of a curriculum based on a Community of Practice model requires nurturing and maintaining a community of scholars composed of both university employees and associates who are practicing in the field. In the Brenau case, the learning community consists of university students and professors and extends to the numerous practitioner educators who provide guest lectures and supervise students in fieldwork experiences. It is a very diffi-cult task to purposefully create and maintain a nurturing community that is sup-portive of an enriched educational environment. Although it may be true that some communities are incidental or happen naturally, to constructively use that environment for instructional purposes is a very purposeful and often labor-intensive enterprise. Before we analyze some of the activities that promote communities of practice, we should acknowledge that the formulation of commu-nities is a natural phenomenon.

Communities Happen

We all participate in communities. All involve learning. Some are formal commu-nities such as the workplace, school, church, and recreation activities. Others are groups that form naturally. Most programs of occupational therapy education can legitimately claim to be a community of practice; some are planned, others more circumstantial. But one would have to ask: Does an incidental community of practice that is based on hierarchy and power have the same potential for stu-dent efficacy? We contend that a community of practice that is unplanned is likely to be less effective than one that is planned and strategically used as a founda-tion for instruction, learning, and reflection.

What we mean by a community of practice is one in which learning is inten-tionally focused and has elements of (a) a group of people pursuing commonly accepted enterprises, (b) negotiated and commonly accepted practices, (c) oper-ational learning strategies to promote meaning among the learners, and (d) mul-tiple opportunities for learners to recognize and develop professional identities (Wenger, 1998). This is not to say that our approach is perfect—far from it. Communities of practice can also be dysfunctional and even subject to Darwinian extinction.

Communities That Go Bad

The purposive instructional use of community is not automatically a good thing. John has often contended that communities that fail have most of the same properties as those that succeed. For example, communities that go bad may fail to adapt to cultural or technological changes that are needed to be relevant to a changing environment. Another reason for organization dysfunction is a lack of direction due to inability to "manage agreement" among members of the community. Jerry Harvey, Professor of Management at George Washington University, describes this phenomenon as the *Abilene Paradox* (1988), in which members end up on a metaphorical trip to Abilene, even though when carefully questioned, no one intended to go there. Faculties, students, and staff often agree on a given educational purpose; but although they may agree to agree, their agreement may be based on entirely different assumptions. For example, one faculty member may agree that a community of practice–type curriculum is important, but uses misaligned instructional practices. Another faculty may also acknowledge a community-based approach, but is much more learner-centered in his or her instructional practice. Even though these two outwardly agree on a community-based curriculum, their instructional philosophies are rooted in very different places. Such unmatched expectations often lead to a dysfunctional organization with no one realizing that superficial agreement is actually the source of intense internal dissonance. The important difference to us is the intentional use of community when matched with philosophically consistent instructional assumptions and practices shared by all faculty.

Delicate Balance Between Learning and Teaching

Philosophically, we have come to believe that higher education instructors who wish to promote professional reasoning must strike a subtle sense of balance between the assumptions that students learn best from their own experiences and the competing perspective that students must digest a vast quantity of professorial knowledge.

Thinking About Thinking 12-2

You cannot learn anything through the efforts of others. The world's greatest teachers can teach you absolutely nothing unless you are willing to apply what they have to offer based on your knowing. Those great teachers only offer you choices on the menu of life. They can make them sound very appealing, and ultimately they may help you to try those items on the menu; they can even write the menu. But the menu can never be the meal.

—Wayne Dyer, 1998 (p. 8)

The research is clear that a teacher's intentional use of authentic contexts for learning can promote active use of knowledge (Brown, Collins & Duguid, 1989). This presumes an expert instructor who understands how adults learn to efficiently guide a novice practitioner through a complex maze of professional content. For example, learners exploring a given topic can be captivated by it, becoming highly motivated through living their experiences. Yet, without suffi-cient reflective guidance from an expert teacher, inappropriate inferences can be drawn, causing long-term negative consequences. This is why we come down near the middle of the controversy with regard to student- and teacher-centered-ness. Drawing from Dyer's "menu of knowledge" metaphor quoted above, it may be true that the learner chooses from the menu, but the menu does provide struc-ture and efficiency to the learning process . . . and in higher education, the instructor is often the chef who creates the menu and prepares the food.

Authentic Experiences in Authentic Contexts

If the intention is to enable learners to apply their knowledge to solve problems in OT clinics or in client's homes or commuter trains, instruction should be authentically situated in clinics, homes and community settings. In Chapter 11, we discussed the nature of abstract and authentic learning contexts. Here, we are making a definite endorsement of the ungrammatical idea: The realer; the better. It is most desirable to provide instruction in authentic practice situations. It is the higher education version of using the natural environment as advocated by early interventionists. You may be saying to yourself, "that's unrealistic!" And we partially agree with you. There are many instructional situations in which it is not practical to provide instruction in the real world. It might even be unethical to use authentic contexts in some instances. That said, instruction within authentic contexts can lead to knowledge that is relevant and connected to real practice (see, for example, Brown et al., 1989). When it is possible and appropriate, we believe that a cornerstone of a community of practice curricu-lum is instruction delivered and received in authentic contexts. If it is not prac-tical to use real-life situations, we advocate the use simulations that closely replicate actual practice.

Reflection on Authentic Experience Is Required

John's research at UGA strongly suggests that context is only one aspect of teaching for expertise. Without appropriate examination, even authentic experi-ences can lead to limited learning outcomes. Reflection and experiences might be thought of as twin dynamics (Schell, 2001). To maximize learning, enrichment experiences must be examined through a variety of reflection activities. The cou-pling of experience and meaning making is not new, as shown in Box 12-2.

BOX 12-2

Education as Emancipation and Enlargement of Experience

Jeffs and Smith (2005) wrote of John Dewey's observation that education is an "emancipation and enlargement of experience." As educators, most of us can identify with these words. For example, we may describe parts of our work in terms of "learning by doing" and of widening opportunities, or giving people new experiences. Yet, Dewey meant something more than this.

BOX 12-2

(*continued*)

When we talk of "enlarging," the meaning is fairly clear. We usually mean that we want to make something bigger, to extend its limits. With regard to experience, this is not just a matter of widening, of encouraging people to do different things, it also involves deepening. By this, we mean that as educators our task is to work with people so that they may have a greater understanding or appreciation of their experiences. Again, the meaning of emancipation need not trouble us; it is a process of setting free. But what does it mean to set free experience? Here, we touch on the profound. It is easy to fall into seeing experiences as things. After all, we often talk of "having an experience," of things "happening to us." We get a picture of being on the receiving end of some event. *Yet this is only half the story.* Experiences are not only "had," they are also "known. In other words, they are thought about at some level, although we may not be conscious of this. We interpret what is going on and this allows us to be set free; we need not be dictated to by, or victims of, experience. We can become not just experiencers but also experimenters—creators as well as consumers. Experience entails thought. It includes reflection. To emancipate and enlarge experience, we must attend to both having and knowing (Jeffs & Smith, 2005 [emphasis added]).

We particularly like their point that experience is not something that is *had* but is also *known*. Dewey (through Jeffs & Smith) reminds us that education frees us to mindfully examine experiences. There are many tools that can be used to help as we attend to the important task of extracting meaning from our experiences (Moon, 1999). Moon describes the use of "concept maps," "artful expression," "identification and analysis of critical incidents," and "systematic review of instructional materials" (1999). We urge instructors to facilitate reflection among learners from many perspectives. Of course, some reflection techniques are effective with some individuals but not for others. For example, some learners respond favorably to keeping a reflective journal; others do not. So, as is true in almost any discussion of instructional methods, many reflective strategies are required and must be a fit with the needs and interests of the individuals within a given community.

At Brenau, reflection is systematic and is a daily part of instructional practice. The clinical reasoning seminar provides an informal context that instructors systematically facilitate as students articulate their newly acquired knowledge, make comparisons with appropriate theoretical assumptions, draw a meaningful lesson, and gain insight into other possible applications of their knowledge. This way of thinking about reflection permits modeling of a variety of learning-teaching strategies. This is a form of reflection "on-action," as suggested by Schön (1990). Clinical reasoning seminars are also natural laboratories for making connections between experiences and meaning-making, as described by Jeffs and Smith (2005).

Power and Trust Within Communities of Practice

Whatever reflection techniques are used, it is critically important to acknowledge that power and trust are inherent in a positive teacher–learner relationship. French and Raven (1960) wrote extensively in their classic works about positional power. Of course, this is a type of power enjoyed by instructors in higher education. All legitimate teaching positions come with some degree of positional power. These powers give license to academic decisions that can dramatically affect the lives of students. Unfortunately, some in higher education are infamous for abuse and mistreatment of students. When John teaches his class on administration and supervision of public schools, he likes to quote Barbara, who often reminds us that "a move into administration is a promotion, not a coronation." We all have experienced professors and teachers who splendidly enjoy their coronation as "philosopher king [queen]"—those who rule their classroom through divine privilege.

To the contrary, positional power is one of those rare commodities that grows richer when given away to the learner. Such a gift to students in the context of high scholarly expectations often returns a much more potent combination of expert and referent powers that may result in a much more desirable mixture of power and "influence" (French & Raven, 1960).

The degree of expert power can be a mere artifact of low supply and high demand. Experts are those with skills appropriate to solve a difficult problem. Professors in higher education are usually hired for their high levels of expertise. Tenure is subsequently granted on the fact that expertise cannot be easily replaced at a lower salary. Professors with validated expertise in the form of tenure do enjoy scholarly recognition. Unfortunately, referent power does not automatically accompany tenure and formal recognition of expertise. Teachers who earn referent power are those with whom students can identify easily, believing in their inspirational leadership. When teachers combine scholarly expertise with good will and mutual respect for learners, the effect can be exponentially effective. Those who successfully combine expertise and referent powers are teachers who can positively influence lives; they place the needs of the student in the forefront. This approach can contribute significantly to an environment of trust, another element critical to the development of a successful community of practice.

Higher-education faculty members often talk about the need for a trusting classroom environment. How trustworthy students perceive faculty members might come as a surprise. John experienced such a surprise as the result of an unintended consequence of a research study he conducted with a graduate assistant. This research examined the degree to which a semester-long simulation could be considered authentically contextualized (Schell & Black, 1997). His graduate assistant that semester, Rhonda (now Dr. Rhonda Black of the University of Hawaii) conducted follow-up interviews with members of a doctoral-level class. The participants in the study found the simulation educationally useful once they trusted the professor (John) to act in their best interests. This probably sounds obvious, but John was surprised to learn that students only gradually learned to trust him. In his words, "I know myself to be trustworthy. I know I have the best interests of learners in my heart. I assumed that students knew and trusted me from the very beginning of a class just because of who I think I am. Unfortunately, some students have had difficult experiences with faculty and were reluctant to take me at my word." Students reported their belief that a successful community of learners is dependent on level of trust in the faculty (Schell & Black, 1997).

ADOPTING THE PRACTICE OF REASONING WITHIN THE COMMUNITY

The ethic of reasoning is nicely symbolized by the ancient writing of the Buddha.

Thinking About Thinking 12-3

Do not believe what you have heard.
Do not believe in tradition because it is handed down many generations.
Do not believe in anything that has been spoken of many times.
Do not believe because the written statements come from some old sage.
Do not believe in conjecture.
Do not believe in authority or teachers or elders.
But after careful observation and analysis, when it agrees with reason and it will benefit one and all, then accept it and live by it.

—Buddha (563–483 BC)(as published in Dyer, 1998)

It is often very difficult to convince youthful learners that it is okay to question and to be skeptical of ideas that are learned as truth from their experiences with family, church, peers, community, and school. Experts argue that countering these beliefs has become even tougher in recent years (Fischhoff, Crowell & Kipke, 1999). Adolescents are increasingly likely to engage in risky behaviors and have a difficult time analyzing the potential negative consequences of such behaviors (Fischhoff, 1992). It is our belief that, to some extent, students are intellectual victims of today's standardized "test and recall" high school curriculum. "There's an enormous difference between memorizing a few key facts and having an authentic grasp of a subject: It's the difference between doing well on a multiple choice test and being able to hold a substantial discussion about a topic. It's the difference between reading about hospitals and being hospitalized for a week . . ." (Jensen, 2000, p. 279). Youngsters who have learned to expertly take multiple-choice tests are those now entering higher education. For many of these students, it is difficult to follow the ancient advice of the Buddha when simplistic truths are deeply engrained and are thought to be indisputable.

The main point is that the ethos of reasoning and questioning is a matter of being socialized to the culture of scholarship. It is nonetheless central to the success of a community of practice curriculum. Without a community ethic of questioning and reasoning, educational activities are one-dimensional and sterile. Faculty and administration must be devoted to nurturing a culture of reasoning among everyone associated with the community.

Systematic interaction of advanced learners with newer ones is a good way to begin this difficult task. Another meaningful strategy is to encourage metacognition by the purposeful use of a framework such as King and Kitchner's reflective judgment (1997). You will recall our conversation on this topic in a previous chapter. I have found that novices often need a mental organizer to help them structure their reflection. Among the aspects of King and Kitchner's work are the twin dynamics of universal to relative "truth" and the "quality of evidence" used to make reflective judgments. The use of evidence to formulate practice is inherently connected to all forms of professional reasoning and is discussed in Chapter 13, which describes how to develop students into practitioners who can find and use evidence effectively in practice.

At Brenau, from the first orientation, the program's philosophies and instructional practices are openly discussed. New members of the community are informed that they will be treated as a colleague with all the expectations and respect suggested by that type of teacher–student relationship. As a foundation to maintaining an ethic of reasoning, students are encouraged to communicate openly and directly. Feedback opportunities are built in throughout the program for both students and faculty. Faculty is encouraged to deal with students collaboratively, and to minimize the power issues that can threaten trust, and therefore community. All these strategies are foundational for promoting an ethos of professional reasoning.

MEANING-MAKING FROM LEARNING EXPERIENCES

"Authentic, meaningful learning requires the student to process information in his/her own way, along his/her own timeline, and in relation to his/her own perceptual maps. Sorting, analyzing, and drawing conclusion in the context of one's own life is the only learning that sticks" (Jensen, 2000, p. 279). Psychologists and sociologists often refer to two types of meaning: reference and sense. Other words for these types of meaning are surface and deeply-felt (Jensen). These concepts are thought to operate within macro- and micro-relationships. Reference meaning is the larger or macro context. You might think of this as you would a state highway map that is useful when driving from state to state. A sense meaning experience might be more like using a detailed (micro) local map to find and experience specific neighborhoods. In OT education, we can learn/teach about disabling conditions among the elderly and draw reference or surface meaning from it. It is only when novice OTs encounter elderly people with disabilities struggling to adapt to difficult conditions in their own home that real sense or deeply felt meaning can be accessed.

Jensen (2000) identified three factors that trigger a sense of meaning: (a) relevance, (b) emotions, and (c) context. What is relevant to a student is a tricky concept. What is relevant to one individual is not to another. Jensen and others view this as a neurological response to other neural fields formulated by prior experiences. Since we all are individuals with differing experiences, our sense of what is relevant is unique to each learner. "There's little doubt about it, emotions and meaning are linked" (Jensen, p. 282). Depending on positive or negative states of mind, emotions can be either a facilitator or an inhibitor of learning. Generally, keeping learning experiences positive suggests a better chance of creating better perceptual maps. The learning context can be as we discussed in Chapter 11, abstract or "of the mind" (p. 287) or somewhere along a continuum leading to real-life authenticity. Based on the assumption that our brains make and discriminate among a collection of patterns, the context in which learning happens is critical to meaning making. Either end of this imaginary continuum context can be useful to learning, depending on how it is skillfully manipulated by the instructor. It is also likely that some students might have strong preferences for abstraction or application. What seems clear is that context, emotion, and relevance are intertwined and critical to how our minds make meaning. Of course, we do have to admit a bias toward learning in authentic practice contexts. It is our belief that real contexts can promote relevance and can evoke strong emotion.

Admittedly, this is a shorthand and simplistic discussion of very complex assumptions with regard to brain-based learning. Regardless, our purpose is to set a framework for discussing teaching practices that engender meaning making among novice therapists.

CHALLENGES TO A LEARNING COMMUNITY OF PRACTICE

We do not want to give the impression that learning and teaching from a community of practice curriculum are easy or a quick fix for a broken curriculum. Honestly speaking, this form of teaching is quite labor-intensive. A period of adjustment on the parts of both instructors and students is often required. At the beginning of their OT program, Brenau faculty had one major advantage when this curriculum was developed: It was an entirely new program. No complicated institutional history existed, no sacred traditions had to be maintained, and there was no established organizational culture. This was blank slate start-up. For once, it was possible to negotiate "buy-in" from college administrators and hire specific faculty members who were a just-right fit for such a program. Another advantage was the importance Brenau places on good teaching. The type of higher education institution can be a determining factor with regard to the type of curriculum that can be offered. A community of practice curriculum may not be consistent with the demands of a Research 1 university, for example.

Privileges Teaching Over Research

It is clear that a community curriculum requires extensive instructional time and maintenance. Although research and publication are respected at Brenau, faculty time is mostly allocated in support of instruction. If the program was provided at the nearby University of Georgia, faculty would view this level of emphasis on teaching as an obstacle to obtaining research grants, publication, and promotion and tenure. In teaching institutions, some faculty understandably would like to spend more of their time in scholarly pursuits that extend beyond their teaching load. This is often a source of dissonance. To give a flavor of the time commitment, consider a class using a web-based bulletin board and discussion groups as a way to promote reflection, as John does. He typically posts questions about upcoming readings on the bulletin board and requires students to post their responses to his questions or to post their own. This is an effective strategy that he has put to productive use for several years. It is a good way to build and maintain a sense of community while it is focused on specific academic content. Unfortunately, the more active the students are with the bulletin board, the more time is required from John. On some mornings two hours are gone even before he answers e-mail, performs administrative duties, prepares for class, advises students, or works on his research.

Frequent Interaction with Students

A community-based curriculum or educational practice is by nature student centered. To be effective, a community of practice is truly a social place. For example, Brenau faculty members go out of their way to make their entire program a warm and inclusive learning experience. But frequent interaction with students can be as challenging as it can be rewarding. As was stated earlier, emotional involvement often plays an important part of learning and meaning-making. This is a positive with regard to learning, but it can mean that instructors are involved in the lives of students. At times students are tearfully in your office with the day's crisis before morning coffee or tea. Of course, crises invariably arise on a variety of fronts. Problems can range from difficulties with boyfriends/girlfriends to childcare to professional ethics encountered in field experiences. For some faculty, this is a natural way to share a nurturing relationship with students. For others, this level of personal involvement can be more taxing. It can also be difficult for students who do not know how and when it is appropriate to share their emotions. At Brenau, group discussion and peer counseling among faculty members are potent approaches to balancing the desire for community against unrealistic or inappropriate demands from students (or the faculty, for that matter). At times, faculty group lunches or "time out" have been built into the schedule to ensure sufficient time for relaxed interactions, away from the pressures of a meeting agenda.

A New Way of Thinking About Learning

Another possible source of complex emotions for students is that in a community of practice curriculum they are asked to think about learning differently. They are asked to take responsibility in a way that is foreign to the way they have previously succeeded in their educational careers. This can be a shock for many students used to a curriculum successfully negotiated via factual recall and objective tests. As in most occupational therapy programs, Brenau students are pretty good at test-taking, which was critical to meeting program prerequisites. However, when they enter the Brenau community of practice, they are expected to actually develop solutions to ill-structured problems set in real-world contexts. Barbara refers to this as "throwing them in the deep end . . . but with a lifeguard." Because so much of the Brenau curriculum is shared with field experiences, solutions to real OT problems are required in addition to book work and difficult tests. These are the kinds of tests in which possible answers are not always conveniently labeled: A), B), C), or D) none of the above. It can take a while for some students to get used to this more demanding and rigorous approach to professional education.

Balancing High Expectations with Loving Support

Some might see this juxtaposition of high expectations within a nurturing environment as paradoxical. It is not at all contradictory. John is known among his students as a very critical grader. They know that when written work is returned, it probably will be marked with many suggestions for improvement. Early in the semester, this can be a shock but they soon learn that he affords many opportunities to "get it right." His objective is to promote a safe environment that aspires to high-level cognition, deep meaning-making, and a chance for a life-changing education. He is not impressed with fast recall of facts. He views this approach to measuring learning as education in "bankruptcy." It is that "safe environment" for learning that eventually wins the day. When together teachers and students achieve reciprocal respect and deep engagement we begin to observe students learning in such a way that potentially changes their lives.

Brenau faculty holds their OT students to a similar high standard of excellence. This is one reason why the "ethic of reasoning" that was discussed earlier in this chapter is so critical to a successful learning community. But a curriculum

Schell, B. A. (1998). Clinical reasoning. In M. E. Neistadt & E. B. Crepeau (Eds.), *Willard and Spackman's occupational therapy* (9th ed.). Philadelphia: JB Lippincott.

Schell, J. W. & Black, R. S. (1997). Situated learning: An inductive case study of a collaborative learning experience. *Journal of Industrial Teacher Education, 34*(4), 5–27.

Schön, D. (1990). *Educating the Reflective Practitioner: Toward a New Design for Teaching and Learning in the Professions.* San Francisco: Jossey-Bass.

Schemm, R. L., Corcoran, M., Kolodner, E., Schaaf, R. (1993). A curriculum based on systems theory. *American Journal of Occupational Therapy, 47*, 625–634.

Wenger, E. (1998). *Communities of practice.* Cambridge: Cambridge University Press.

ADDENDUM A

Brenau University OT Program: A Working Community of Practice

Here we discuss how the philosophy described in the "Philosophical Basis for an Occupational Therapy Curriculum based on a Community of Practice" Case Study is used to design and implement the curriculum. Notice that implementation decisions must be sensitive to the timing of courses and fieldwork, sequencing of learning opportunities, as well as how courses are named and framed to promote desired mental frameworks.

At Brenau University, professional preparation programs require undergraduates to complete two years of prerequisite coursework before beginning a three-year course of study culminating in both BS and an MS degrees. Similarly, those with prior degrees complete a comparable three-year course of study, culminating in an MSOT. The occupational therapy program was initiated in 1996 and is fully accredited by ACOTE, most recently receiving a 10-year accreditation with no areas of deficiency. The following discussions reflect both founding principles illustrated in the "Philosophical Basis for an Occupational Therapy Curriculum based on a Community of Practice" case study, along with lessons learned in the implementation of the program.

Founding Principles

Guiding assumptions when designing the new occupational therapy educational program reflected Barbara's deeply held beliefs about occupational therapy as a profession, and therefore what students needed to learn (or not learn) to be highly functioning occupational therapists. These beliefs were shared by those joining the faculty and were revised and reaffirmed as the program evolved.

The Brenau faculty believes that occupational therapists need to practice in a holistic manner and focus on the person's ability to perform meaningful occupations. Occupational therapy practice requires an appreciation of the many personal and environmental facets that interrelate in occupational performance.

Developing practitioners require extensive opportunities for recognizing the complexities associated with performance, as well as selecting and combining interventions likely to be effective in solving these problems. By understanding and developing different aspects of clinical reasoning, students will be better prepared to implement the principles of occupational therapy.

Another belief is that novice occupational therapists need to counteract the problem of insufficient supervision early in their OT career. In other words, they have to be ready to hit the ground running. At Brenau, the initial emphasis is on the development of professional skills required of entry-level professionals functioning within a variety of practice contexts. OT practice is viewed as a problem-solving profession, which includes direct service and the use of educational and consultative strategies. It is also viewed as a social activity in which practitioners must function in a variety of practice cultures, requiring understanding of the legal, ethical, and fiscal variables that influence practice.

The undergraduate portion of the program emphasizes the development of knowledge, skills and attitudes necessary to professional practice at the entry level. The early parts of the professional preparation phase require the student to focus on occupational performance throughout the lifespan, and to appreciate the effects of health conditions on that performance. This lifespan approach is intended to help students appreciate the relationship between development and occupational performance. Further, it supports clinical reasoning that is grounded in problem finding related to occupational performance rather than impairment.

A fundamental belief is that knowledge for use requires action (Cervero, 1992). Therefore, students (or very inexperienced practitioners, as they are called) engage in weekly Level I Fieldwork, which lasts throughout each semester. The Level I Fieldwork opportunities permit students to use their professional knowledge in authentic situations and to understand service delivery in a variety of practice contexts. Small group clinical reasoning seminars also occur weekly and are designed to help students understand and reflect on the clinical reasoning process as they actually experience it in their field activities. Both open discussion and structured metacognitive activities are used in these seminars. All the strands of clinical reasoning described earlier in the book (see Unit II) are systematically addressed over the course of four semesters.

As students gain competence in service delivery, they explore educational and administrative aspects of practice. Research coursework is also started early. Students have the opportunity to practice aspects of the research process throughout their second year, including a directed data collection project either concurrent with their first Level II experience or immediately adjacent to it.

The graduate portion of the program continues to build on earlier understandings of practice, service management and research. Advanced coursework on theory and research heighten student abilities to critically select and evaluate therapy options. Other coursework builds skills in population-based approaches to health promotion, as well as administrative, legal, political, and ethical issues in service delivery. Students are provided with the opportunity to select advanced practice electives that serve to deepen skills in areas of special interest and to augment their program with graduate electives. All students engage in a group thesis, and the communication of thesis findings in the form of a manuscript suitable for journal publication and/or conference poster.

Aligning the Philosophies of OT and Education

The philosophic footing for the Brenau OT program is found in the traditions of progressive education. Rooted in pragmatism, this philosophy presupposes that through experience humankind must continuously progress toward more effective solutions to problems while acknowledging the relativistic nature of both problem finding and generation of solutions to complex problems. The situated cognition approach was congruent with Barb's desire to prepare professionals who are critical thinkers and solvers of complex problems within the context of OT practice.

This progressive educational position proved to be a nice fit with the philosophical base of occupational therapy (AOTA, 1979). A harmony between the tradition of progressive education and the philosophy of the American Occupational Therapy Association was well articulated by Christiansen (1991): the client as the agent of change, the therapist as a teacher-facilitator, intervention as a laboratory for development of life skills, and occupation as the foundation for therapy. This led naturally to the adoption of a context-based teaching and learning approach.

ADDENDUM B

Key Teaching Practices: Promoting Community

Faculty at Brenau often go to extraordinary lengths to create a social network among faculty, students, and the OT community. The social network is designed to enhance and promote higher-order learning and socialization of novice OTs. For example, Brenau faculty strives to maintain a warm and welcoming community of practice through a variety of strategies.

- Planned social events such as swimming parties welcoming new students, potluck meals organized by the Brenau Occupational Therapy Student Association, class luncheons, and faculty and student skits at graduation parties.
- Acknowledgement of larger parts of self, such as sharing challenges in balancing different life roles. This "humanizing" of the professor helps to create trust and open doors to the development of mentoring.
- Being family-friendly by allowing children to accompany parents to class on school holidays or when daycare problems arise; working around life events such as weddings, babies being born, and caregiving of those who are ill.
- Providing recognition of those important in the student's lives, by providing PhT (Putting her Through) certificates at graduation open house events for families, significant others at graduation reception.

Each of these approaches has to be balanced against professional behavior expectations and the need for boundaries. For instance, as this is being written, there is a discussion going on about whether it really okay for parents to bring children to the classroom. Although the occasional school-aged child is generally considered acceptable in the circumstances noted above, there is controversy about the appropriateness of having infants in the classroom at all. Is this too distracting for both the mother and the rest of the class? Are there unacceptable liability issues? How can we support our returning adult learners and not compromise learning for the larger group? Ongoing communication is required to maintain the culture of mutual respect and support that is critical to creating trust and openness.

13

Curricular Approaches to Professional Reasoning for Evidence-Based Practice

Wendy J. Coster

OBJECTIVES

After reading this chapter, the learner will be able to:

1 Identify the elements of evidence-based professional reasoning.
2 Understand the difference between evidence-based practice (EBP) as a course and as a curriculum thread, and the implications of the latter for instruction.
3 Understand how well-formulated questions help guide the clinical reasoning process.
4 Generate examples of PICO (Person, Intervention, Comparison, Outcome) questions that address different types of practice decisions.
5 Understand the importance of searching for negative as well as positive evidence.
6 Distinguish focused EBP appraisal of evidence from traditional approaches to critiquing research.
7 Become familiar with the format for writing a critically appraised topic (CAT).
8 Become familiar with a format for teaching how to construct a balanced synthesis of evidence.
9 Understand the importance of developing effective skills for communicating about evidence to diverse audiences.

Evidence-based practice (EBP)

Enablement/disablement model

PICO question

Randomized clinical trial (or randomized control trial) (RCT)

Threat to validity

Levels of evidence

Research notation

Clinical bottom line

Critically appraised topic (CAT)

Evidence-based practice (EBP) is a relatively recent addition to the curriculum vocabulary in occupational therapy. It was first included in the revised Accreditation Council for Occupational Therapy Education (ACOTE) Standards adopted in 1998 (American Occupational Therapy Association, 1998), and efforts to define EBP and incorporate it into occupational therapy education are ongoing. Many discussions in the field have focused on controversial issues such as the appropriateness of using medicine's levels of evidence for occupational therapy research or whether EBP is inherently unfriendly to individualized clinical decision making. This emphasis is unfortunate because it distracts from more careful consideration of the broader paradigm shift represented by the EBP approach. This chapter focuses on those larger issues and their implications for curriculum design. In the sections that follow, I attempt to illustrate the benefits of adopting an EBP "framework," particularly the ways in which this approach directly supports sound and ethical professional reasoning.

WHAT DO WE MEAN BY AN EVIDENCE-BASED PRACTICE (EBP) FRAMEWORK?

The classic definition of EBP (evidence-based practice) remains that given by Sackett (Sackett, Straus, Richardson, Rosenberg & Haynes, 2000, p.1): ". . . The integration of best research evidence with clinical expertise and patient values." This definition emphasizes three important elements that must each be considered: the best scientific evidence available, the values and preferences of the client, and the clinician's expertise gained through practice. Furthermore, as the discussion in the text of Sackett and colleagues makes clear, this process is guided by the specific clinical decision that is required at the moment for a particular client (or group of clients). Although the definition appears relatively straightforward, implementation is not. This is particularly true as professions such as occupational therapy attempt to "translate" the guidelines and methods that were originally developed in and organized around the context of medicine. The translation effort is complicated by the many differences between occupational therapy and medicine, including the paucity of clinical studies in occupational therapy that meet optimal criteria for scientific rigor, the relative imprecision of our assessment methods (compared with medical diagnostic tests), and occupational therapy's strong client-centered philosophy (compared with the role of physician as expert) (Law, 2002). These differences must be acknowledged and appropriate responses developed. If not, we risk adopting methods that distort or provide poor guidance for our practice or risk providing inadequate responses to increasing demands by payers and consumers for evidence to support what we do. However, with some modifications of the guidelines and vocabulary and clarification of basic principles, the EBP approach provides excellent guidance for professional reasoning in occupational therapy.

The Underpinnings of EBP

Values and Attitudes

Integration of EBP into a curriculum and eventually into practice begins with careful examination of the values and attitudes that support EBP and their congruence with current occupational therapy education. EBP is first and foremost about asking good questions. Our professional training prepares us well to ask questions regarding the client: What are his or her needs and goals? What factors are currently limiting the client's participation in important occupations? To answer these questions, we draw on what we were taught in our professional curricula and what we have learned since then in other educational activities and from our clinical experience. How comfortable are we asking questions about that knowledge? Typically, once we have an "answer" that appears to fit the situation—whether it is a definition of the client's problem, a frame of reference to guide our intervention decisions, or an expectation regarding likely outcomes for the client—we tend to stop asking further questions. After all, we have a lot of other work to get on with. However, asking questions regularly about the knowledge underlying our practice is an essential habit for the evidence-based practitioner. Thus, one of the important skills needed to implement EBP is a way of formulating good questions, that is, questions that direct our attention to important issues and that guide our reasoning productively.

There are two important premises that are embedded in this emphasis on asking questions. The first premise is accepting that our clinical knowledge at any given moment is imperfect and therefore it will need constant refinement. The second is that ongoing self-directed learning is an essential aspect of ethical practice. The first premise is not likely to receive much argument given the pace of scientific advances in recent years. And yet, it is worth asking ourselves: How recently were the theories and techniques in our practice repertoire developed? Have they been substantially modified since then? If not, why not? What is the major focus of current research in our area of practice and with our primary client population, and how have the findings of this work been integrated into what we do?

We have an obligation to our clients to locate and use the most updated information possible. However, in the past, practitioners have not found research reports to be a particularly useful resource for this purpose (Dysart & Tomlin, 2002). Research studies rarely focus on the specific concerns or involve samples that are exactly similar to those of individual practitioners. Traditional approaches to reading the literature often lead to frustration and the unfortunate perception that research is "not relevant" to practice in the real world. In addition, because relatively few studies have directly tested occupational therapy interventions, practitioners may come to the conclusion that "there isn't much evidence in occupational therapy." They may conclude that EBP is not possible in occupational therapy or that time spent reviewing research will not be very productive. These perceptions also contribute to anxiety that payers will increasingly refuse to cover our services because we cannot support our recommendations with evidence.

Perhaps the problem is not with the research literature, however, as much as with how we have approached it. This is one of the important arguments made by Sackett and his colleagues (Sackett et al., 2000; Strauss, Richardson, Glasziou & Haynes, 2005), the developers of evidence-based medicine. One of the most valuable contributions of the EBP approach is that it offers an alternative way to investigate and apply science-based information in practice, one that is organized around decisions that the clinician faces. Implementation of this approach, however, requires commitment from the practitioner to ongoing, self-directed learning because the needs of each practitioner dictate the evidence that is needed at a given moment.

Self-directed learning does not have to be an isolating process. The final important element of the approach stressed in this chapter is collaborative effort. The originators of EBP were grappling with the same realities of clinical practice that occupational therapists face today: The scientific knowledge base is vast and practitioners have limited time to spend searching for useful, valid information. The methods of EBP were designed to work in that context. EBP is optimized when practitioners share the effort, so that no one wastes time "reinventing the wheel." This means that preparation for EBP should always include exploration and practice in collaborating with colleagues to distribute the work that needs to be done, and in sharing the results of the search for evidence with others who could benefit. Fortunately, collaboration is something occupational therapy practitioners are especially comfortable with.

A Curricular Approach

An increasing number of papers, texts, and websites describe the steps of EBP and teach the various skills required to carry out each step (e.g., Law, 2002). The purpose of this chapter is not to duplicate that information, but rather to invite reflection and discussion about how instruction in each of these steps can contribute to the development of effective professional reasoning. Much of this material is based on my experience over the past several years teaching EBP in a variety of formats to hundreds of entry-level students and practitioners.

In the interests of full disclosure, I should reveal my biases up front. (As is typical with biases, my experience has mostly confirmed them.) Here are three beliefs that have shaped my approach to teaching EBP:

- Research suffers from an overly stuffy image. Students need to discover that inquiry into the scientific basis of practice can be dynamic and fun as well as helpful. I often liken the search for evidence to an archeological dig: You *know* there is something of value there, but you're not sure just where it is or what it will look like.
- If the students don't "get it," my instructional scaffold was inadequate. Students need to learn practical techniques to carry out each step of the EBP process and they need to practice them until they can implement them efficiently. The techniques also need to be easily transportable into practice. Instructional activities and assignments should take into account the realities of a practice environment as much as possible to help facilitate this process.
- Students don't need to know everything about research methods and statistics to be effective evidence-based practitioners. It is most important to learn how to find and evaluate the most important elements of a study rather than to learn how to examine every detail exhaustively. In a critical appraisal, thorough examination of the methods, tables, and figures may be more critical than taking apart the researcher's rationale.

The most important point to stress is that EBP is a curricular thread, not just a course. Although an academic course (or sequence of courses) may be used to teach the basic skills, the outcomes of this instruction will be limited if the rest of the curriculum does not support the basic premises and methods of EBP. EBP must be treated as integral to all clinical reasoning, not as a set of rules to be followed in limited circumstances, for example, for one particular assignment. This requirement poses a challenge to both faculty and students. Because EBP is grounded in constant questioning, it is incompatible with instruction that emphasizes "received knowledge" from textbooks. It requires that curricula emphasize assessment and intervention approaches that have the soundest scientific basis, rather than those that may currently have the most adherents in the field. It requires that both students and faculty develop a high tolerance for decision making under uncertainty (Tversky & Kahneman, 1974), as the nature of clinical practice, in which evidence comes in shades of gray and rarely offers clear-cut answers. These are difficult challenges, especially for student practitioners who are anxious to *know* what is good and right to do in practice and for whom the answer "it depends," can feel intolerably vague. Therefore, it is critically important to provide a solid scaffold to support development of EBP as an element of clinical reasoning.

ASKING GOOD QUESTIONS: A CRITICAL ELEMENT OF REFLECTIVE PRACTICE

In everyday life, we applaud those who have the answers, but in EBP one of the most important skills is to ask the right questions. Good questions are like a road map of where we want to go; without them, we are likely to waste time and energy on the wrong route. Good questions come from systematic reflection in practice, in particular reflection about the decisions we need to make. Typically, we receive much more instruction focused on "answers" than on asking good questions. Much of the content we learn is organized around what is generally true of a particular group (for example, people with stroke). However, in practice we must apply this knowledge to an individual situation, which never exactly resembles the typical case examples used for instruction. This translation process is helped if we start by specifying the decisions we need to make and the questions we need to answer to make those decisions.

Practice can be thought of as a series of decisions. What method would be best to gather information about this client? Should I use an alternative method, given his or her (cultural, clinical, age-related) characteristics? What should I do if some of the information I have obtained is contradictory or does not fit into a pattern I have seen before? Given the client's goals and current situation, is intervention A or intervention B the more appropriate choice? What should I do if I have not seen the expected changes from this intervention? Is this the appropriate point to stop intervention, or to switch to another approach? The decision that needs to be made, and its clinical context, dictates the type of evidence we want.

Ideally, when first considering a practice decision, we draw on existing theories, models, and frames of reference as a guide. Our theories and models provide guides for understanding a given practice situation and considering the appropriate options for assessment and intervention. They also provide the basis for the design of intervention and the method and timing of delivery of the intervention. Framing questions at the level of the broader theory or model (e.g., "what is the evidence that sensory integration treatment works?") is not optimal. These questions are too far removed from the situation of an individual client to provide much direction for the practitioner, and are so global as to become easily overwhelming.

As a first step toward a better alternative, it is valuable to have students map out the model of the intervention being considered for a specific client or group of similar clients to look at the causal relationships proposed to exist among the important components of the approach (see Box 13-1 for a sample of a relevant student activity). This process is very similar to developing a "logic model" (as done in program evaluation; Conrad, Randolph, Kirby & Bebout, 1999), or "concept map," as described in tutorials on instruction and critical thinking tutorials (a search on the Internet will turn up a plethora of examples and free programs). The process helps to make our clinical models and hypotheses more explicit. For example, which elements of a given intervention are most important to achieving change (the "active ingredients")? What are the immediate effects expected to be? How will we recognize (measure) these effects? What will the longer-term effects be? How will we recognize (measure) them? What client or contextual factors may moderate the effect of the intervention? What are the intermediate steps in the change process (what does the "input" of the intervention cause to happen, in what sequence)? (For an illustration, see Tickle-Degnen, 1988.)

BOX 13-1
Mapping a Model

---

1. Think of a recent clinical encounter (e.g., a fieldwork experience) or, if not available, use a case example from a text. Use Table 13-1 to formulate an example of each type of question, along with the decision for which one would be seeking information. Prioritize the questions on the basis of immediate need for evidence.
2. Draw a map of the model of enablement/disablement and/or intervention that underlies one of the priority questions. Evaluate the logic of the model, and its consistency with general scientific knowledge.

We can also map our models of the **enablement/disablement** process. What is our model of the client's current condition? What interaction of impairments, person factors, and contextual factors has led to his or her specific limitations in activity and participation? Answering this question may actually require several maps, since the pathways to the different limitations may be different. Why are these maps important? These theories guide practitioners' consideration of particular interventions and expectation of likely outcomes; however, the theories about the relation between impairment and disability are often implicit. The theories must be made *explicit* so that the evidence supporting them we can be evaluated systematically.

We can use both kinds of maps in two important ways to guide professional reasoning. First, we can evaluate whether a model that has been laid out is logically coherent and consistent with general knowledge. For example, is it reasonable to expect that a half-hour practice session with the therapist will have widespread impact on the client's skill development? Is that *consistent* with what we know about the relation between practice and skill? Is it *logical* that fine motor coordination problems will have a direct impact on an elementary school child's friendships, apart from the child's personality, instruction, and community opportunities? Is such a model consistent with what is known about children's peer relationships? This kind of mapping and reflective analysis is an important part of professional reasoning, whether in school or in clinical practice. If the disablement or intervention model doesn't make sense and doesn't fit with what we know, then we must modify our model.

Second, once a map has been created, it is much easier to see what kind of evidence would be relevant to validate (or disconfirm) each aspect of the model. For example, although there may be limited research that has investigated an intervention approach, there may be studies that have investigated one or more of the elements or "ingredients" of the intervention. The results of these studies could provide either positive or negative evidence about this element of the model. As another example, even if studies have not examined longer-term outcomes of the intervention, studies of short-term outcomes provide some indication of whether changes in the direction expected are seen or not. Finally, examining the hypothesized relations between the steps in the change process will clarify what types of research studies would provide appropriate tests of each step. For example, if a model hypothesizes that engagement in meaningful occupation improves perceived quality of life because it improves positive mood, then we would look for studies showing that engagement in occupation is associated with an immediate increase in positive mood, and that this increase is related to improved quality of life over time (*Figure 13-1*).

As described, mapping of models helps to clarify the kind of evidence that might be relevant, for example, if one is trying to decide whether to adopt a

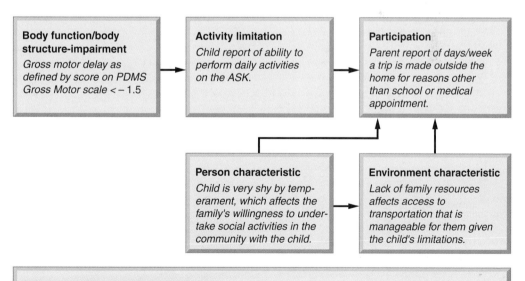

Figure 13-1   An example of a simple disablement model. The information in italics provides possible operational definitions or descriptions of that factor. (PDMS = Peabody Developmental Motor Scales)

TABLE 13-1

A Guide to Focusing Your Clinical Questions

	Person	Intervention (or Issue)	Comparison Intervention (if necessary or appropriate)	Outcomes
Tips for building	*Ask:* "How would I describe a group of clients similar to mine?"	*Ask:* Which main intervention (or assessment or predictive variable) am I considering?	*Ask:* What is the main alternative to compare with the intervention (or assessment)?	*Ask:* What do I hope to accomplish, what do I need to know, or what kind of change do I want from the intervention?
Example 1: Defining the problem	"In kindergarten-age children who participate in population-wide screening programs . . ."	". . . does the First Step . . ."	". . . compared with the Denver II . . ."	". . . more accurately identify children who are diagnosed with learning disabilities later in elementary school?"
Example 2: Predicting outcomes	"In persons who experience their first episode of schizophrenia before age 18 . . ."	"does prior level of academic and social functioning . . ."		". . . predict likelihood of sustained employment at age 21?"
Example 3: Intervention	"In ambulatory 6- to 8-year-old children with mild to moderate cerebral palsy . . ."	". . . does weekly functionally focused movement intervention"	". . . compared to standard neurodevelopmental treatment intervention . . ."	". . . result in greater gains in functional movement activity performance?"

Used with the permission of Wendy J. Coster.

particular intervention approach. It also helps to formulate more precise EBP questions because it forces one to define precisely what the intervention is and what the expected outcomes are. This specificity, in turn, supports application of the **PICO** (Person, Intervention, Comparison, Outcome) template for question formulation recommended in EBP texts and tutorials and illustrated in *Table 13-1*.

Another prompt that may be helpful for generating questions is given in *Table 13-2*. This chart (loosely based on material from Sackett et al. (2000)) illustrates different types of questions that may arise in occupational therapy practice for which we might be seeking evidence. The sample questions have been formulated using the PICO template.

TABLE 13-2

Types of Questions

Broad Focus	Specific Focus	Examples of Questions
Defining or describing a clinical problem	*Prevalence/presentation* How often and when does a particular clinical disorder or impairment cause the profile I see in my client?	(Broad) What is the prevalence of substance abuse in adolescents with disabilities? (Focused) Are adolescents (13-18) with ADHD more likely to use illegal drugs than adolescents without ADHD?
	Clinical assessment What is/are the best (most reliable, valid) way(s) to gather and interpret information about my client's concerns, strengths, and difficulties?	(Broad) Which developmental screening tests are the most accurate to identify young children with mild to moderate motor or cognitive delays? (Focused) For this 3-year-old who has scored in the "typical" range on the Denver II, what is the likelihood that further testing would identify mild to moderate cognitive difficulties?
	Causes What is/are likely causes of the problem my client is having? Of the possible causes of my client's difficulty, which are those that are most likely? Which methods are most accurate in distinguishing between possible causes of this problem?	(Broad) What is the best method to determine whether a child's difficulty completing daily tasks is due to cognitive rather than coordination deficits? (Focused) For this 3-year-old with Down syndrome, would the Vineland ABS scores clarify the extent to which communication delays are limiting social interactions?

(continued)

TABLE 13-2 (continued)

Broad Focus	Specific Focus	Examples of Questions
Effectiveness of interventions	*Therapy* Of the available intervention options, which do more good than harm and therefore are worth the effort and cost? Are there specific factors that identify those most likely to benefit from the intervention?	(Broad) Is peer-mediated social skills intervention effective for increasing social initiations by young children with autism/PDD? (Focused) For young children (age 2-3) with severe mobility limitations, does provision of powered mobility result in more self-initiated interactions with peers?
	Prevention Can the chance of future problems be modified by a particular intervention directed at one or more risk factors?	(Broad) Does participation in community programs by preschool-age children with disabilities increase their likelihood of having sustained friendships during elementary school? (Focused) For this 75-year-old woman with osteoporosis, would participation in the Fit for Life program reduce her risk for falls in the next year?
Understanding the client	*Experience and meaning* Which methods are best for understanding my client's experience? How does the client's understanding or meaning influence participation and outcome?	(Broad) What are the most common concerns of families of young children with cerebral palsy? (Focused) Does use of the COPM to establish goals with families of young children with motor disabilities result in greater client satisfaction with services compared to use of a standard problem checklist?

Used with permission of Wendy J. Coster. ADHD = attention-deficit hyperactivity disorder.

SEARCHING FOR EVIDENCE

Electronic access to information has made it increasingly easy to locate research evidence, even for practitioners who don't have immediate access to a university library. However, the internet has also made it more difficult sometimes to distinguish between true scientific evidence and popular sources of information that may be based more on testimonial, opinion, or unsystematic synthesis of findings. Thus, before we send students or practitioners to search for evidence, some evaluation or discussion of what is encompassed by the term *evidence* is in order, as well as an examination of the various sources of information, their strengths and limitations.

This is a point at which it is especially critical for all participants in the educational program (whether academic faculty or practitioner supervisors) to be in agreement and consistent with one another. If students are learning (or have learned) about doing systematic searches of the literature in their EBP course, but faculty in other courses give assignments that simply require them to "find a research article" on a given topic, then the curriculum is not supporting the application of EBP. The definition of "evidence" and what type of information is acceptable to present when students are asked to present evidence will need to be consistent across all participants in the curriculum.

In this regard, it is a good idea to emphasize that a systematic search for, and consideration of, evidence includes negative as well as positive evidence (Box 13-2 shows a sample of a relevant student activity). In other words, the search for evidence must be unbiased by the searcher's preferences for a particular theory, frame of reference, or method. This requirement can be difficult for novices to uphold because they may be especially anxious to find information that validates their professional choice and their current textbooks. It can also be difficult for experienced practitioners who may become defensive in the face of challenges to methods that have been integral to their practice. For these reasons, specific activities may need to be designed to ensure that negative evidence is included in instruction and that discussion of this evidence includes attention to emotional reactions and consideration of ethical and constructive responses to it.

BOX 13-2

Balancing Positive and Negative Evidence

1. Read two reports on the same intervention, one positive and one negative or critical of the intervention. Discuss whether the authors of the positive report have addressed the questions or shortcomings identified in the negative report or, if not, what would be required to do so.
2. Evaluate the strength of the negative evidence, and how it should be incorporated into an overall evaluation of the intervention's effectiveness.

   Suggested topics: constraint-induced movement therapy; neurodevelopmental treatment (NDT) for children with cerebral palsy; fall prevention programs for the elderly.

APPRAISING EVIDENCE: DECISION MAKING UNDER UNCERTAINTY

The standard approach to appraising research evidence is to critique every element of the study. This leads to a thorough, but very generic, critique, because it is undertaken as a relatively abstract enterprise. After completing such a critique, the reader may come away with a comprehensive list of the strengths and weaknesses of the study, but little sense of how to apply the findings. The final evaluation of the study may be based on a "box score" summary: If the strengths "outscore" the weaknesses, the study is deemed useful. The extreme form of this approach is to dismiss research that doesn't meet the most rigorous criteria for sound design (i.e., is not a **randomized clinical trial,** in the case of intervention studies). However, the requirement for EBP is to use the *current best evidence*, which does not provide an escape clause if we do not find evidence from ideal studies.

It is actually relatively easy to identify shortcomings in a research report. In its simplest form, this involves matching the features of the study against a checklist of desirable features, often described under the term "controls." If the appropriate control does not appear to be in place, we put an "X" in the corresponding space: A **threat to validity** has been identified. Unfortunately, this approach often leaves the students with a sense of "so what?" A sound EBP appraisal goes beyond identifying that a potential threat *exists* to evaluate whether or not this threat may have a significant impact on interpretation and application of the findings to the clinical question. In other words, a "threat" may or may not be a "problem," depending on the question that prompted the original search for evidence.

When we are appraising evidence for possible application to a specific clinical context, the threats must be considered in relation to that context (Boxes 13-3 and 13-4 show samples of relevant student activities). For example, if a study used a sample with limited racial or ethnic diversity, it is standard to critique that study because of uncertain application to the general population. However, if the client population of the reader matches that of the study sample, then this limitation to generalization does not really apply; that is, it is not a problem. Because it is rare that any study precisely matches one's own client population or practice setting, students need to become skilled at thinking through the implications of differences to judge the validity of the evidence for their current purpose. See *Figure 13-2* for a sample evaluation form.

BOX 13-3

Can This Evidence Be Applied?

For each of the following situations, think through whether or not you would apply the evidence to the given clinical scenario and why. Discuss your conclusions with a partner to see if you agree.

Example 1: The sample in the study consisted of 12 classes of first-grade students, randomly selected from a large urban school system in New England (no more than one class from each school); classes were randomly selected to receive one of two different handwriting instruction methods (new method versus standard methods).

Your clients are kindergarten and first-grade classes in a rural elementary school in New Mexico.

Can/should you generalize the findings? What specific factors would you weigh?

Example 2: The sample in the study was a convenience sample of 30 older women (mean age = 72.4) living in a supported housing facility in Boston (criteria for entrance = low-income; walking—with or without devices) who participated in a structured strengthening program.

Your clients are a group of older women (mean age = 70), ambulatory with a cane or walker, who are recovering from surgery or illness that caused general loss of strength from immobility.

Can/should you generalize the findings? What specific factors would you weigh?

BOX 13-4

Appraising the Evidence

Select a study with an intervention and sample that you are familiar with. Formulate a PICO question that the study addresses. Next, conduct a standard appraisal of the validity of the study. For each validity issue or limitation you identified, evaluate *how* that feature may have affected the outcome of the study and *how* the feature will affect your use of the evidence.

Internal Validity		Potential Impact
Was the assignment of persons to treatments randomized? Were the groups similar at the start of the intervention period?	Y N	
Were all participants who entered the trial accounted for at its conclusion (i.e., is there a problem with attrition)?	Y N	
Were participants and clinicians kept "blind" to which intervention was being received?	Y N	
Aside from the experimental intervention, were the groups treated equally?	Y N	
Was an appropriate form of the intervention applied (i.e., was it carried out for the appropriate period of time, by appropriately trained people)?	Y N	
Were appropriate controls in place to assure the intervention was carried out as intended (fidelity)?	Y N	
Were the outcome measures used reliable and valid for this purpose and population?	Y N	
External Validity		**Potential Impact**
Were the selection criteria and process described clearly enough so that you know who was included in the study?	Y N	
Was the sample described in detail, e.g., by providing a table of relevant demographic characteristics?	Y N	

Figure 13-2a

Was there an investigation of whether subjects who differed in certain characteristics responded differently to the intervention?	Y N	
Does the sample include a sufficient number of subjects who are similar to those in your question to warrant applying these results?	Y N	
Statistical Validity		
Was a justification for the sample size provided (e.g., was a power analysis reported)?	Y N	
Were appropriate descriptive statistics (e.g., mean, SD, range) provided?	Y N	
If data were manipulated before subjecting them to analysis (e.g., creating composite variables, transforming a continuous outcome measure into categories), is what was done clearly described and is there adequate justification for these procedures?	Y N	
Were the methods of statistical analysis appropriate for these kinds of data?	Y N	
If there were multiple outcomes or if multiple analyses were done, was that taken into account for the statistical analysis (e.g., by adjusting the P-value)?	Y N	

Figure 13-2b Guiding questions for appraisal of intervention evidence. These questions can help students examine the internal, external, and statistical validity of intervention studies. Note that not all questions apply to every study, and there may be other relevant issues for certain studies that are not included in this list. This template can be used to prepare the information needed for the appraisal section of a critically appraised topic (CAT).

Using Clinical Understanding as Part of the Appraisal Process

Much of this discussion has focused on how consideration of scientific evidence contributes to clinical understanding. However, the converse is also true: it is important to apply one's clinical knowledge when appraising research. Interactions with clients, familiarity with clinical disorders, and experience with intervention and the service delivery context provide practitioners with important information with which to evaluate the features of a study. We also may have first-hand experience with the measures used to evaluate client outcomes. This clinical knowledge can raise important questions about the evidence we review.

For example: "My clients have trouble understanding the questions on that assessment. Did the researchers verify that their subjects were interpreting the questions accurately?" Or, "I can't believe that they got subjects to complete a one-hour testing session so soon after their brain injury. Did they check to see if the subjects were really attending throughout that time?" Or, "The authors have mixed children with cerebral palsy, children with muscular dystrophy, and children with juvenile rheumatoid arthritis in their sample just because they all have 'physical disabilities,' but the causes and consequences of those disorders are so different. I wonder if that's why they didn't find anything conclusive in their comparison with typically developing children. They gave means and standard deviations for each subgroup; let me calculate effect sizes as a check."

What About Those Levels of Evidence?

The reader should not conclude that there is no role for the levels of evidence approach for classifying designs. **Levels of evidence,** whether Sackett et al.'s (2000) or other similar classification schemes, are a useful rubric for classifying available research according to the type of design that was used, and provide a global guide to appropriate interpretation of findings. If one is fortunate enough to find multiple studies addressing an intervention question, clearly those with the strongest designs should get our immediate attention. However, it does not follow that studies with weaker designs have nothing valuable to offer. Sometimes the question addressed in a less well-controlled study, or one with a smaller sample, is closer to the question that prompted the inquiry or has other features (such as the sample composition) that make it more applicable to the current situation. In this case, those studies may provide the "best evidence."

Appraisal as Scholarly Dialogue

The perspective I advocate is that appraisal is a scholarly dialogue between the practitioner and the evidence. A dialogue implies exchange of information that is cumulative over time, in which the goal is increased understanding, but not necessarily complete agreement. From this perspective, research is not a set of artifacts, frozen in stone, but something more dynamic, which one can explore multiple times and perhaps argue with. We are not bound to interpret findings exactly as the authors did, and we can even calculate additional statistics (such as effect sizes) to look at the data in a different way. We can raise questions based on our own knowledge and experience. The evidence can also oblige us to consider questions that challenge our current understanding, to revise our models of change, or even to revise our methods.

Literature from other disciplines is especially valuable for encouraging this dialogue. It is essential for students to become aware of and comfortable exploring the literatures of other disciplines if they are to be truly evidence-based practitioners. This literature does not come couched in familiar terminology, however, and often addresses issues relevant to occupational therapy from a completely different theoretical perspective. Going to that literature with a specific question in mind provides a road map for the unfamiliar territory because the searcher knows specifically what he or she is looking for (provided a good PICO question has been constructed). Many of the potential "active ingredients" that are part of occupational therapy interventions have been studied by other disciplines, such as supportive therapeutic relationships (Cruz & Pincus, 2002), caregiver education (Kalra, Evans, Perez, Melbourn, Patel, Knapp & Donaldson, 2004), elements of successful supported employment (Twamley, Jeste & Lehman, 2003). This literature provides another powerful source of evidence, provided that students are prepared to engage with it.

One strategy I have used is to model the process of "unpacking" an unfamiliar research report. I select an article in a completely unfamiliar area of rehabilitation-relevant research (kinematic studies from movement sciences work well for me) and, with the students, set out to try to understand what was done, what the results mean, and their implications. This format enables the experienced reader to share various strategies he or she has developed over time, many of which are not particularly obvious to the novice. For example, novices may read the abstract, but not think to use it actively to create an outline of the main features of the study. The outline, in turn, helps to identify a set of questions for which further information will be sought by reading the rest of the paper: Why was this study important? How was this study different from what had been done before? What made them choose those particular methods, and what kind of data do those methods yield? As they go through the rest of the article, the instructor-guide can also help keep students focused on identifying the key information and avoid getting stuck on unfamiliar technical details.

Constructing a map of the research design is another strategy used to help understand what was done in a research study, particularly one that has a complex, or less familiar design. I introduce students to my own modified version of **research notation** and illustrate how this shorthand can be used to translate a text description of randomization processes, multiple measurement points, etc., into a more digestible form. My modifications include adding details such as the number of participants in each group, the time points when measurement was done, and perhaps the names of the measures so that my map gives me a more complete picture of the essential features of the study (*Figure 13-3* for an example).

Working openly with unfamiliar material also gives the instructor an opportunity to model acceptance of uncertainty and ignorance. It can be extremely valuable for students to hear "You know, I really can't figure this part out, and it seems pretty important, so I would probably go ask Professor Smith for help because she's an expert in this area," or to brainstorm with students about other sources where one might look for clarification. This is also an excellent context to talk with students about the peer-review process, to point out the value of certain elements of a good report (i.e., one that helps even a relative novice to understand key points), and to share frustration over authors who don't communicate clearly or who leave out important details. Students often assume that if they cannot understand something in a research article, it is because they are ignorant rather than that the authors have failed to write clearly.

Perhaps the hardest part of the appraisal process is one that is not mentioned nearly as often, which is resisting the temptation of our biases. We want to find evidence that occupational therapy is effective and supports our theoretical models, and it is hard not to let those preferences color our consideration of the evidence. This point was addressed earlier when the importance of searching for negative—and positive—evidence was stressed. However, there are other ways in which our biases slip in. As acknowledged, relatively few of our intervention studies have been true randomized clinical trials. Many of our research findings are derived, instead, from studies that

Standard Notation Format

R = random assignment to groups

- - - - = non-random assignment

X = intervention

O = observation

Modified Notation Applied to Outline a Study Design

$R_{n=31}$ O	X_1 — clinic only	?	?	O_{28}
$R_{n=22}$ O	X_2 — home only	?	?	O_{20}
$R_{n=25}$ O	$X_{1,2}$ — home + clinic	?	?	O_{25}
Baseline		12 wk	24 wk	1 yr

Interpretation of the Study Design

68 participants were randomized into three intervention groups:
1 = clinic program only
2 = home program only
1, 2 = clinic + home program

Participants were assessed at baseline, before beginning their intervention. The paper reports they were seen again at 12 weeks and 24 weeks; however, no results from these assessments are reported. Participants were assessed again 1 year after the end of intervention. The results from these assessments were compared and reported in the article.

At 1 year, three participants from group 1, two from group 2, and none from group 1, 2 were missing from follow-up assessment.

Figure 13-3 Mapping a research design.

examine the *associations* among variables, not the *causal relations* between them. However much we might wish to, we cannot interpret a study, finding a positive relation between amount of occupational therapy and functional status at discharge from rehabilitation as establishing that more OT caused greater improvements. The greater our investment in a particular theory or method, the greater is the temptation to go beyond the data and to view the results in a way that best confirms our beliefs.

Complex or unfamiliar statistical methods in a research report may make it easier to succumb to these biases. With methods such as regression analysis, structural equation modeling, or hierarchical linear modeling, even the researchers slip into causal-sounding language with such phrases as "the effect of X on Y" to describe regression results. Thus, students need to be reminded over and over again, through practice with relevant research examples, that the research *design* dictates the appropriate inferences that can be drawn from the data, not the statistical analysis used (Box 13-5).

BOX 13-5

Reference Materials

Ensuring access to good practical reference materials on statistics is one way to help students appraise studies that use less familiar methods. Two very useful books for this purpose are:

Grimm, L. G. & Yarnold, P. R. (1995). *Reading and understanding multivariate statistics*. Washington, DC: American Psychological Association.
Grimm, L. G. & Yarnold, P. R. (2000). *Reading and understanding more multivariate statistics*. Washington, DC: American Psychological Association.

Although the discussion in this section has focused primarily on appraisal of the research evidence, this focus should be balanced by explorations of the susceptibility of clinical observation to bias as well. There is a significant, growing literature on cognitive, motivational, and social biases in human information processing that bears on this issue. One very accessible introduction to this literature is a review by Huebner and Emery (1998) examining a controversial intervention-facilitated communication. The paper introduces some of the literature on sources of erroneous belief and how these biases may lead to belief in the effects of an intervention despite lack of scientific support.

SYNTHESIS: ORGANIZING COMPLEXITY

One of the more valuable features of Sackett and colleagues' approach to appraising evidence is their emphasis on deriving the **clinical bottom line**. Thus, after the appraisal is done, one must finally come to the point of deciding what is the best answer to the question that was originally posed and what clinical decision should be recommended. This component is what differentiates the EBP approach to the research literature from the more traditional study critiques, which included no requirement to address the "so what?" question with regard to practice. Deriving the clinical bottom line is the point at which students come to grips with the complexities of practice and the need to make decisions under uncertainty. Thus, it is an incredibly important context for developing clinical reasoning, and, for that reason, it is especially important to have effective scaffolding to support students to manage this complexity successfully.

A variety of methods have emerged from EBP that we have found helpful in our instruction. One of the very best is the **critically appraised topic***, or CAT,

---

*Note that CAT, the term used by Sackett and colleagues (2000), is frequently applied to a summary of a single study. However, AOTA now uses the term CAP (critically appraised paper) for single papers, and reserves CAT for summaries of multiple studies. Because much of the material in this chapter references Sackett et al., their broader definition is used.

format. The CAT is a structured, brief summary of evidence on a specific question that includes the clinical bottom line derived from the appraisal (Fetters, Figueiredo, Keane-Miller, McSweeney & Tsao, 2004). The format was designed to support easy, quick access to the relevant information by practitioners; hence it is both concise and informative. We teach students to use the CAT format to report their appraisal results for single studies; they find it straightforward to learn and highly useful. Thus, the CAT provides one piece of the scaffolding to help students begin to manage information from research.

Typically, however, the best answer to a clinical question is derived from a synthesis of multiple studies. Although the first step in the learning process may be to have students complete a CAT on each relevant study, they need additional strategies to help them integrate all of the results. Thus, the next step we have them complete is a summary table, in which key elements of each study (e.g., subjects, design, procedure, results, other relevant factors) are entered (in brief, bulleted-list format) so that they can be compared more readily. Although this process may sound straightforward, selection of which information should be entered in each column requires students to reconsider the key elements that will affect their overall interpretation (and application) of results. Published critical reviews and meta-analyses provide examples of summary tables.

Even with an excellent summary table, however, the overall clinical bottom line does not make itself crystal clear. Sometimes, a student's first reaction to the table is to become overwhelmed by the differences across the studies and not to see the common threads. This is probably the point at which effective supports are most important to help them achieve a true, balanced synthesis. In my experience, collaborative practice in a group on several examples is far more effective to move this process forward than sending students off on their own immediately.

It can be helpful to start by revisiting the clinical decision that led to the question initially. What are the alternatives the practitioner faces? Is there an option to do nothing, and if so, what is the potential for harm? What is the potential for harm if one makes the wrong choice among the alternatives being considered? Reconsideration of the options and their potential consequences at this point brings up discussion of issues such as cost (human and financial) and ensures that students are focused on the ultimate goal for the client as they approach the evidence.

Next, it is useful to consider what the conclusions (bottom lines) were from each separate study, while looking for common themes. This approach can be especially valuable when the studies that were located seem very different from one another in terms of subjects, or specific details of the intervention, or the outcome measures used. As an example, a group of students investigated the effect of seating devices on functional performance of manipulative tasks by children with cerebral palsy. They found a small number of studies, each of which had used a different device and none of which produced consistent effects across all children. The students focused on the differences across studies, but during our discussion we identified a common thread: Although no device produced improvement for all children, each device demonstrated positive impact for certain students. In fact, several of the authors noted that the match between student profiles of physical functioning and device seemed to be a key factor in the results obtained. We then focused on the implications of this conclusion for practice. Is there a valid reason to think that developing modified seating for a child with cerebral palsy might improve task performance? Yes, there *is* some evidence that seating devices can improve functional performance of manipulative tasks for at least some children with cerebral palsy. Should we recommend the same seating device for all children with cerebral palsy? No, currently available evidence does *not* support use of a single device with all children. The evidence that exists suggests that positive impact depends on the individual match between student needs and device design.

In the context of helping students to frame clinical bottom lines, I have found it helpful to use the concepts of "confidence intervals" and "boundaries." Like the results of a statistical analysis, appraisal conclusions always should be thought of as having a degree of uncertainty. If we have found strong, clear evidence, then the confidence intervals we need to set around our conclusions are smaller. That is, we are relatively sure that our answer is correct. If the evidence is limited or if the studies have significant limitations, then our confidence intervals are wider. That is, we may have a general sense of an answer, but there is great room for variation from that answer. Thus, part of our work in constructing a synthesis is to define the "boundaries" around our answer. These boundaries, of course, reflect the results of our appraisal: the uncertainty introduced by small samples, or less well-controlled designs, limitations in the outcome measures used, or limits to generalization because of differences in age, clinical characteristics, etc.

Identification of the boundaries leads the discussion into consideration of the final major element of the synthesis, which is consideration of additional factors that are relevant to the clinical decision. Up to this point, our discussion of the appraisal and synthesis process has focused on the first component of the definition of EBP: the best available scientific evidence. Two additional elements need to be integrated into the discussion: clinical expertise and the client's values and preferences. The importance of clinical expertise was addressed earlier in the context of appraisal of individual research studies. At the synthesis stage, clinical expertise helps address issues such as the practicality of implementing the intervention in a manner that preserves its key components and the clinical relevance of the degree or type of improvement reported in the research. Clinical expertise may also provide some preliminary evaluation of the likely acceptability of the proposed intervention to one's clients.

Ultimately, however, the client's preferences and values determine whether or not the intervention with the "best evidence" is the one that will be best for the client. This evaluation can be made only in collaboration with the client, as discussed in more detail below. However, an instructional context (even without a client present) can be used effectively to prepare students for this element. What if the client rejects the intervention option that the research evidence supports most strongly? What if it requires a commitment of time, energy, or financial resources that the client doesn't have? True client-centered occupational therapy requires that we respect the client's decision; however, this poses a challenge: How can I be an evidence-based practitioner if the client does not accept my evidence-based recommendation?

Linda Tickle-Degnen (1998a,b, 2000, 2002) has written several valuable papers on communicating about evidence with clients. The important point she stresses is to enable the client to make an *informed* decision. Our task is to present the available evidence about why we are recommending a particular option to the client and what is reasonable to expect as an outcome from that intervention (both benefits and problems that might result). If there is more than one reasonable option for addressing a particular problem (i.e., two options that each have some evidence to support them), then we need to be knowledgeable about both options. The critical point is that we need to inform the client so that he or she can participate in the decision making as a true partner with the practitioner.

This point raises important issues around ethics in clinical decision making, which also need to be addressed during discussions of evidence and the application of evidence (Box 13-6). What does the ethical practitioner do if there is no clear scientific support for a preferred intervention approach? Is the situation different if there is *no* evidence (i.e., an absence of research altogether) rather than negative evidence (i.e., evidence that the intervention yields no significant improvement)? What if the client insists on an intervention that has little to no research support? What if the most effective intervention method (according to the evidence) is one that the practitioner has not been trained in or that is provided by another professional? These discussions can evoke powerful emotions and reveal biases that continue to operate outside of consciousness, such as the belief that doing something is better than doing nothing, or that clinical experience should always trump research ("I know the study results were negative, but I've seen results in my clients"). Classroom discussions of these issues help introduce strategies for responding to these situations so that students or practitioners are better prepared when the issues arise in practice.

BOX 13-6
Ethics and Evidence

Faculty responses to student questions about conflicts between evidence and clinical practice are crucial for influencing how learners will implement EBP. When controversial discussions about evidence versus experience occur, it is important to help students identify ethical responses.

An example of a possible strategy is to negotiate a trial period of the controversial intervention with the client that is set up like a single-case study so that the effects can be monitored. If, after an appropriate interval (established a priori) an expected degree of improvement (also established a priori) has not been achieved, then the practitioner and client agree that they will stop that intervention and negotiate a different approach. Sometimes the research evidence can provide some guidelines in this situation, such as when a study may identify a time point by which those participants who did have a positive outcome had begun to show improvement (for a more detailed discussion see Backman & Harris, 1999).

Faculty should be prepared that these discussions around evidence and ethics may lead students to question why certain assessment or intervention approaches are being taught in their professional curriculum, given the status of the evidence about them. Faculty response to this challenge is critical in determining whether students will continue to incorporate an EBP approach into their clinical reasoning or not. If student questioning is viewed as problematic or distracting in the context of "clinical" courses, then students are likely to abandon the demands and uncertainties of EBP in favor of the greater apparent certainty of established methods.

It may be helpful to view these challenges as an expression of students' anxiety about becoming practitioners. They want to be the best practitioners they can be, and now they are confronted with what seem to be irreconcilable definitions of what that means. From an EBP standpoint, they draw the conclusion that many accepted practices have not been supported by research and thus may not constitute best practice. Then, their texts or discussions with experienced practitioners contradict this conclusion. Who are they to believe? What are they to do? If they don't use the standard approaches, what WILL they do in practice?

Students often tend to view these contradictions in stark, either-or terms. It is up to the faculty to help them reason through these apparent contradictions and come to a solution that is acceptable. They need help to create an understanding of practice that is built on evidence, but that does not leave them paralyzed when the evidence is uncertain or the better alternative isn't clear. They need to develop a set of strategies they can apply when they need to make a practice decision under uncertain conditions so that they do not opt for the familiar just because it is easier. Learning this kind of reasoning is a recursive process because the knowledge and skills required need to be revisited over time in multiple contexts for them to become well established. Thus, this is one more place where the commitment of the faculty as a whole to the EBP approach is critical for success.

COMMUNICATING ABOUT EVIDENCE

As noted, from its beginning EBP has stressed communication with clients and with colleagues. Effective communication with different potential users of evidence requires skill translating the evidence into the language that is most clear and appropriate for the particular group. This can be difficult to do "on one's feet" without prior practice, so it is useful to incorporate this requirement in EBP assignments.

For example, after students have identified the clinical bottom line for a CAT, ask them to summarize the results in language appropriate for a clinical audience of colleagues, and then again in language appropriate for clients. The same could be done with the "boundaries." Students need to reflect on what they know about the context and about the recipients of the information and make appropriate choices of language and emphasis. (See Tickle-Degnen, 2002, for an excellent discussion and examples.)

Communication is one essential component of a larger process of collaboration that provides a foundation for EBP. Consistent application of an EBP approach is supported when a professional community shares resources and workload to enable best practice. The potential evidence base is already vast and is increasing daily. Time is limited, which makes it impossible for a single practitioner to examine the evidence on all the questions she or he may formulate during practice. Nor is it necessarily beneficial for each practitioner to work solo, since such an approach can leave one open to influence by personal biases. Although each client's situation is unique, there are also many common questions that arise among practitioners and it is inefficient for each to search for evidence individually. Thus, an additional skill that students need to learn is how to think creatively about distributing the effort of searching for and appraising evidence, and how to disseminate the results of their work to others who could benefit.

Students learning EBP have already benefited from the collective efforts of others if they have used materials such as *OTSeeker*, or AOTA's *Evidence Briefs*, or if they have accessed any of the myriad tutorials and evidence reviews that are on the web. It is important for them to see themselves as part of this larger professional community and to make contributions to it. This may require a shift in attitude because students are used to thinking of things like course assignments as a private enterprise, that is, one dedicated to their own learning. However, given the opportunity, our students have always been pleased when an assignment in which they have invested a lot of time has some value beyond the classroom. Thus, from the start, we try to identify situations in which information generated in the context of an EBP course or assignment can be shared with the professional community. For example, we have disseminated a student-compiled annotated list of internet resources through our program newsletter for fieldwork supervisors; we had students share the results of their evidence searches with faculty who teach content related to the questions posed; and we had students prepare an EBP notebook with course handouts and readings they could share with others at their Level II Fieldwork site (see Coster & Schwartz, 2004, for additional discussion).

SUMMARY

This chapter advocates for including search, appraisal, and application of scientific evidence as a thread throughout the occupational therapy curriculum. The habits of thinking stimulated by the appraisal of evidence in relation to clinical questions enrich and support sound clinical decision making. Far from replacing clinical expertise, EBP engages that expertise, along with knowledge about research, to provide optimal appraisal of the quality of evidence and its application in a given clinical situation. When applied appropriately, EBP fundamentally supports our philosophy of client-centered practice. By insisting that the client be informed about his or her options and the best available evidence on them, the client is engaged as a full partner in decisions about which path to pursue toward his or her goals. Finally, preparing students to be questioners and active seekers of information is an important way to develop the involvement in lifelong learning that will keep them—and the profession—healthy and growing.

LEARNING ACTIVITY 13-1

EBP and Curriculum Planning
Barbara A. Boyt Schell

Purpose

The purpose of this activity is to help learners consider how to build curricular models that incorporate evidence-based practice.

Connections to Major Clinical Reasoning Constructs

Requires learners to make use of information provided in previous chapters on learning as well as curricular approaches used in this chapter to promote evidence-based practice.

Directions for Learners

1 Select a curriculum that you are interested in evaluating in terms of how well evidence-based approaches are being taught.

2 Based on the information provided in Chapter 13, assess the following:

- Is there attention to evidence-based practice in the curriculum?
- Is there attention to EBP across courses in the curriculum?
- How are learning strategies introduced?
- How are they contextualized within real-life demands of practice?
- What, if any, changes should be considered to improve student ability to engage in EPB?

REFERENCES

American Occupational Therapy Association. (1998). ACOTE standards for an accredited educational program for the occupational therapist. Bethesda, MD: AOTA.

Backman C. L. & Harris S. R. (1999). Case studies, single-subject research, and N of 1 randomized trials: comparisons and contrasts. *American Journal of Physical Medicine & Rehabilitation*, 78(2), 170–176.

Conrad, K. J., Randolph, R. L., Kirby, M. W. & Bebout, R. R. (1999). Creating and using logic models: four perspectives. *Alcoholism Treatment Quarterly*, 17(1/2), 17–31.

Coster, W. & Schwarz, L. (June, 2004). Facilitating transfer of evidence-based practice into practice. *Education Special Interest Section Quarterly*, 14(2), 1–3.

Cruz, M. & Pincus, H. A. (2002). Research on the influence that communication in psychiatric encounters has on treatment. *Psychiatric Services*, 53, 1253–1265.

Dysart, A. M. & Tomlin, G. S. (2002). Factors related to evidence-based practice among U.S. occupational therapy clinicians. *American Journal of Occupational Therapy*, 56, 275–284.

Huebner, R. A. & Emery, L. J. (1998). Social psychological analysis of facilitated communication: implications for education. *Mental Retardation*, 36, 259–268.

Fetters, L., Figuieredo, E., Keane-Miller, D., McSweeney, D. & Tsao, C. C. (2004) Critically appraised topics (CATS). *Pediatric Physical Therapy*, 16, 19–21.

Kalra, L., Evans, A., Perez, I., Melbourn, A., Patel, A., Knapp, M. & Donaldson, N. (2004). Training careers of stroke patients: randomized controlled trial. *British Medical Journal*, 328, 1099–2004.

Law, M. (Ed.) (2002). *Evidence-based rehabilitation: A guide to practice*. Thorofare, NJ: Slack.

Sackett, D. L., Straus, S. E., Richardson, W. S., Rosenberg, W. & Haynes, R. B. (2000). *Evidence-based medicine* (2nd ed.). Edinburgh: Churchill Livingstone.

Strauss, S. E., Richardson, W. S., Glasziou, P. & Haynes, R. B. (2005). *Evidence-based medicine* (3rd ed.). Edinburgh: Churchill Livingstone.

Tickle-Degnen, L. (2002). Communicating evidence to clients, managers, and funders. In M. Law (Ed.), *Evidence-based rehabilitation: A guide to practice* (pp. 221–254). Thorofare, NJ: Slack.

Tickle-Degnen, L. (2000). Evidence-based practice forum: Communicating with clients, family members, and colleagues about research evidence. *American Journal of Occupational Therapy*, 54, 341–343.

Tickle-Degnen, L. (1998a). Communicating with patients about treatment outcomes: The use of meta-analytic evidence in collaborative treatment planning. *American Journal of Occupational Therapy*, 52, 526–530.

Tickle-Degnen, L. (1998b). Using research evidence in planning treatment for the individual client. *Canadian Journal of Occupational Therapy*, 65, 152–159.

Tickle-Degnen, L. (1988). Perspectives on the status of sensory integration theory. *American Journal of Occupational Therapy*, 42, 427–433.

Tversky, A. & Kahneman, D. (1974). Judgment under uncertainty: Heuristic and biases. *Science*, 185, 1124–1131.

Twamley, E. W., Jeste, D. V. & Lehman, A. F. (2003). Vocational rehabilitation in schizophrenia and other psychotic disorders. *Journal of Nervous & Mental Disease*, 191, 515–523.

Facilitating Clinical Reasoning in Fieldwork

The Relational Context of the Supervisor and Student

Ruth S. Farber and Kristie P. Koenig

CHAPTER OUTLINE

Theoretical and empirical background
  OT fieldwork: Learning in context
  Supervisory relational context
  Information processing and problem solving
Supervisory reasoning and problem solving
  Development of supervisory reasoning
  constructs
  Problem elements and problem naming
  Problem naming and problem solving
  Reflection: Supervisor's expectations and
  supervisory role schemata

Facilitating clinical reasoning in fieldwork
  Developmental aspects of teaching clinical
  reasoning
  Clinical reasoning emerging within the
  supervisory relationship
**The relationship of affect and clinical
reasoning in supervision: Importance
of reflection**
  Summary
  Postscript

OBJECTIVES

After reading the chapter and reflecting, the learner will be able to:

1 Understand the importance of professional reasoning within the context of the
   student-supervisor fieldwork relationship.
2 Gain a qualitative understanding of the variety of the novice to expert fieldwork
   supervisor's experience.
3 Understand the fieldwork supervisor's reasoning process, including knowledge
   representation, problem naming, and problem solving and reflection.
4 Identify the parallels between supervisory and clinical reasoning.
5 Articulate the processes the supervisor uses to facilitate and foster clinical
   reasoning in their students.
6 Understand the relationship of affect and clinical reasoning in supervision, and
   the importance of reflection.

Fieldwork education	Facilitating clinical reasoning	Problem elements
Fieldwork educator		Mismatch
Problem solving	Supervisory reasoning	Reflection

Fieldwork education is an integral part of the professional development of future occupational therapists and an essential link between the academic world and practice (Cohn, 2003; Cohn & Crist, 1995). According to the Accreditation Council for Occupational Therapy Education (ACOTE), "fieldwork experience shall be designed to promote clinical reasoning and reflective practice; to transmit the values, beliefs that enable ethical practice, and to develop professionalism and competence as career responsibilities" (American Occupational Therapy Association, 1999, p. 58). The fieldwork educator has a "crucial" role in facilitating the students' clinical reasoning through discussion of clinical situations (Paterson & Adamson, 2001). In spite of how central the process of facilitating and developing quality clinical reasoning is to future occupational therapists, there is relatively little research examining the actual processes of doing this in fieldwork (Sladyk, 1997).

Thinking About Thinking 14-1

You cannot acquire experience by making experiments. You cannot create experience. You must undergo it.

—Albert Camus, French existentialist author and philosopher (1913–1960)

In health professions such as occupational therapy, cognitive processes and skills (including decision-making, reasoning, problem solving, and critical reflection) are essential for fulfilling the therapeutic role. Problem solving, and clinical reasoning in particular, have been the basic pedagogy for many occupational therapy curricula. As students move from classroom to clinic, the importance of clinical reasoning and problem solving is paramount to successful performance. How do fieldwork supervisors foster the development of these cognitive processes and skills necessary for success as an occupational therapist? How do fieldwork supervisors think, feel, and respond to the students within their complex multifaceted relationship? Are there parallels between the reasoning of the supervisor ("supervisory reasoning") with their students and the clinical reasoning of their students with their patients? How does the expert supervisor facilitate the kind of environment necessary for reflective practice to emerge?

The purpose of this chapter is to describe and reflect on the various dimensions these questions raise, including the fieldwork supervisors' reasoning process with their students, their direct role in facilitating clinical reasoning, as well as their role in creating the optimal affective environment for their students' best reasoning to emerge. This chapter integrates background from educational theory on learning in contexts such as fieldwork, counseling psychology supervision theory on the importance of the supervisory relationship, problem solving and information-processing conceptualizations, the relationship of affect and reasoning, and the actual "lived" experiences of occupational therapy fieldwork educators.

THEORETICAL AND EMPIRICAL BACKGROUND

Recent clinical reasoning research has broadened the focus beyond the analysis of the therapist's thinking to including the examination of contextual factors (Hooper, Farber & Schell, 2002). Theoretical work in the area of problem solving, reasoning, reflection, and learning in context or "situated cognition" provide the orientation to discern how students learn to reason and supervisors problem solve during the fieldwork experience. The theory of situated cognition has its roots in constructivist learning. This approach emerged as a result of dissatisfaction with behavioral and informational approaches to learning, devoid of the rich human interaction and context that shape learning and see such learning and knowledge as resulting from "processes that occur in a local, subjective, and socially constructed world" (Kirshner & Whitson, 1997, p. vii). Situated cognition supports the idea of authentic activity such as what occupational therapists actually do, in context. Assessment of learning and performance must be based on similar contexts. A seminal article by Brown, Collins, and Duguid (1989) identified the problems that arise from assessment of students without authentic activity, concept, and culture. They write:

> **Communities of practitioners are bound by socially constructed webs of belief . . . unfortunately students are often asked to use tools of a discipline without being able to adopt its culture . . . learning is then a process of enculturation . . . the learner can then enculturate as an apprentice or enter school as a student (p. 33).**

The context may include national or sociopolitical change that affects treatment structure (Kouloumpi, Ryan & Savaris, 2002), reimbursement changes, type of care provided, as well as the type of practice setting. Schell and Cervero (1993) describe how the individualized context of the practice environment contributes to pragmatic reasoning, which makes examination of therapists' reasoning "more anchored in the daily realities of clinical practice" (p. 609). Fieldwork provides this reality context for the student to apply knowledge and skills within an actual occupational therapy setting.

OT Fieldwork: Learning in Context

The fieldwork experience requires the student to not only use the tools he or she has learned throughout professional education, but also adopt the culture, norms, and values that define the profession. This enculturation happens as the result of the ambient culture. In the classroom, a student is socialized into the process of examinations, simulated case-based learning, group projects, and so on. Students may be proficient at passing examinations but may have difficulty using the domain's conceptual tools in practice. The student needs the experiences to be in situ to observe and practice the behaviors of the culture, use the jargon, imitate behavior, and act in accordance with the norms of the culture. Fieldwork provides the context to transmit the culture, including how to reason, problem solve and reflect.

The epistemology articulated by situated cognition suggests the importance of activity, apprenticeship (Rogoff, 1990), and enculturation to the learning processes seen in the education of health professionals, specifically occupational therapists.

Brown and colleagues (1989) also articulate the developmental process that is seen via this enculturation process:

> Apprenticeship and coaching in a domain begin by providing modeling in situ and scaffolding for students to get started in an authentic activity. As students gain more self-confidence and control they move into a more autonomous phase of collaborative learning, where they begin to participate consciously in the culture. The social network within the culture helps them develop its language and belief systems and promotes the process of enculturation (p. 39).

Through collaboration and discussion, students' "situated understanding" can be generalized and conceptual knowledge solidified.

Collins, Brown, and Newman (1989) suggest a sequence for an apprenticeship model (which parallels the fieldwork experience) that includes increasing complexity and diversity of skills, as well as a focus on global before local skills. In addition to the enculturation process, fieldwork students must demonstrate the ability to reason, problem solve, and reflect. Greeno, Collins and Resnick (1996) describe a situated view of learning in which "reasoning, remembering, and perceiving is understood as an achievement of a system, with contributions of the individuals who participate, along with tools and artifacts" (p. 20). Inherent in the fieldwork system are the student, the supervisor, the clients or patients, and the tools and artifacts of occupational therapy practice. The fieldwork supervisor plays a key role in providing the student feedback and modeling these processes. In addition, the supervisor must not only engage in clinical reasoning with his or her own caseload, but may also have to problem solve and reason within the context of student supervision if the student is not demonstrating adequate performance. The supervisor must also demonstrate the ability to reflect on his or her supervision and its ability to foster clinical reasoning and problem solving. As Lave and Wenger (1991) point out, an apprenticeship relationship can be unproductive for learning if the apprentice is not afforded opportunities for legitimate participation in the community of practice. The supervisor must be able to foster reasoning, problem solving, and reflection in order for the student to be a central participant. This process is likely to develop out of a supervisory relationship in which the trainees feel respected and safe. A sense of safety is critical to having learners be open for authentic reflection.

Supervisory Relational Context

In addition to pedagogical perspectives, other paradigms of clinical learning describe the primacy of the supervisory relationship for facilitating learning. These evolved from disciplines such as counseling psychology and social work. In a seminal conceptual paper on supervision, Loganbill, Hardy, and Delworth (1982) proposed a complex developmental model that described supervision as "an intensive interpersonally focused, one-to-one relationship in which one person is designated to facilitate the development of the therapeutic competence of the other person" (p. 4). They include four primary supervisory functions: (a) monitoring client welfare, (b) enhancing growth [of the supervisee] within stages, (c) promoting transition from stage to stage, and (d) evaluating the supervisee.

Holloway (1995) describes the goal of clinical supervision as "the enhancement of the student's effective professional functioning and the interpersonal nature of supervision provides an opportunity for the supervisee to be fully involved toward that end" (p. 6). His model examines the "supervisor's challenge to create a learning context that will enhance the supervisee's skill in constructing relevant frames of reference from which to devise effective strategies in working with clients" (p. 1). Holloway further emphasized the importance of the relationship to be "mutually involving" and empowering for the supervisee (p. 6). Examination of both content and process of supervision are important to learn from. Based on this model, the supervisor can facilitate the learning environment by his or her way of being with the student, by modeling, and by direct instructive processes.

Despite the theoretical and empirical importance of the supervisory relationship (Christie, Joyce & Moeller, 1985a), there are potential tensions inherent in this relationship that may complicate the learning alliance between student and supervisor (Bonello, 2001). From the supervisor's perspective, she or he is expected to balance the responsibility for the patient's care and welfare with the responsibility for the students' training needs. These potential role conflicts contribute to anxiety in the supervisor, especially for novices (Ellis & Douce, 1994). The occupational therapy fieldwork supervisor is expected to foster the development of potential colleagues and yet is responsible to gate keep for the quality of the profession as a whole. Often the conflict about this is captured by the colloquial criterion: "Would I want this person to treat my mother?" In addition, the supervisor may be working side by side, co-treating patients with the student, and may subsequently (or concurrently) have to evaluate or give corrective feedback. Sweeney, Webley, and Teacher (2001a) found that many supervisors experienced difficulty (and distress) being direct with students, because of a desire to be liked, or fear of a defensive reaction by the student.

There are complications from the students' perspectives as well, although there is less evidence in the literature from this viewpoint (Sweeney, Webley & Teacher, 2001b). For students, fieldwork is the last step of a long journey toward a professional career and having an adult livelihood. Sweeney, Webley, and Teacher found that students worked hard to manage the impression they made. They found that students presented a "professional face" to protect a "fragile sense of competence" (p. 380). This is particularly problematic with the belief in the importance of an honest and open interaction in facilitating the highest level of reflective practice. Sweeney, Webley, and Teacher (2001c) studied both perspectives (individually and collectively) and found discomfort from both sides. They suggest that the nondisclosure on the supervisees' part could inhibit the process of supervision, and that the nondisclosure of the supervisor could potentially "damage an open and reflective relationship" (p. 427).

Martin (1996) also found evidence of incongruence between espoused supervisory beliefs and practice in a small qualitative study. Although the supervisors believed in "active, student–centered learning" (p. 229), Martin found supervisory sessions moved at a fast pace, with little time for reflection of the students' feelings and ideas, and the supervisors were primarily in control of the session. Therefore, opportunities for the reflective aspect of processing information and more creative problem solving might be missed in the complexities and challenges of this type of relational context.

Stoltenberg (2005), the originator of the Integrated Developmental Model of supervision, suggests that advances in knowledge about cognitive theories maybe a useful addition to supervision theories, to better understand the development of complexity and expertise. Further information is needed about the cognitive models, including the nature of information processing and problem solving, to integrate this into the intricacies of the supervisory relationship.

Information Processing and Problem Solving

Cognitive theory developed in the 1970s and 1980s included information processing models of problem solving and reasoning. As discussed in Chapter 2, information processing has provided ways to look at an individual's ability to handle information. Theories of problem solving are dominated by the work of Newell and Simon (1972, Newell, 1990), using an information-processing paradigm for the study of problem solving and "problem space." A key principle was that problem-solving behavior involves means-ends-analysis in which the individual breaks down the problem into subcomponents or subgoals and works to resolve the problems systematically. Earlier, Wertheimer (1959) conducted research on problem solving and emphasized understanding the structure of the problem. The essence of successful problem-solving behavior according to Wertheimer is being able to see the overall structure of the problem. In addition to the structure of the problem, Bruner (1990) has identified learning as the active process in which the learner selects and transforms information, constructs hypotheses, and makes decisions relying on a cognitive structure to organize and provide meaning. Examples of cognitive structures include schemas, pattern recognition, mental models, and concept maps.

Thinking About Thinking 14-2

A certain region in the field becomes crucial, is focused; but it does not become isolated. A new, deeper structural view of the situation develops, involving changes in functional meaning, the grouping, etc. of the items. Directed by what is required by the structure of a situation for a crucial region, one is led to a reasonable prediction, which like the other parts of the structure, calls for verification, direct or indirect. Two directions are involved: getting a whole consistent picture, and seeing what the structure of the whole requires for the parts.

—Frederiksen, 1984, p. 212

Problem solving alone does not define the professional. Professional education has embraced the use of reflective practice as a legitimate base to ground practice beyond the technical or technician perspective. As Boud and Walker (1998) outline, a theory of reflective practice serves educators well. It elevates a simplistic technical problem-solving approach to an art of practice. Reflection, reflective thinking, and reflectivity are synonymous terms that highlight a careful consideration of alternatives (Dewey, 1910), the mind's ability to turn a subject over (Schön, 1983), and use of a knowledge base to make decisions that influence practice (McAlpine, Weston, Beauchamp, Wiseman & Beauchamp, 1999). Reflection is not simply a cognitive insight but rather leads to praxis, a change, and an alteration in perspective. Dewey (1933) believed that reflective thought was something that arose when there was a felt difficulty, a forked-road situation. He advocated a logical five-step process to address that difficulty which included (a) the problem, (b) its location and definition, (c) generation of solutions, (d) thoughtful considerations of the solutions, and (e) experimentation. Schön (1987) extended Dewey's forked-road metaphor to include the "messy swamp" that professionals face as they examine their practice and problem solve. Researchers in a variety of fields have found key differences in the way novices versus experts use cognitive structures to problem solve and engage in critical reflection.

Key aspects of novice to expert differences include cognitive schemas that are used, which have their base in the amount of relevant domain specific knowledge the individual possesses and the ability to demonstrate reflective practice. Experts have highly organized schemata, are adept at pattern recognition, and demonstrate more counterhypotheses, defining the problem space more richly (Schön, 1983; Schön, 1987; McAlpine et al., 1999; Newell, 1990). The schemas that experts use to solve problems are influenced by past experiences and contain problem elements, constraining factors, and solution procedures. Similarly, Robertson (1996) looked at novice to expert differences in occupational therapists' clinical reasoning and found that expert clinicians had a highly organized knowledge base, which allowed them to see meaningful patterns. Experts were able to demonstrate cognitive schema that could lead to implementation and solution procedures.

Although there is a growing literature on expertise in occupational therapy, there is relatively little research about expertise in fieldwork supervision. For the future of the profession, the fieldwork supervisor needs to strive toward facilitating the students' best clinical reasoning regarding the loosely structured problems of clients and to promote relevant problem solving strategies. However, the need for this type of problem-solving process is not unique to clinical practice itself. In addition, ambiguous, unclearly defined problems can emerge between the fieldwork supervisor and student as well, and these need to be responded to adeptly so as to not adversely affect the learning process.

Good supervision contributes to a transformation and development of thinking, which fosters cognitive complexity, which in turn leads to more advanced comprehension and problem solving (Granello, 2000). Within the supervisory relationship, variation exists in the ways supervisors interact and solve problems with students, and it facilitates clinical reasoning development. By understanding both of these processes more fully, the supervisor can gain expertise in fieldwork supervision with both the clinical education activities and the relational foundation that will foster student development. The following sections describe the variations in actual reasoning (supervisory reasoning) and interpersonal problem solving of fieldwork educators with students. This will be followed by their description of their experience facilitating clinical reasoning.

SUPERVISORY REASONING AND PROBLEM SOLVING

In our work exploring the thinking of fieldwork supervisors, we found that the structure of supervisory reasoning and problem solving with students paralleled the structure of clinical reasoning (Farber & Koenig, 1999; Koenig & Farber 2000; Farber & Koenig, 2002). The following sub-section will describe these processes which we identified as **supervisory reasoning** and the related problem-solving processes in more depth. However, some background may be helpful. Case Study 14-1 below describes the situation that prompted this line of study.

CASE STUDY 14-1

What's Up With Joseph? The Start of a Research Agenda on Supervisory Reasoning

The inception of this line of research began when I (Ruth S. Farber) overheard a problematic fieldwork situation from our fieldwork coordinator at that time, over a decade ago. I was a new PhD who had studied counseling supervision, including a class in the "supervision of supervision" as part of my doctoral program. Joseph, a mild-mannered student I knew from class, was reported to be putting his feet up on the table, reading the newspaper, and playing with the therapeutic putty at his fieldwork site. The supervisor was very upset and wanted to "fail" him. I did a double-take and wondered what was going on with this situation. I first wondered what Joseph was thinking. What was contributing to his informal and unfocused behavior in the clinic? Quickly, I wondered more about the meaning this supervisor was making of his behavior. Did she talk to him? Was she comfortable setting limits or providing boundaries? Was she so upset that she was unable to think about other options beside failure?

Joseph's behavior was interpreted as a lack of interest and engagement, and as what could be considered "unprofessional behavior." During this time period, more problems seemed to be reported regarding these unprofessional behaviors. Historically, this was a period of increased caseloads for therapists, and although these problems did not occur frequently, they were seen as requiring a disproportionate amount of time and energy to resolve, as well as being stressful to the supervisor (Farber, 1998). Operationalizing professional behaviors became a primary focus of fieldwork discussion lists, workshops, and conference presentations. The problematic behaviors that a supervisor sees today tend not to be as be as simplistic, like putting one's feet on the desk, but may be rooted in more complex ambiguous attitudinal conflicts that affect the supervisor-student relationship. Thus began the journey to understand the systemic interpersonal problem solving that occurs in the fieldwork supervisory relationship. This research began with the first fieldwork coordinator and continued primarily with the next fieldwork coordinator and my current co-author who adeptly brought her knowledge of reasoning to the ongoing process of this research.

Through a series of studies (qualitative and quantitative), we discovered that the problem solving and reasoning of the fieldwork supervisors had parallel structures and processes with that of clinicians. The supervisory reasoning process included the way fieldwork supervisors understood and interpreted the students' behavior (named or represented the problem) (Robertson, 1996), their ability to generate and entertain competing hypotheses (Fleming, 1991), problem solve (decide action), and reflect and revise to make ongoing changes (continuous reasoning) to individualize their approach with students in an educational context.

In addition, we noticed that some supervisors (usually novices) relied more on *procedural reasoning*. (One newer supervisor even brought the book of procedures she developed for students. She showed them proudly to us after a focus group.) Supervisors also used *interactive reasoning* (Bailey, 2001) to understand the students' perspective with other methods of reasoning. In addition, we found that some (expert) supervisors seem to take pride in helping the students create their professional story by asking them questions and helping them envision (imagine) what kind of therapists they would like to be after fieldwork (*narrative reasoning*).

Development of the Supervisory Reasoning Construct

At first, problem identification and intervention strategies were explored and identified (Farber & Weiss, 1996, 1997; Farber, 1998; Farber & Koenig, 1999). Although we conceptualized a systemic model in which the problem to solve was between the student and the supervisor, we initially focused on the fieldwork educators' perception of problematic student situations (n = 218). It was found at first that behaviors that were perceived as most problematic were (Farber, 1998):

1. attitude toward fieldwork (critical, detached, or disinterested) (10%)
2. interpersonal difficulties (with staff or patients (8%)
3. difficulty using feedback constructively (6.5%)
4. difficulty integrating theory and practice (6.5%)

Following our systematic assumptions, we then examined the supervisors' responses. It was found that supervisors either responded to the student directly using "student-centered interventions' (Box 14-1) or sought further education, reflection, or support to be more effective using "supervisor-focus interventions" (Box 14-2), or they pursued structural changes in the relationship using "environmental interventions" (Box 14-3).

BOX 14-1

Student-Centered Interventions: Interventions Directed Toward the Student or Those the Student May Engage

Proactive (student orientation and preparation):
- Clearly state expectations and responsibilities of student (sometimes in writing).
- Facilitate activities which orient student to staff.
- Go over safety/infection control check list with student.

Reactive (immediate or timely direct action):
- Identify and directly approach student about problematic behavior.
- Address safety or hygiene concerns immediately or as soon as possible.
- Address student for being judgmental toward patients or staff.
- Set direct expectations for time sensitive written records.

Active problem solving:
- Set up a contract (with specific goals, behaviors or learning objectives) and timeline.
- Mid-term evaluation by student to clarify expectations/concerns.

BOX 14-1

(continued)

- Maintain, improve, and open communication (in general or with specific techniques).
- Increase general feedback, as well as positive feedback to build self-esteem and efficacy.
- Use active strategies to foster students' competence (role playing, or group problem solving).
- Plan physical unavailability (when safe) for students who hold back.

Reflective:

- Understand cause.
- Get more information and discuss issues with student. Seek student's solutions.
- Suggest self-monitoring (student sets weekly goals and reports back informally).
- Build empathetic understanding of patient.

Facilitating student supports:

- Providing student groups for support and problem solving.
- Pairing with person from another discipline.
- Call faculty or fieldwork coordinator as student advocate.
- Promote a village orientation and opportunity for multiple learning experiences.

BOX 14-2

Supervisor-Centered Interventions: Interventions Provided for or Pursued by Supervisors for Support, Education, or Professional Development

Proactive:

- Develop Fieldwork II supervisory preceptorship, supervisory orientation, and training.
- Supervise Level I students before Level II. (Balance types of students.)

Active problem solving:

- Gather information (observing student in other situations with other staff).
- Learn different communication strategies and changing style of feedback.

Reflective:

- Self-examination or self-monitoring. (Am I modeling what I am asking student to do?)
- Depersonalize behavior and feedback (not intentional).
- Readjust expectation. (This person is a student.)
- Learn from experience and adjust behavior for the next student.

Seeking support:

- Get feedback regarding perceptions from colleague.
- Call or arrange meeting with academic fieldwork coordinator for collaboration or support.
- Develop collaborative training network (versus solo responsibility) for student.

> **BOX 14-3**
>
> **Supervisory Structure Changing Interventions: Structural Changes in the Supervisory Relationship**
>
> Changing ratio of supervision:
>
> - Pair more and less experienced supervisors to clarify expectations.
> - Bring in additional supervisor (co-supervise).
> - Bring in additional student(s) (for peer support).
> - Increase structure and/or provide additional informal supervision.
>
> Changing clinical settings (improve the goodness of fit):
>
> - Transfer student to a clinical setting with a different pace of practice
>
> Changing supervisors:
>
> - For entrenched personality conflict (after other approaches are tried thoroughly but unsuccessfully).

Although we started with a linear model, we later discovered that the reasoning behind the supervisors' intervention choices appeared to be governed by the quality of their reasoning and problem solving about it (versus the actual problem). Since differences in the quality and types of the reasoning (problem identification) and problem solving and reflection were found to show parallels to clinical reasoning, it was named *supervisory reasoning* at that time (Farber & Koenig, 1999). We also noted qualitative differences related to the development of expertise. Our most recent research, described in the next section, examined the quality of the supervisor reasoning (problem solving) with experts (nominated as having a high degree of expertise in supervising fieldwork II students by four fieldwork coordinators) and novices (having had no more than three students).

To capture the differences in thinking and problem solving, we piloted an actual (disguised) student vignette of an ambiguous, potentially problematic student-supervisor situation at two large regional meetings of fieldwork educators. The vignette is shown in Case Study 14-2 below.

CASE STUDY 14-2

Student Vignette Used to Research Supervisory Reasoning

You are supervising an occupational therapy student on week 4 of his/her second Level II rotation in a fast-paced outpatient clinic. The student is able to interact with the patients appropriately, establish treatment plans and document progress. You notice that the student does not seem to initiate during his/her downtime and is not as enthusiastically involved as your other students have been. You pride yourself on running a "tight ship" and having high standards, and this student is not meeting your expectations. Rather than writing notes you think the student should be observing treatment. You have repeatedly corrected the student throughout the day regarding this behavior, but he/she is still not responding. You are very frustrated and the student appears very frustrated.

The supervisors were asked to answer the following questions:

1. What are the problem elements?
2. How would you solve the problem(s)?
3. What do you see as the issues that you would reflect upon?

You might want to take a moment and jot your thoughts down to see how your thinking compares with others. The actual situation will be revealed at the end of the chapters.

Problem Element and Problem Naming

The fieldwork supervisors attending the large regional meeting had a wide variety of responses to the problem element(s) presented in Case Study 14-2 (Student Vignette), ranging from a focus on the student whom they either saw sympathetically (stressors in their life, uncomfortable with the situation) or as having deficit (having motivational or organizational problems, or being disrespectful). Some supervisors saw this as a transactional problem, between two people (problems of communication; differences of opinion; differences of needs, priorities or expectations). Last, some participants saw this as primarily the supervisor's problem (having too high standards, difficulty accepting the student, misreading intention, or having unclear expectations or communication *(Figure 14-1)*.

Problem naming or representation may be one of the most important aspects of good problem solving (Ferry & Ross-Gordon, 1998).

Ferry and Ross-Gordon (1998) found that reflective educators "sought to know as much as possible about the problem and what clearly defined its unique parameters. It is not through a simple act of naming and framing, but rather within a dynamic, ongoing interaction with the situation that the problem takes life and becomes constructed in a way to be addressed" (p. 103). The process of the reflective educators was in contrast to the non-reflective educators, who wanted to name the problem more simply, and fix it and move on.

In our study, the nominated expert fieldwork supervisors described rich complex schemata, which were contextually situated, stimulated by Case Study 14-2

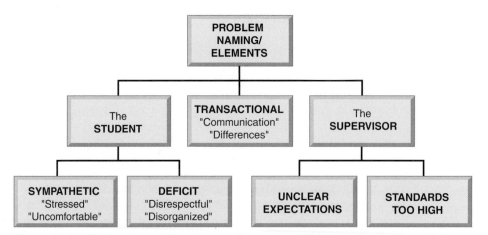

Figure 14-1   Fieldwork supervisors can each generate different understandings of the same student behavior.

(Student Vignette) earlier in the chapter. For instance, one expert shows both the transactional representation of the problem (communication) and a schema of temporal student performance expectations (when to expect or not expect which behaviors):

> Somewhere there's a lack of communication; what the student expects and what the supervisor thinks she may have communicated to that student may be two separate things. But I also have a question. Which Level 2 rotation is this? Is this their first or their second Level 2?
> Interviewer: Why would it make a difference?
> Because with the third question, what issues would I reflect upon, it would make a difference if it is the first Level 1 experience for the student and it's only week 4; I might think that the knowledge base of the student might not be as secure so the student might not feel as secure, but if it's a second Level 2 experience, then I would begin to think some other things.
> Interviewer: Let's say this is a Level 2, second rotation, what might you start to think?
> If the student had a solid background, from previous experiences, whether Level 1 or Level 2, then I would think if there were other students in the same clinic, if they are stronger, maybe the student feels intimidated. Or, it could be the other staff people who might be around that might not be as open to having the student come over and see what else they're doing. The third thing I was thinking, that it could just be that particular student's supervisor's style.

This expert began to expand both a sympathetic understanding of the student and the contextual possibilities contributing to the problematic situation, very smoothly and rapidly.

Thinking About Thinking 14-3

If the first button of one's coat
is wrongly buttoned,
all the rest will be crooked.

—Giordano Bruno

Problem Naming and Problem Solving

These multiple hypotheses about the nature of the problem influenced the problem-solving method used. Using interactive reasoning, another expert supervisor took the information that this was the student's second fieldwork and saw it as an opportunity for more dialogue to understand the larger picture of this student, in time.

> In communicating with the student, I think I could reflect more on his past experiences when I know somebody has been through a 12-week field work.

> This [past fieldwork experience] gives me a lot more to work with, in reflecting back and forth and problem solving and talking about expectations. It's just a different base to work from.
>
> I would start to ask the student what he or she thought . . . And, here we are, and I've talked about this, so tell me what you see is happening. As we sort of talked, to be less threatening about it and more educationally based about it—[I'd ask] so what have you done in the past? Suppose the student says, well, I'm scared to go over there. I feel uncomfortable. Well, how was it the last time for you? What kinds of personalities had you worked with and, just kind of draw from their experience to kind of develop into the new one. But basically to problem solve, I would start with the student in saying, what do you see happening . . . you look kind of frustrated. I was looking for this and, you know, kind of figure out whether it's clearly understood and there's a hesitancy or whether it was just misunderstood what the expectation was from the beginning.

Again having an opportunity to understand the larger (educational) context of the student's life (through dialogue) may help the supervisor understand the ambiguous or potentially problematic situation more fully and to address it more appropriately.

In contrast, the problem solving (regarding the same Case Study) varied greatly among the general sample of supervisors initially studied. Approaches ranged from (a) directive approaches (telling) using confrontation (doing) and using procedurally oriented processes (including giving more structure, working on time management), to (b) clarification of communication (negotiating a learning contract), to (c) a dialogic or uncovering approach (Koenig & Farber, 2000) (*Figure 14-2*). This last approach used more advanced interactive reasoning with an exploration and uncovering of larger issues that were influencing the situation.

In the case of supervisors with higher levels of expertise, problem solving begins almost simultaneously with problem identification. When knowledge and skill become more solidified, fluency between these two processes occurs quickly. This phenomenon was named as automaticity in Chapter 3 of this book. Experts in our study shared more complex and organized schemata to call upon, which made problem solving smoother as well.

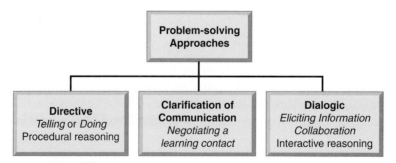

Figure 14-2   There are a variety of problem-solving approaches used by fieldwork supervisors.

From their experiences, the expert supervisors described complex schemata for individual student differences including demographic and geographic cultural specificity (being from India and the South), age, and life span developmental issues (i.e., being perimenopausal with memory issues). In contrast, novice supervisors had variations in problem identification, but included more limited general behavioral description, interest, learning style, personality, etc. The following is an example of the experts' schemata for individual differences, as well as the perception of the student being "off-time" for the supervisors' schemata for temporal performance expectation. The therapist describes the process of problem solving, seamlessly continuing through interaction around a series of interventions:

> She was an older student and she was very organized. But when it came to actually dealing with the patient one on one like that, she'd get all flustered and forget everything. So we sat down and talked and I wasn't exactly sure what it was at that time. So I said everything else is falling into place, I just don't understand what's happening here— putting the blood pressure cuff on the wrong way and pumping it up and saying—I can't get a blood pressure reading.
>
> By week 6, when the patient is talking about their interests, [and] she wasn't paying attention to what the patient was saying...[She'd say] I'm going to test your strength and your range of motion and then she comes back to the interest question. So what do you like to do? And it's [should be] pick up on what the patient is saying and go from there. Don't keep it checkbook [cookbook].
>
> So we sat down and talked and I said, you know, tell me what it is exactly. And I also had her keeping a journal. I said, if you don't feel comfortable talking to me about it, write it in your journal and that way we can discuss it. Well, she was very verbal. She was good at that.
>
> And she said, well, you know, my husband is very sick and I'm going through premenopausal situations right now. So, okay, that made it easier for me to understand what was going on. So then we were able to problem solve. Okay, how can we work this out so that you're going to get the most out of this affiliation?
>
> By this time we were coming close to the midpoint. I said we don't normally do this, but I'm going to take the AOTA evaluation form that we're supposed to fill up at the end of the year, [and] we're going to do a midpoint evaluation so . . . we have a comparison from midpoint to the end to make sure that you're going to be okay. And I gave her a copy of it and I said I want you to fill it out also, so that we can see whether we're both on the same line. So I did . . . when I presented it to the student, she actually rated herself a whole lot lower than I had.
>
> After that, she started listening more to what patients were saying. She started forcing herself to listen more and then things started to flow a lot more smoothly. I think she felt more comfortable.

The latter demonstrates how an expert fieldwork supervisor was able to uncover the source of the students' real difficulties (problem elements) through interactive reasoning. The fieldwork supervisor had a better understanding of the life of this student; by helping the student express her anxiety and pressure, she was freed up to perform more effectively.

In addition to having complex schemata for diversity of students' contexts, expert supervisors provided rich descriptions of working with students' problems of initiation or freezing when the supervisor was present. They described these schemata as having a way to move the "birds out of the nest." One supervisor had clever ways to make herself "physically unavailable" for the previous student.

> I would also have her come up with treatment plans and backup treatment plans in case what she had planned wasn't going to work . . . I physically spaced myself farther away from her and out of her sight. I was still in the room because I didn't feel secure with her being left alone with a patient at that particular time.
>
> And then the way that the rooms are set up, I just hid behind the bathroom door [adjacent to the room the client was being treated in] . . . so she would feel more comfortable.
>
> I would tell her, you know, I'm going to go check on a chart on someone else whom I needed to see. I'd step out and then I'd just hang around right in that area and hear her talking, and she sounded a lot more comfortable and more at ease and things seemed to flow a lot better.

Another supervisor described a similar technique.

> There are pictures in each patient's room . . . to start getting them used to going and doing ADLs. I can hang out behind the curtain, stand there. I can watch everything that's going on [in the reflection].

The supervisor in these cases had a plan to promote the comfort of the supervisee's possible self-consciousness, but stayed close enough to be a safety net to monitor their clients' welfare. The novices we spoke to described being more tentative and perplexed by students who were reticent initiating patient activity.

Reflection: Supervisor's Expectations and Supervisory Role Schemata

Supervisors varied on what they reflected on. When presented with the ambiguous vignette, the reflections of the general sample ranged from could this be me, or is it them? They sometimes focused on the individual student or referenced their reflection on their norms of students past. Their transactional reflections focused on the possibility of a mismatch of personality, style or setting, or miscommunication of expectations. Also they wondered if their expectations were clear or fair (Koenig & Farber, 2000).

Another specific area many supervisors wrestled with and reflected on was their expectations of students just passing rather than optimizing their learning experience in fieldwork. "The students want to do just what they need to do. I have to be able to pass and this is what I need to do to be able to pass, rather than looking at the more global experience and increasing their knowledge base and just general experience."

Coming to terms with what was adequate for an entry level therapist, rather than optimal, was something that many of the expert supervisors voiced and accepted. One expert described how she gave ownership of professional goals to the student. She used narrative reasoning, helping the student write their professional story. "They can be okay at what they do, or they can be really good at what they do, or they can excel at what they do." She asked the student "So what kind of therapist did they want to be?"

Although some novices demonstrated clear reflection about their expectations of the student, one novice supervisor struggled more with what to expect and was more reactive than reflective. She said in an irritated way "when is enough, enough!" The following is her perception of the problem, which reminded her of a student she had. There was more personalization and distress associated with her response.

> It's easier for her to write, easier for her to do the treatment plan or— because it doesn't seem like she's having trouble with the basics. It seems like she's having trouble with the extracurricular . . . observing someone else treating someone. She's not effectively getting the most out of her 8-hour day. Just try to discuss what are your goals for this affiliation? I know that there's no perfect affiliation and it really gets me when it seems like they are interested in [another area like] pediatrics, well, you have 12 weeks to impress me. And you're going to learn how to transfer a big person just like a little person. I think a lot of people think well, this isn't the perfect affiliation, but you have to get something out of it. So a lot of times I'll talk to someone, well, what do you want to get out of this? I mean, you're not going to sit here for 12 weeks.

This supervisor's distressed affect seemed to be associated with her perception of the student (in the vignette) as being disinterested or critical toward the fieldwork setting. Drake and Truital (1997) discuss the importance of clarifying ambiguity in problem fieldwork placements. They found dramatic signals (safety of patient) were likely to be managed well, whereas more subtle "petty" signals such as "floating through" fieldwork could escalate if not clarified and resolved in a timely way.

Also, the same novice supervisor saw these issues as "extracurricular." This may be related to her newly forming supervisory role schemata and could contribute to some additional complications. The responsibilities in the schemata for the supervisory role were more expansive for many of the experts interviewed. Their schemata included the importance of a thorough orientation and anticipation of expected areas of student anxiety (regarding the chart, adding clients with new diagnoses, adding more patients, and interacting with other professionals, especially physicians) as part of their supervisory role. A supervisor in an acute setting described this anticipation aspect of her role.

> I take them through a simple process. They don't have to go through the whole chart, but these are the important pages in the chart to know to go, to understand this information. It is best to understand what's going on with that patient overnight and the last notes the day

> before, the nurses' notes . . . And once they get comfortable, with me observing them, once they get comfortable with the chart, then walk them through the first couple of SOAP notes, you know, 'cause they're afraid of this chart. This chart is really a scary thing, you know.

The same supervisor also had schemata for helping students with becoming comfortable with the team.

> If I find that students are a little timid when they talk to other authority figures such as doctors and physical therapists and speech pathologists . . . I try to get them over the fear factor by walking around with the doc . . . and I'll [gently] push them toward the doctor and they say, who are you? And I'll let the student speak.

This schema of supervisory role performance, which anticipated the normative occurrence of student's anxiety, was believed (by the supervisor) to prevent some potential complications (such as the ones in the extracts above) from occurring. The way in which the supervisors interpret the ambiguity of the supervisee's behavior, conceptualize their supervisory role, and reason (procedural, interactive, narrative, continuous, conditional) collectively contribute to the quality of the process of problem solving and outcome with the student. This in turn could influence the student's meta-learning about problem solving in helping relationships by both observing positive models and experiencing the reasoning and approach being utilized. Arling (1998) found the importance of this type of meta-learning phenomenon occurring in psychotherapy supervision. The process and type of problem solving utilized with the student could either facilitate or inhibit the development of student reflection and reasoning. The next section describes the larger picture of how clinical reasoning, including reflection, is facilitated in fieldwork.

FACILITATING CLINICAL REASONING IN FIELDWORK

Clinical reasoning encompasses "knowledge of procedures, interactions with patients, and interpretation and analysis of the evolving situation" (Cohn, 1989, p. 241). This thought process is not a set of skills to be taught, but "a complex process dependent upon years of experience" (Cohn, p. 241). In fieldwork, Cohn suggests there is a tension between the developmental necessity to teach standard routine skills and procedures, and facilitating complex clinical reasoning, which takes more reflection and experience. Cohn suggests that it is unrealistic "to expect students to emerge from a 3-month fieldwork experience with clinical reasoning firmly established." She believes the fieldwork experience will more likely "serve as a foundation or preparation for clinical reasoning" (p. 241).

Clinical reasoning is a cognitive process and, therefore, not directly visible. We can only learn about it by asking people to describe their reasoning (Cohn & Czycholl, 1991), or we can infer it from their behavior. Similarly, it is somewhat challenging to teach directly or didactically. Generally, there is a need to set up the right circumstances for the learner to be an active participant. In a review of research, Norman (2005) identified the importance of practice on clinical reasoning. The student must be allowed to practice a "think aloud" process in context of fieldwork. Thinking while doing is also context-specific, since the agent is responding to and affecting the specific context. Having some knowledge base and experience is needed to more accurately name the problem and to engage in more advanced problem solving and go beyond the data for a creative individualized solution, which is essential for good clinical practice. There are a variety of ways in which clinical reasoning is taught in the classroom and in fieldwork situations.

In an international study (five United Kingdom countries), Paterson and Adamson (2001) found a number of strategies in occupational therapy curriculums used to facilitate clinical reasoning. This included "case studies (92%), to experiential learning (83%), seminars (76%), and didactic teaching 68%" (p. 403). Other methods, such as clinical story telling, reflective diaries, role playing, and other active exercises, were mentioned. It is not clear whether these were used in the classroom or fieldwork exclusively, although they concluded that the discussion of cases with the fieldwork supervisor was "crucial" for learning related to clinical reasoning. Also, the interpersonal aspect of learning was mentioned often across the various methods described.

Developmental Aspects of Teaching Clinical Reasoning

It is important for fieldwork educators to have realistic expectations for students' development of clinical expertise. Expert clinical reasoning is a consequence of an extensive and multidimensional knowledge base (Norman, 2005); therefore, the student will not have access to a high level of reasoning. Krammer (1998) suggests that fieldwork educators may at times have unrealistically high expectations for student performance and mastery and that the supervisor, in turn, may need more time for clinical mastery to develop. Cohn (1989) also underscores the importance of the supervisor having reasonable expectations for the level of clinical reasoning processes of the student, since real expertise in which the therapists can truly individualize their response to the particular client takes years. She suggests that there are developmental aspects of this process (Cohn 1989) that provide a "foundation for clinical reasoning (p. 241)." There are a number of considerations for setting the foundation for clinical reasoning development. These include explicitly identifying what clinical reasoning is, integrating theory and practice, sharing scripts, questioning, and fostering activity in obtaining resources.

One supervisor described how she helped the student identify what his clinical reasoning was, as well as fostering flexibility of planning. Flexibility is also one of the dimensions of professional expertise posited by Van der Heijden (2002). One of the experts describes how she fosters flexibility with treatment planning.

> Let's say that they're trying to show someone how to put on socks and they'll go straight to a sock donner. I'll say, oh, well, that's interesting. Could you think of a different way to do this?
> You know, what if, what if we'd forgotten a sock donner downstairs. You can't use the elevators because the elevators take forever to come. You'd have to run from the 6th floor down to the ground

level and then come back up. We're going to lose a lot of time; what's another way that we can work on this? Then they'll say, well, I guess I can have them cross their legs over. And then they'll start problem solving, so then I'll say, okay, well, you know what? *That was clinical reasoning that you just did.*

The supervisor went on to explain how she was integrating her theoretical framework, as well.

Using the Rehab model . . . we're very much into trying to [get the client to] regain normal function and we get orthopedic [patients] sometimes and knees. I mean, they came to bend the knee, so if you give them a sock aid, are they going to bend their knee? Okay, so, what can you do to get to that point where they can then put their sock on without that sock aid?

This supervisor demonstrates what Holloway (1995) believes about the role of the supervisor. That supervisors can articulate "the layers of thinking and understanding, conceptualizing" and application, as well as to be "the translator of theory and research to practice" (p. 2).

Clinical reasoning is facilitated by the ability to meaningfully chunk information into a collection of patient scripts (Bruning, Schraw & Ronning, 1999) to pull from. Supervisors share their scripts and thinking with their students initially. Expert supervisors talk aloud about their thinking.

I talk out loud, from my past experience. In general, I have this formulation and then when I did this, I'm taking into consideration that this man doesn't get dressed himself so he's not going to do that. And they need to know how I modify my thinking, to change, and to re-prioritize.

Most [students] don't know. They don't have the experience. They are not familiar with the diagnosis. They are not sure. They kind of know I should range that arm every day, but the choice of activities that goes into it and all the reasoning part of it, they are not quite sure of. In the beginning I share my stories. They ask questions. I pull up a patient I had in the past . . . I choose this technique or that or give them generalities regarding knee patients.

As they are telling me [about their cases] and justifying it [what they did] to me, they start building stories. And we reflect back to other patients. So they can start developing their own reasoning, based on their own learning.

Another way to foster clinical reasoning is to set up a series of carefully guided questions. This increasingly gets the student to learn more about the client, as well as plan more comprehensively for the client's treatment. Cohn and Czycholl (1991) suggest that there is a developmental sequence to these questions. They believe that the supervisor should initially start out with specific questions regarding diagnostic information and then generalize to the population of patients with the condition, such as: "What problems will a patient present following a cerebral vascular infarct?" (p.175). These authors believe that this encourages the student to develop a "pre-assessment image of the patient" based on diagnosis. Secondarily, the supervisor can evaluate the student's knowledge base on this topic. Once the student understands the relationship between the diagnosis and the patient's functional abilities, she suggests the focus of the questions is expanded to learning about the big picture, and what is meaningful to the client. Questions can be asked such as: "What does the patient care about?" or "What is this patient's hope for the future?" (p. 176). At the same time, the supervisor can assess how much the student can observe and integrate multiple pieces of information. These authors believe that the fieldwork supervisor should avoid being "overly concerned with covering all aspects of a clinical problem. Rather the emphasis should be on expanding students' views of patients' problems as additional information becomes available or the learner is able to integrate more complex information" (p. 177).

Once the students are doing treatment planning, the expert supervisors in our study described preparing the groundwork for why questions. They tell the student, "I'm going to be mean" or "You could be right or you could be wrong, but I want to know why you're doing what you're doing, why you're proceeding, and why did you choose that activity?"

They had two basic rationales for the why questioning. One was to help the student clarify, consolidate and strengthen his or her clinical reasoning.

> **We always do this in real life. You're going to need to explain this to people, families, and doctors, and they are going to come up and ask you questions and you need to be able to articulate and come up with a concrete basis [for what you are doing] and how you went about and came to the conclusion.**

The other rationale was to see that they were not guessing. Helping students be solid in their thinking, planning, and performing client treatment is crucial. There were varied perceptions of the student using outside resources to back up their thinking based on the expertise of the supervisor. Some of the novices were concerned about the students being too "textbook." And that could be problematic because of the need to put theory into action very spontaneously. However, experts tended to encourage the student to foster investigative activity of outside resources, to strengthen treatment planning and think on their own.

> **They [the students] come up to me with questions like, How do you do this? or How would I treat a rotator cuff. Well, let me see, how would you treat a rotator cuff? Let's look on the Internet. Or, there are some books there. You know, I let them problem solve to do it, with any kind of problem. Instead of just giving them the answers, I try to do a dialogue. You know, let's problem solve this. Let's see what we can come up with. Well, that's a good idea. Let's [hear your] strategy, you going to look on the Internet? Okay, well, when you, when you find that stuff, come in and we'll talk about it tomorrow morning before the patient comes, and we'll see what you found, how your plan and treatment are. You know. I let them come up with . . . the answers.**

> I encourage them to think. What I say all the time is, 'You're going to be a therapist and I'm not going to be there with you.' You know, you're going to be a therapist. Just the kind of thinking that you have to do when you're out there by yourself. And don't be afraid; you can even call another therapist if you have to . . . You know, but you've got to get the information. You've got to know what you're doing before you're doing it.

In general, there are many ways to facilitate clinical reasoning through questioning and encouraging active participation of the student. Many of these techniques that the fieldwork supervisors used were found in the theoretical literature regarding facilitating clinical reasoning in fieldwork. These included probing questions, reflective journal writing, reviewing case studies, videotaping treatment, and using consistent populations and role modeling (Sladyk, 1997; Cohn, 1998). Although increasing the quality of clinical reasoning skills is essential for the future of the profession, there is relatively little written about this topic, and most articles are theoretical papers or descriptive studies. In her doctoral research, Sladyk (1999) studied this phenomenon quantitatively. One of her interesting findings was that there was an inverse relationship between the number of clinical reasoning activities in which students participated and their clinical reasoning skills. This suggested that the "depth of processing activities is more important than number of activities to which the student is exposed" (p. 246). Also she found that students reported "reflective dialogue activities" as most effective in building analogue maps, which are believed to refine abstractions and strengthen clinical reasoning skills. Fieldwork supervisors are in a unique position to facilitate this dialogue and to modify the learning environment to maximize clinical reasoning development in students. The next section describes more fully the interrelationship of clinical reasoning and the supervisory relationship.

Clinical Reasoning Emerging Within the Supervisory Relationship

In counseling education, "Supervision provides an opportunity for the student to capture the essence of the psycho-therapeutic process as it is articulated and modeled by the supervisor, and to recreate it in the counseling relationship" (Holloway, 1995, p. 1). This may occur in the occupational therapy fieldwork supervisory context as well, with unique characteristics related to the professional role of the occupational therapist. Two general aspects that influence this implicit process are described: the intersubjective experience and parallel process.

O'Byrne and Rosenberg (1998) posit that the supervision could be seen as "intersubjective processes that revolve around solving ambiguous and ill-structured problems; key features include the co-construction of shared meaning, framed by a continuous cycle of reflection and action, and the emergence of a professional identity" (p. 39). Current research on clinical supervision has included qualitative methods, which have allowed a greater examination of supervision from this systemic contextual perspective. This fits with the contemporary interest in constructivist theory development (O'Byrne & Rosenberg, 1998; Neufeldt, 1997). Constructivist perspectives permit the opportunity to examine the skill development of the supervisee in context and the shared construction of practice knowledge that occurs within the supervisory relationship. A significant part of this shared knowledge for the occupational therapist is the process of clinical reasoning.

This is similar to the goal of achieving the intersubjective for occupational therapists. Crepeau (1991) described this process as the occupational therapist "enters into her patient's life-world and simultaneously controls and manages the treatment process" (p. 1016). She believes that this capacity to understand the other is developed through formal education and fieldwork. How this is accomplished in fieldwork is important to understand. It appears that fieldwork supervisors who can empathize, join with their students (where they are), and foster mutuality, may be more likely to be able to participate in the co-construction of knowledge through cycles of reflection and action (*Figure 14-3*).

There is a concept described as parallel process in the supervisory literature, primarily from counseling psychology; however, it may have implications for occupational therapy supervision. Doherman (1976) did a seminal study describing the parallel process between Client, Supervisee, and Supervisor. This is also known as a "mirroring" process in which the dynamics in one relationship mirror the dynamics of the other (Carrol, 1996). It is heuristically useful, yet somewhat of an elusive process. Originally, this was conceptually linked to psychoanalytic treatment, and it was believed that unconscious behavior (transference) of the client affected the supervisee and supervisor relationship. Now, it is used by other schools of thought, including systems theorists, and is seen as a more broad-based, multidirectional process. This includes the transfer of learning from the supervisory relationship to the therapy relationship. It has been found to be especially useful with more advanced supervisees. This fits with the intersubjective aspect of supervision mentioned earlier.

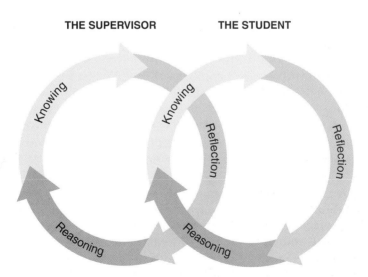

Interaction: Co-construction of meaning

Figure 14-3   Fieldwork supervision is an intersubjective process in which supervisors and student co-construct clinical reasoning.

Regarding occupational therapy fieldwork supervision, there were a few possible ways this process may occur. These emerged from the fieldwork supervisors' description of their relationship with their students. Although this is posited to be multidirectional, the scope of this chapter describes the supervisors' perception of their role in this process. The ways this occurs in occupational therapy fieldwork were characterized by our participants as "being the OT." "Being the OT" involved both maximizing students' functioning, and fostering mutuality and collaboration (which is what we want to see in our students' relationships with their clients). When asked about an ambiguous potential problematic student situation, a supervisor gave this response.

> I think part of it is just because we're OTs. You see what a problem is, how it presents itself, and then you try to come up with all the possibilities as to why the person has that problem. And then when you're dealing with patients, you come up with ways; if Plan A doesn't work, what's your backup plan? And if Plan B doesn't work, what's another way that you can probably combat the problem? So I think I just transfer that over to student affiliations. If something's not working with the student, what could be the possible reasons for it and what could be possible options to address so that you can have it a successful experience for the student and for the supervisor.
>
> That what's now becoming more common, you know, thinking outside the box. You just try to brainstorm every possible situation that you can come up with. You know, you have to think outside of the traditional way of thinking. Yeah, I like being able to come up with different solutions or different options.
>
> And then, of course, running it by the student, but I like that creativity part of it. I normally ask them how they see themselves—in the situation. And if they don't come up with some of the things that I've come across that might be problem areas, I'll say, well what do think about this? I tend to leave it more open-ended so they can do a self-evaluation.
>
> When asked: What if they don't come up with it?
>
> Then if they don't come up with it, I'll just be point blank with it and say, well, what about this? I'll say, well, let's brainstorm or problem solve. I won't necessarily say, well I've come up with solutions. Because what I come up with might be totally displeasing to the students. I don't know what the past history has been with that student, you know. So I'll ask them to, well, let's come up with solutions.

Other expert supervisors talked about finding the "just right challenge." A supervisor described the way she attempted to maximize functioning of the student as she did with her patients. This supervisor would ask the student: "How can I help you do your job best?" Many of the expert fieldwork supervisors described building of common ground for collaborative goal setting, with students, which also epitomizes qualities of best practice in patient care. This sets the positive affective tone for reasoning to emerge. Since the knowledge process is embedded in the relationship, it may be important to consider how the affective state of the individual affects this process.

THE RELATIONSHIP OF AFFECT AND CLINICAL REASONING IN SUPERVISION: IMPORTANCE OF REFLECTION

In recent years, psychologists have been recognizing the influence of affect on thinking (Forgas, 2001). In addition to the cognitive processes, affective processes occur in supervision. The role of affect is also described in the supervision literature. Tickle-Degan and Puccinelli (1999) explored the role of students' nonverbal negative expression on fieldwork outcomes. It was found that students rated as expressive of negative emotionality (by their peers) were more likely to be evaluated as less clinically skilled by their fieldwork supervisors (than non-negatively expressive students).

In an extensive study of occupational therapy supervision, Sweeney, Webley, and Teacher (2001c) found discomfort on the part of both the student and the supervisor. Ronnestad, Skovholtz, and Thomas (1993) described the new supervisees' anxiety as intense and pervasive. Sweeney, Webley, and Teacher also described beginning supervisors as having "equivalent anxiety." New supervisors can worry about their performance and what the student thinks of them. The novice supervisor might be mastering his or her clinical skills as well. This is relevant to learning, since both student and supervisor must feel comfortable to disclose their concerns and questions. All this affects student disclosure versus saving face, which makes it more difficult to say what one really thinks and authentically reflect on practice, which is essential for the development of clinical reasoning (Sweeney, Webley & Teacher, 2001c). With this lack of disclosure, the "image of professionalism" covers "frail competence." If so, how does the student begin an authentic dialogue with a mentor and allow him- or herself to reflect in a supportive environment?

For reflective practice to occur, it may be necessary for the fieldwork educator to share his or her thinking and uncertainty to provide a safe environment for the fledgling therapist to share newly developed thoughts (Cohn & Czycholl, 1991).

A supervisor who works in home health in an impoverished area described her thinking:

> She's going to be with me for 3 months . . . So I do talk a lot [in the beginning] . . . I'm trying to build a real comfort level with not knowing things and, and being repulsed by things, and to set a base for that so that they, too, would feel free to talk about things that are tough for them in trying to work in that environment. . . . So I, I talk a lot about how uncomfortable those things are and, and how difficult the reasoning is, cause it all looks so smooth and so fast.
>
> [I talk about] how I got there because it looks so simple whenever you're trying to be smooth with people. I mean, I can walk up a flight of stairs. I can be counting the stairs. I can be checking if their railing is solid and I can be carrying on a conversation. You know, and it, you really have to explain that—all that was going on. I'm only trying to just create a sense of what my clinical reasoning is and how it goes and how complex it can be and how I'm not always sure. And then, and then to start them practicing with that and trying to talk to me about the same issues that I've talked with them.

Another way in which expert supervisors in our study created a supportive tone (appropriate to promoting reflection) in the relationship was the thoughtful way they gave feedback. The supervisors were consciously aware of the responsibility to give corrective feedback, but to do it in a respectful way. Two supervisors had an especially well thought-out schema for doing it, which they characterized as "the sandwich."

> Well, because you want to start off with something good because as soon as you start to talk with someone and say, we've got a problem here, right away, it's like panic sets in the student, who only half listens to what you're saying. So you tell them something good to begin with. You give them the thing that you want them to improve on.
>
> And then you don't want them to walk away with feeling, well, that was kind of like a backwards compliment. Okay? So then you finish with something positive and then the student feels good and walks out and usually is motivated to try to work on the area that you've addressed. Yeah, you don't like the pat, pat, smack. You don't want to end with that. You want to end on a more positive, open communication note.

Another supervisor added specifics about the student in the Case Study.

> I would take the student aside if I really believed that this person needed to jump in a little bit more. You give the good thing. You give the bad things. And you end with the good things. Right. So I would tell them, you know, you've taken the initiative, you're getting the work done and everything, but what I'd like to see now is for you to take the initiative a little bit further and this time go and jump in—pick up a chart the night before, review it, and come up with a treatment plan for when this person comes in. And then end it with, I read your last note and it was perfect. Your goals were measurable, your plan was good.

She also explained that she would find an opportunity to discuss the student's frustrations and explore situational solutions, such as other staff encouraging reaching out to the student. Similarly, in literature from other fields, the induction of positive affect was found to improve "integration of information, problem solving, decision making and cognitive organization in a wide variety of settings" (Estrada, Isen & Young, 1997, p.118). In their study of physicians' clinical reasoning, Estrada and colleagues found that conditions of positive affect facilitated the integration of information and clinical reasoning of physicians (1997). Physicians who were in the induced positive affect group diagnosed the condition significantly sooner, and there were fewer distortions or less inflexibility of thinking observed.

The same experience can occur with occupational therapy supervisors who may deal with the complex range of feelings that may be a part of the supervisory relationship. If positive affect facilitates better reasoning, anxious affect may inhibit it. For instance, uncomfortable affect may intensify by not feeling comfortable with the role inherent in supervision, or not having administrative support (Sweeney, Webley & Teacher, 2001), or feeling inadequately prepared for the complexities in the relationship (Christie, Joyce & Moeller, 1985b). According to Forgas (2001), these affective states can provide a significant influence on an individual's thinking, including his or her perception and interpretation of social situations (the ambiguous swampy lowlands), and his/her resultant planning and execution of further interaction.

Without careful reflection and appropriate support, the supervisor might inadvertently act out his or her misperception with the student, personalize the student's behavior, or internalize a stressful affect related to their perception of the situation. On an earlier survey, when asked what the supervisor did when she perceived a problematic student situation, she answered in jest "I eat chocolate" or "I take a Xanax" (Farber, 1998).

The supervisor may ask a colleague for a "reality check" or may call in the academic fieldwork coordinator (which was jokingly referred to in the group of supervisors as calling in the "National Guard"). This was usually found to be very helpful in giving the supervisor an opportunity to vent, get support and perspective, and then to constructively problem solve.

There is an importance of reflecting in general, but especially when affect is high. Gladwell (2005) describes the importance of trusting our rapid cognitions (knowing and without knowing) or tacit knowledge or processing of information. This smooth thinking and doing are seen in experts, and Gladwell believes it is important to trust this much of the time. However, when there is interference (beyond consciousness) of high affect states, further reflection versus action is called for.

A fieldwork supervisor described the following scenario in which she had an initial perception that changed with time and further reflection. Subsequently, the fieldwork educator (in mental health) was willing to change the course of her behavior with a student who had been at her facility for one week.

> **I first thought she was blowing things off. I thought I needed to take immediate action and confronted her. I basically gave her an ultimatum to think . . . about making a decision . . . is this the setting for you . . . It was Friday and I told her to think about it over the weekend (Farber & Koenig, 1999, p. 99).**

The supervisor subsequently thought about it as well and was worried about being "too quick" to react or hurting her potential "supportive role." The supervisor also realized that the pressures she (herself) was under influenced her sense of urgency. In a subsequent discussion that was more mutually reflective, she discovered that what she originally perceived as "unconcern" was actually that the student felt "really paralyzed" in a psychiatric setting. The student wasn't used to the expectations of this setting or the population and had personal life issues that became "stirred-up" (Farber & Koenig, 1999). The importance of self-reflection when affect is high is particularly important to be clearer and more effective in the exchange with students. The supervisor's willingness to reconsider her initial hypothesis (even in nonaffectively charged perceptions) and change her response (Farber & Koenig) is similar to the continuous reasoning that clinicians do, which entails a "continuous stream of small decisions or temporary hypothesis" (Fleming, 1991, p.992). This contributes to supervisors' ability to make ongoing changes and individualize their approaches with students.

SUMMARY

Fieldwork is the context for cognitive processes related to transitioning from classroom to actual therapy practice. It also is a time of significant professional enculturation. The student supervisor's reasoning during this process is critical on several levels. First, the fieldwork educator must be able to facilitate reasoning in a novice therapist and create appropriate and graded situations for its development to occur. An important aspect of this is the interpersonal environment fostered by the fieldwork educator, which affects the further unfolding of the student's development. When challenges occur in the relationship, the fieldwork educator uses supervisory reasoning to identify the problem, problem solve and reflect effectively to maximize successful student transition to practice. We contend that supervisors model reasoning through their interaction with their students as well as with their clients.

Being able to reason and respond in the moment, with continuously changing client feedback is challenging for novice practitioners. Novice supervisors are similarly challenged by working with students from diverse backgrounds and abilities. This situation is compounded when relatively novice practitioners become supervisors, assuming the dual responsibility to both their students and their clients. This chapter focused on the complexity of developing clinical reasoning within the supervisory relationship in fieldwork.

The expert fieldwork supervisors described in this chapter are like expert practitioners everywhere, in that they used complex schemata that are context-driven and highly organized. They were adept not only at pattern recognition but also at the generation of multiple hypotheses and responses. With their advanced thinking, expert supervisors easily individualized their interaction with students with diverse needs and abilities, as expert therapists do with clients. Supervisors do this in the way they facilitate clinical reasoning with each student directly, as well as the way they perceive and respond to ambiguous student situations.

Within the supervisory relationship, variation exists in the ways supervisors interact and solve problems with students, as well as with the ways they foster the development of clinical reasoning. By understanding these complex processes, the fieldwork supervisor can become more adept at facilitating the student's reasoning and professional development. Fieldwork education occurs within a relational context. The supervisory relationship substantially shapes the learning environment in which the transformation from student to practitioner occurs. Because of the importance of the supervisory role for the development of future occupational therapists, both training in supervision and ongoing support for supervisors is recommended.

BOX 14-4
Postscript: Student Vignette Used to Research Supervisory Reasoning

As in an actual fieldwork situations, there are many ways to think about and approach a student–supervisor dilemma, such as the one described in Case Study 14-1 earlier in this chapter. However, here is what actually transpired.

BOX 14-4
(continued)

Background

The student in the vignette had first been placed in a Level II Fieldwork at a busy rehab facility, which had been canceled because of last-minute staff changes. His fieldwork was changed to an Outpatient Hand Center. The supervisor was known for being an excellent supervisor, and all of her students had given her positive feedback on the Student Evaluation of Fieldwork assessment. However, this student did not share the same interest in hands as the previous students, who had requested a placement at that type of facility.

The student felt that he was doing a "good job," which was very different from the supervisor's perception. This was creating conflict and frustration. The supervisor's previous experience with students involved a level of motivation and "passion" for the practice area that she was not seeing with this student.

Problem Elements

Problem elements were identified by the following:

1. Discussions between the academic fieldwork coordinator and fieldwork educator regarding the background and **"mismatch"** between the student's motivation and her expectations, specifically what the "tight ship" looked like in her clinic
2. Discussions with the student about the difference between his perception of his performance and what she was expecting
3. A meeting between the fieldwork educator and the student

Problem Solving

The problem was solved by first creating a safe/neutral environment for both the student and the supervisor to reflect on the situation, and second by identifying student behaviors that the supervisor expected that would show initiation and interest.

Reflection by the supervisor was about the initial interest that students may have and to consider "performance versus passion" as an indicator of progress. The student passed his Level II Fieldwork rotation with a good recommendation from his supervisor.

LEARNING ACTIVITY 14-1

Taking Home the Message

Purpose

To analyze an actual fieldwork supervisory situation in light of the materials in the this chapter

Connections to Major Clinical Reasoning Constructs

Relates to supervisory reflection and the co-construction of reasoning between the fieldwork supervisor and the student

Directions for Learners

1 Think about a student whom you are currently supervising or have supervised in the past. (If you are currently a student, you can reflect on how your supervisor functioned within a given fieldwork situation.)

2 Read through the Take-Home Messages provided below.

3 Reflect on the degree to which the actions that occurred in the fieldwork situation you have identified are consistent with the suggestions in the Take-Home Messages.

Take-Home Messages

1 The relationship between a supervisor and a fieldwork student is a critical one, which will be remembered. (Remember your Level II supervisors?) Engage in the relationship, realize the importance of it to the student, and foster a safe environment for change and growth to occur.

2 Like a mortgage, front-end loading pays off later. Take time to make sure the student is oriented to the chart, the procedures, the population treated, and the staff of the department and team.

3 Remember, things may not always be what they seem with students. Expert supervisors can recognize patterns, but when things seem elusive, they also have the ability to generate competing hypotheses, check with the student, and reflect in order to more appropriately name and frame the actual problem. This leads to more effective and student-grounded problem-solving.

4 Experts draw upon positive or negative past experiences. One difficult experience with student supervision should not define your skills as a supervisor (or with most students). Look at the meaning that was created, how you reflected on the situation, and then consider the proverbial . . . "next time I would do this differently." You will be a better supervisor and your students will be rewarded.

5 Think of it as a strength to ask for support or "a reality check." Sometimes you may need to vent your initial frustration or disappointments before you accurately sort out the problem situation. Support or perspective from a trusted peer, fellow supervisor, or the fieldwork coordinator can be extremely helpful in understanding the situation more fully and fairly. This can make a big difference in problem solving with your student.

6 Safety first! This is paramount with our clients and patients. It is the most important concept for fostering clinical reasoning as well. Just as you want to "lock the brakes" on the wheelchair for your patient to safely physically transfer, you need to create a safe environment for dialogue and reflection to occur, which minimizes anxiety so the student can activate the learning needed to move from student to clinician.

7 While directly fostering clinical reasoning, expert supervisors use "subtitles" while they work so that they can articulate the layers of their thinking that go into complex clinical reasoning and actively translate theory into practice. Identify what your clinical reasoning is and underscore how the student is doing this.

8 When fostering clinical reasoning, expert supervisors share scripts and treatment stories from their own experience. The students may borrow these initially and build on them with their own stories to build their own clinical schemata to apply to new cases.

9 Supervisors should use developmentally sensitive questioning, building from specific diagnostic knowledge to broadening to the larger view of the particular patient's life. Expert supervisors set the groundwork for the purpose of asking "why" questions about their interventions so that students do not become defensive about their newly developing ways of thinking and doing.

10 Expert supervisors, like expert clinicians, talk about finding the *just right challenge* for their students. They try to maximize functioning of the student and bring out the best in them, as they do with their patients.

REFERENCES

American Occupational Therapy Association (1999). Standard for an accredited educational program for the occupational therapist. *American Journal of Occupational Therapy, 53*(6), 575–582.

Arling, M. (1998). Supervision in Psychotherapy: An educational experiment in integrative metalearning. *Transactional Analysis Journal, 28*(3), 224–233.

Boud, D. & Walker, D. (1998). Promoting reflection in professional courses: The challenge of context. *Studies in Higher Education, 23*, 191–206.

Brown, J. S., Collins, A. & Duguid, S. (1989). Situated cognition and the culture of learning. *Educational Researcher, 18*(1), 32–42.

Bruner, J. (1990). *Acts of meaning*. Cambridge, MA: Harvard University Press

Bruning, R. H., Schraw, G. H. & Ronning, R .R. (1999). *Cognitive psychology and instruction* (3rd ed.). Columbus, OH: Merrill.

Carr, M. & Shotwell, M. (in press). In B. A. Schell & J. W. Schell (Eds.), *Clinical reasoning in occupational therapy*. Philadelphia: Lippincott Williams & Wilkins.

Carroll, M. (1996). *Counseling supervision: Theory, skills and practice*. New York: Cassell.

Christie, B. A., Joyce, P. C. & Moeller, P. L. (1985a). Fieldwork experience, Part I: Impact on practice preference. *American Journal of Occupational Therapy, 39*(10), 671–674.

Christie, B. A., Joyce, P. C. & Moeller, P. L. (1985b). Fieldwork experience, Part II: The supervisor's dilemma. *American Journal of Occupational Therapy, 39*(10), 675–681.

Cohn, E. (1989). Fieldwork education: shaping a foundation for clinical reasoning. *American Journal of Occupational Therapy, 43*, 240–244.

Cohn, E. (2003). Interdisciplinary communication and supervision of personnel. In E. B. E. S. Crepeau, E. Cohn & B. A. Schell (Eds.), *Willard and Spackman's occupational therapy* (10th ed.). Philadelphia: Lippincott Williams & Wilkins.

Cohn, E. & Czycholl, C. (1991). Facilitating a foundation for clinical reasoning. In L. A. Crepeau & T. La Garde (Eds.), *Self-paced instruction for clinical education and supervision (SPICES)*. Rockville, MD: America Occupational Therapy Association.

Cohn, E. S. & Crist, P. (1995). Nationally speaking- Back to the future: New approaches to fieldwork education. *American Journal of Occupational Therapy, 49*(2), 103–106.

Collins, A., Brown, J. S. & Newman, S. E. (1989). Cognitive apprenticeship: Teaching the craft of reading, writing, and mathematics. In L. B. Resnick (Ed.), *Knowing, learning, and instruction: Essays in honor of Robert Glaser*. Hillsdale, NJ: Lawrence Erlbaum Associates.

Costa, D. M. & Burkhardt, A. (2003). The purpose and value of occupational therapy fieldwork education (2003 statement). *American Journal of Occupational Therapy, 57*(6), 644.

Crepeau, E. B. (1991). Achieving inter-subjective understanding: Examples from occupational therapy treatment session. *American Journal of Occupational Therapy, 45*(11), 1016–1025.

Dewey, J. (1933). *How we think: A restatement of the relation of reflective thinking to the educative process.* Lexington, MA: D.C. Heath.

Dewey, J. (1910). *How we think.* Lexington, MA: D.C. Heath.

Doherman, E. (1976). Parallel processes in supervision and psychotherapy. *Bulletin of the Menninger Clinic, 40,* 3–104.

Drake, V. & Truital, V. (1997). Clarifying ambiguity in problem fieldwork placements: Picking up and dealing with problem signals. *Australian Occupational Therapy Journal, 44,* 62–70.

Estrada, C. A., Isen, A. M. & Young, M. J. (1997). Positive affect facilitates integration of information and decreases anchoring in reasoning among physicians. *Organizational Behavior and Human Decision Processes, 72*(1), 117–135.

Ellis, M. V. & Douce, L. A. (1994). Group supervision of novice clinical supervisors. *Journal of Counseling & Development, 72*(2), 521–525.

Farber, R. S. (1998, March). Supervisory relationships: Snags, stress, and solutions. *Education Special Interest Section Quarterly, 8*(1), 2–3.

Farber, R. S. & Koenig, K. (1999). Examination of fieldwork educators' responses to challenging fieldwork situations. *Innovations in Occupational Therapy Education,* 89–104.

Farber, R. S. & Koenig, K. P. (2002, May). *Supervisory reasoning in fieldwork: Connection and implications for the development of clinical reasoning.* Paper presented at the meeting of the American Occupational Therapy Association, Miami, Florida.

Farber, R. S. & Weiss, D. (1996, May). *Clinical educators' perceptions of problematic Behaviors of fieldwork students and supervisory intervention variables.* Paper presented at the meeting of the Faculty Research Symposium, Temple University, College of Allied Health Professions, Philadelphia.

Farber, R. S. & Weiss, D. (1997, April 11). *Perceptions of problematic fieldwork behaviors and supervisory intervention.* Paper presented at the American Occupational Therapy Association Conference, Orlando.

Ferry, N. M. & Ross-Gordon, J.M.(1998). An inquiry into Schön's epistemology of practice: Exploring links between experience and reflective practice. *Adult Education Quarterly, 48*(2), 98–112.

Fleming, M. H. (1991). Clinical Reasoning in medicine compared with clinical reasoning in occupational therapy. *American Journal of Occupational Therapy, 45*(11), 988–996.

Forgas, J. P. (2001). Feeling and doing: Affective influences on interpersonal behavior. *Psychological Inquiry, 13*(1), 29 (EPSOT, downloaded, August 5, 2003).

Frederiksen, N. (1984). Implications of cognitive theory for instruction in problem solving. *Review of Educational Research, 54*(3), 363–407.

Gladwell, M. (2005). *Blink: The power of thinking without thinking.* New York: Little, Brown & Company.

Granello, D. H.(2000). Encouraging the cognitive development of supervisees: Using Bloom's taxonomy in supervision. *Counselor Education & Supervision.* (EHOST, retrieved 7/9/03)

Greeno, J. G., Collins, A. M. & Resnick, L. B. (1996). Cognition and learning. In D. C. Berliner & R. C. Calfee (Eds.), *Handbook of educational psychology* (pp. 15–46). New York: Simon & Schuster.

Holloway, E. (1995). *Clinical supervision: A systems approach.* Thousand Oaks, California: Sage.

Hooper, B, Farber, R. S. & Schell, B. B. (2002, June). *Emerging concepts in clinical reasoning: Implications for teaching and research.* Paper presented at the meeting of the World Federation of Occupational Therapy, Stockholm, Sweden.

Hummel, J. (1997) Effective fieldwork supervision: Occupational therapy student perspective. *Australian Occupational Therapy Journal, 4,* 147–157.

Kirshner, D. & Whitson, J. (Eds.). (1997). *Situated cognition: Social, semiotic, and psychological perspectives.* Mahweh, NJ: Lawrence Erlbaum Associates.

Koenig, K. P. & Farber, R. S. (2000). *Components of supervisory reasoning: Implications for fieldwork educators' development.* American Occupational Therapy Association Annual Conference, Seattle, WA.

Kouloumpi, M., Ryan, S. & Savaris, I. (2002). *From psychiatric asylum to mental health hospitals: Clinical reasoning in transition.* (2002). Paper presented at the meeting of the World Federation of Occupational Therapy, Stockholm, Sweden.

Kramer, P. (1998). Questions (but no answers) about clinical reasoning and student supervision. *Education Special Interest Newsletter 4,* 6.

Lave, J. & Wenger, E. (1991). *Situated learning: Legitimate peripheral participation.* Cambridge, England: Cambridge University Press.

Loganbill, C., Hardy, E. & Delworth, U. (1982). Supervision: A conceptual model. *The Counseling Psychologist, 10*(1), 3–42.

Martin, M. (1996). How reflective is student supervision? A study of supervision in action. *British Journal of Occupational Therapy, 59*(5), 229–232.

McAlpine, L., Weston, C., Beauchamp, J., Wiseman, C. & Beauchamp, C. (1999). Building a metacognitive model of reflection. *Higher Education, 37*, 105–131.

Morrow, K. A. & Deidan, C. T. (1992). Bias in the counseling process: How to recognize and avoid it. *Journal of Counseling & Development, 70*(5), 571–577.

Neistadt, M. E. (1998). Teaching clinical reasoning as a thinking frame. *American Journal of Occupational Therapy, 52*(3), 221–229.

Nelson, M. L. & Neufelt, S. A, (1998). The pedagogy of counseling: A critical examination. *Counselor Education & Supervision, 38*(2), 70–89.

Neufeldt, S. A. (1997). A social constructivist approach to counseling supervision. In T. L. Sexton & N. L. Griffin (Eds.), *Constructivist thinking in counseling practice, research and training.* New York: Teachers College Press

Newell, A. (1990). *Unified theories of cognition.* Cambridge, MA: Harvard University Press.

Newell, A. & Simon, H. (1972). *Human problem solving.* Englewood Cliffs, NJ: Prentice-Hall.

Norman, G. (2005). Research in clinical reasoning: Past history and current trends. *Medical Education, 39*(4), 418–427.

O'Byrne, K. & Rosenberg, J. I. (1998). The practice of supervision: A sociocultural perspective. *Counselor Education and Supervision, 38*, 32–42.

Paterson & Adamson. (2001). An international study of educational approaches to clinical reasoning. *British Journal of Occupational Therapy, 64*(8), 403–405.

Robertson, L. J. (1996). Clinical reasoning, Part 2: Novice/expert differences. *British Journal of Occupational Therapy, 59*(5), 212–232.

Rogoff, B. (1990). *Apprenticeship in thinking.* Oxford: Oxford University Press.

Ronnestad, M. H. & Skovholt, T. M. (1993). Supervision of beginning and advanced graduate students of counseling and psychotherapy. *Journal of Counseling & Development, 71*(4), 396–405.

Schell, B. (2003). In E. B., Crepeau, E. S. Cohn & B. A. Schell (Eds.), *Willard & Spackman's occupational therapy* (10th ed.). Philadelphia: Lippincott Williams & Wilkins.

Schell, B. A. & Cervero, R. M. (1993). Clinical reasoning in occupational therapy: An integrative review. *American Journal of Occupational Therapy, 47*(7), 605–610.

Schön, D. (1987). *Educating the reflective practitioner.* San Francisco: Jossey-Bass.

Schön, D. (1983). *The reflective practitioner.* London: Temple Smith.

Sladyk, K. (1997). *Clinical reasoning and reflective practice: Influence of fieldwork.* Dissertation, University of Connecticut.

Sladyk, K. & Sheckley, B. (2000). Clinical reasoning and reflective practice: Implications of fieldwork activities. *Occupational Therapy in Health Care, 13*(1), 11–22.

Stoltenberg. C. (November 2005). Enhancing professional competence through developmental supervision. *American Psychologist,* 857–864.

Sweeney, G., Webley P. & Treacher, A. (2001a). Supervision in occupational therapy, Part 1: The supervisor's anxieties. *British Journal of Occupational Therapy, 64*(7), 337–345.

Sweeney, G., Webley, P. & Treacher, A. (2001b). Supervision in occupational therapy, Part 2: The supervisees dilemma. *British Journal of Occupational Therapy, 64*(8), 380–386.

Sweeney, G., Webley, P. & Treacher, A. (2001c). Supervision in occupational therapy, Part 3: Accommodating the supervisor and the supervisee. *British Journal of Occupational Therapy, 64*(9), 426–43.

Tickle-Degan L. & Puccinelli, N. M.(1999). *Occupational Therapy Journal of Research, 19*(1), 18–39.

Van der Heijden, B. I. J. M. (2002). Individual career initiatives and their influence upon professional expertise development throughout the career. [references]. *International Journal of Training and Development, 6*(2), 54–79.

Wertheimer, M. (1959). *Productive thinking.* New York: Harper & Row.

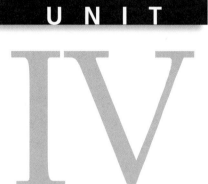

UNIT

IV

Professional Reasoning Research

Review of Methodologies for Researching Clinical Reasoning

Carolyn A. Unsworth

CHAPTER OUTLINE

OBJECTIVES

After reading this chapter, the learner will be able to:

1 Understand the differences between a qualitative and quantitative approach to researching clinical reasoning and decision making.
2 Describe a range of approaches that a researcher may take when collecting and analyzing clinical reasoning data.
3 Articulate some of the advantages and disadvantages of different approaches to data collection and analysis.
4 Describe several of the qualitative theoretical frameworks that could guide a clinical reasoning study, and describe the associated techniques used to analyze data.
5 Reflect on the methods that he might choose to adopt in future studies of clinical reasoning.

KEY TERMS

Concurrent report	Grounded theory	Phenomenology
Retrospective report	Ethnography	Action research

I n a delightful book on the "wisdom of crowds" when making decisions, James Surowiecki (2004) recounts the tale of Francis Galton, a British scientist. Galton believed that people were generally not very intelligent. In 1906, Galton attended the West of England Fat Stock and Poultry Exhibition, which included a competition to guess the weight of a plump ox on display after being slaughtered and dressed. A total of 800 people tried their luck. Although many of the competitors were farmers and butchers who could be considered experts in the field, many others had no knowledge of livestock at all. Interested in how the competition results could be used to further support his hypothesis, Galton borrowed the tickets from the organizers and ran a series of tests with the 787 legible tickets. Among other things he calculated the mean weight guessed by the crowd. Galton assumed that this combination of a few good guesses with a lot of mediocre guesses and many stupid ones would be way off the mark. However, Galton was wrong. The average guess of the crowd that day was 1,197 pounds. The actual weight of the slaughtered and dressed ox was 1,198 pounds. Surowiecki (2004) used this story (among many other detailed examples) to support his thesis that a crowd's judgment can be almost perfect. However, what is also illustrated is that human decisions can be readily studied and that judgments can be scored and analyzed mathematically. What is not so apparent is how the individuals arrived at their guess of the ox's weight. In other words, what was their *reasoning*, and how can we *study* an individual's reasoning.

Thinking About Thinking 15-1

As the mind learns to understand more complicated combinations of ideas, simpler formulae soon reduce their complexity; so truths that were discovered only by great effort, that could at first only be understood by men capable of profound thought, are soon developed and proved by methods that are not beyond the reach of common intelligence. The strength and the limits of man's intelligence may remain unaltered; and yet the instruments that he uses will increase and improve, the language that fixes and determines his ideas will acquire greater breadth and precision and, unlike mechanics where an increase of force means a decrease of speed, the methods that lead genius to the discovery of truth increase at once the force and the speed of its operations.

—*Marie Jean Antoine Nicolas Caritat*
Marquis de Condorcet, 1743–1794

Guessing an ox's weight for sport is a long way from the clinic and the importance of the reasoning processes and decisions made by clinicians on a daily basis. Throughout this text, the complexity of clinical and professional reasoning has been explored. The purpose of this chapter is to examine some of the methods that can be used to study clinical reasoning.* The chapter is unique in the field, since an overview of all the frameworks, data collection methods, and analysis techniques used in clinical reasoning research are co-located. The chapter opens by examining the differences between studying clinical decision making and clinical reasoning. From there, methods of accessing what clinicians are thinking are documented, such as the think-aloud procedure, written notes, free recall, and audio- and video-assisted recall. A novel method when using video involving a head-mounted camera is then described, and details are provided on a modified approach to debriefing using video-assisted recall. Research

---

*The term "clinical reasoning" is used here, as it is the term found in the literature being summarized in this chapter.

examples, together with anecdotes from the author's experience of using these methods, illustrate the text. An overview is then provided of the kinds of theoretical frameworks for conducting qualitative research and the kinds of data analysis approaches used with these frameworks. Although information on the theoretical frameworks for clinical reasoning research usually precedes a discussion of data collection techniques, in this chapter this material comes last so that the reader is familiar with the kind of data that might be collected before considering the ways these data can be treated. No single method is advocated; rather it is proposed that research using a variety of methods will build the most comprehensive understanding of clinical reasoning. The chapter concludes with a series of worksheets that the reader can use to further develop knowledge of the material covered.

ASKING QUESTIONS TO EXPLORE WHAT *IS* CLINICAL REASONING

Before thinking about what methods may be used to study clinical reasoning, the researcher must first ask what is being researched and develop either the area for study, or pose specific questions to be answered. The research questions we need to answer to fully explore and understand clinical reasoning and decision making are endless, including the following examples:

- How do clinicians reason in everyday practice concerning assessment, interventions, and discharge with their clients?
- What is the thinking that guides a therapist to select which splint to manufacture for a client with rheumatoid arthritis?
- How do a therapist's personal beliefs and ethics shape clinical reasoning?

In the area of clinical reasoning and decision making, the researcher may use a quantitative approach with a very focused research question, such as "What information do occupational therapists use when determining referral prioritization for clients with mental health problems?" (Harries & Harries, 2001; Harries & Gilhooley, 2003a, 2003b). On the other hand, using a more qualitative approach, the researcher may simply ask, "What is clinical reasoning," as posed in one of the foundation studies in the field (Mattingly & Fleming, 1994). The nature of the questioning or the topic for study guides the selection of methodological framework and specific data collection and analysis techniques. Quantitative approaches are useful when the question is concerned with measuring something and quantities or amounts are compared, or when information provided as data can be numbered in some way. Qualitative approaches are favored when there is a need to investigate human behavior, and data take the form of descriptions sometimes referred to as "thick description." When using a qualitative approach, Morse and Field (1995) suggest that questions relating to meaning (eliciting the essence of experience) are best explored using a phenomenological approach; this was the approach adopted by Mattingly and Fleming (1994). Descriptive questions in which the researcher attempts to access questions of values, beliefs, and practices of a group are best studied using ethnography. For example, research that examines how a therapist's personal beliefs and worldview impact or influence reasoning can be studied from this perspective (Unsworth, 2004). Process questions that examine individuals' experiences over time may be studied using grounded theory, and questions regarding verbal interaction and dialogue are best studied using techniques such as discourse analysis (Morse & Field, 1995). Throughout this chapter, the reader will be able to consider the different kinds of methods used (predominantly in the qualitative research tradition) to study clinical reasoning and thus be in the best position to select the most suitable approach when conducting his/her own research on clinical reasoning.

STUDIES OF MEDICAL DECISION MAKING VERSUS CLINICAL REASONING

The focus here is on methods supporting research on clinical reasoning. However, to contextualize these approaches, an overview is initially provided of the quantitative types of methods used in medical decision making. A basic knowledge of how diagnostic and other medical decisions are studied enables the reader to compare and contrast these approaches and consider the advantages and disadvantages of the qualitative approaches primarily used in the study of clinical reasoning.

A Quantitative Approach: Methods for Investigating Medical Decision Making

Clinical practice is driven by decisions. Every day health professionals, including occupational therapists, make important decisions such as which assessments to use with a client, identification of client occupational performance difficulties (referred to as a diagnosis in medical decision making), what interventions to offer, when to offer these, and when to stop treating. Decision making refers to the process of arriving at a resolution to behave in a certain way and involves making a choice between alternatives through the use of judgment. Decision making is generally viewed as objective and scientific; hence, research in this field is often quantitative and involves mathematically mapping decisions that were made so they can be examined and debated.

There is a long history of studying medical decisions (diagnosis in particular) using decision-making theories (Klein, Orasanu, Claderwood & Zsambok, 1993; Hammond, McClelland & Mumpower, 1980), and entire journals such as *Medical Decision Making* are devoted to the topic. In these kinds of studies, clinicians are generally presented with carefully constructed written case vignettes that describe the client and with relevant information about their medical and social status. Hence, the research environment and the kinds of information presented are controlled by the researchers and can therefore be more easily dissected for analysis (e.g., see Elstein, Shulman & Sprafka, 1978; Fonteyn & Fisher, 1995; Unsworth, Thomas & Greenwood, 1995). There are essentially two theoretical approaches to studying medical decision making: *prescriptive* and *descriptive*. Prescriptive approaches are primarily concerned with prescribing how decisions ought to be made and focus on the outcomes and results of decision processes. Using a Bayesian approach, researchers investigate how clinicians acquire and manipulate probability information. In an extension of this approach referred to as Psychological Decision Theory, researchers examine how individuals use probability information to make decisions. Behavioral Decision Theory attempts to investigate decisions by combining information about the chances of certain outcomes and their desirability (Thomas, Wearing & Bennett, 1991).

In contrast, descriptive approaches are concerned with describing how decisions are actually made. Social Judgment Theory, for example, investigates how decision makers combine and weight information when making judgments. Social Judgment Theory has been used in occupational therapy research investigating discrete decisions such as my own research investigating housing recommendations made for clients following stroke (Unsworth & Thomas, 1993; Unsworth, Thomas & Greenwood, 1995; Unsworth, Thomas & Greenwood, 1997) and rehabilitation admission decisions for these clients (Unsworth, 2001a). Studies using both descriptive or prescriptive approaches usually involve collecting response data which are easily scored, mostly concerned with input-output connections and do not usually involve direct examination of the reasoning processes supporting these connections (Patel & Arocha, 2000). In addition, as in the example of judging the weight of an ox as described in the chapter introduction, there is often an attempt to obtain a gross average across individuals making the judgment rather than study individual thought processes in detail. However, relatively few isolated decisions in occupational therapy lend themselves easily to such quantitative methods of study. Of far more usefulness to our profession are the more qualitative theoretical approaches and methods developed to study clinical reasoning.

A Qualitative Approach: Methods for Investigating Clinical Reasoning

Clinical reasoning has been explored in detail in this text, but it may be simply defined as the thinking processes of therapists when undertaking a therapeutic practice. Although occupational therapists have written extensively about clinical reasoning over the past 20 years, we are still just at the beginning of understanding what clinical reasoning is and its importance to practice (Unsworth, 2004). Mattingly and Fleming (1994) describe clinical reasoning as being a practical know-how that puts theoretical knowledge into practice and as a complex (yet often common sense) way of thinking to find what is best for each client. Clinical reasoning encompasses how therapists think when planning to be with a client, when with a client, and afterward when reflecting on therapy. It involves intuition, judgment, empathy, and common sense (Unsworth, 2004). The kinds of quantitative methods that have traditionally been used to study medical decision making have limited application in occupational therapy research, since our profession is more interested in how therapists "think-in-action" rather than diagnose. Accessing therapists' clinical reasoning is no easy task because these cognitive processes can be studied only indirectly. Hence, research on clinical reasoning is often qualitative.

Before the 1950s, a more behavioristic approach to understanding reasoning was taken. Emphasis was placed on developing instruments to assess a clinician's performance rather than describing the clinician's actual reasoning. From the late 1950s on, researchers such as Newell and Simon (1972) and Elstein, Shulman, and Sprafka (1978) aimed to characterize clinical reasoning and to describe the knowledge and processes used in reasoning. Hence, researchers wanted to access the clinician's cognitive processes and thus based their research on an information-processing approach. In fact, an information-processing approach, which views human cognition as a "... sequence of internal states successively transformed by a series of information processes" (Ericsson & Simon, 1993, p. 11), forms the basis for most clinical studies of reasoning and thinking today (see Chapter 3 for an in-depth discussion of information processing). The information-processing model assumes that recently acquired information (e.g., in a newly completed clinical session) is kept in short-term memory and is directly accessible for processing, for example, to produce verbal reports. Within this tradition, researchers have also emphasized the study of interactions (as occurs between client and clinician) as a form of reasoning. This interpretive tradition forms the basis for well-known research by Benner (1984); Benner, Hooper-Kyriakidis, and Stanard (1999); and Benner, Tanner, and Chesla (1996) on clinical reasoning and the development of expertise in nursing. This research approach has also given rise to studies of situated cognition, which is concerned with interpreting cognitive functions such as clinical reasoning as part of an interaction between a person and his/her environment.

Although different methods may be used to collect and analyze data, a common approach used by researchers in the field is to compare the clinical reasoning of novices and experts. Through such contrastive methods, patterns of thinking can be most clearly juxtaposed and therefore understood. In particular, educators can use information arising from such research when training novices. Research examples comparing the clinical reasoning of novices and experts include the work of Benner (1984) and Greenwood and King (1995) in nursing; Unsworth (2001b), Strong, Gilbert, Cassidy, and Bennett (1995), and Gibson et al. (2000) in occupational therapy; and Embrey et al. (1996) in physical therapy. Although the methods used to study clinical reasoning are detailed below, the reader should note that researchers often add the methodological dimension of contrasting novice and expert clinician reasoning.

METHODS FOR ACQUIRING CLINICAL REASONING DATA

The assumption is usually made that professionals in a number of fields know more than they can say (Schön, 1983). However, as shown by Schön (1983), among others, when confronted with an account of their performance these practitioners often reveal a capacity to articulate this tacit knowledge (Schön, 1983). This section of the review outlines five methods suitable for eliciting therapists' reasoning. Two of these methods are described as concurrent, since they collect data as the clinician reasons in relation to a real or simulated client. These two approaches are asking therapists to write notes as they solve a problem and use the think-aloud technique in which the therapist provides a verbal commentary during a therapy session. The remaining three approaches are described as retrospective because they demand the clinician to recount reasoning after it has occurred. These approaches are known as free recall (in which the therapist presents his or her reasoning about a therapy session afterwards from memory), audio-assisted recall (in which the therapist listens to an audiotape of the therapy session and uses this to aid recall of his or her reasoning processes), and video-assisted recall (in which video footage is used to prompt recall of his or her reasoning processes).

Advantages and limitations of these approaches are provided, and the text is illustrated with examples from occupational therapy and other allied heath research. Finally, information is provided concerning the use of interviews to ask clinicians for information about and descriptions of their reasoning.

Concurrent Reports

Written Notes Using Vignettes

One of the simplest methods of accessing a therapist's clinical reasoning is to ask her/him to write notes about what s/he is thinking while reviewing a written case vignette. For example, Roberts (1996) examined the reasoning processes of 38 occupational therapists by asking them to write their thoughts in response to a written referral for a new client. This approach has the advantage of requiring very little setup, and the researcher has complete control over the problem environment by selecting which information variables to include in the vignette.

Think Aloud

The term "think aloud" is a straightforward description of this method in which the therapist is asked to talk while thinking, when working with a real or simulated client or with written case notes. This method of capturing clinical reasoning data was first described by Newell and Simon in 1972 and is presented in detail in Ericsson and Simon (1993). Although this method can be used concurrently in the clinic, think aloud is more commonly used by researchers as a retrospective approach in which the clinician talks through their reasoning directly after the therapy session ends. Ericsson and Simon (1993) describe three different levels at which subjects may verbalize thought processes, and their content:

Level 1 verbalizations—the therapist undertakes a usual therapy session with the client, but is instructed to verbalize the thoughts and intentions that are within his or her "current sphere." An advantage of this approach is that the therapist need expend no special effort to communicate his/her thoughts; however, since complete sentences may not be used and idiosyncratic statements may be made, it may be difficult for the researcher to fully comprehend exactly what the therapist is saying. It is important that therapists are requested to focus on the therapy session as a whole when verbalizing rather than explaining verbally each part of the session. Most researchers using the think-aloud approach aim to attain Level 1 verbalizations from their subjects.

Level 2 verbalizations—refers to the situation in which the therapist is required to translate information in the therapy session into language before thinking out loud. This occurs when the therapist has to process information that is nonverbal, such as odor, sounds, or movements. Level II verbalizations do not bring new information to the subject's attention, but explicate information that is held internally by the subject (Ericsson & Simon, 1993). For example, when describing the movements of a client with Huntington's chorea, the therapist has to process information about the movements and then translate these into language.

Level 3 verbalizations—refers to requests to verbalize specific information such as explanations or reasons (Ericsson & Simon, 1993). For example, the therapist may be asked to explain the positioning of a client during fabrication of a splint. Because therapists usually position the client automatically, requests to reason about this require additional processing. Level 3 verbalizations require the therapist not only to articulate current ideas and hypotheses, but to link these with stored thoughts and information. Requesting Level 3 verbalizations can change the subject's cognitive processes and thus may alter his or her performance.

When using the think-aloud method, the researcher needs to be present to transcribe the therapist's commentary verbatim, or a video or audiotape is made of the session and transcribed at a later point. The think-aloud method was not developed specifically for clinical use, and Ericsson and Simon (1984) provide many examples of the technique being used when subjects solve mathematical problems or make retail choices. Therefore, using this method to capture clinical reasoning data is limited to the few situations in which the therapist can speak in an uncensored manner in front of the client. This may be possible when manufacturing a splint or when working with clients who are in coma, although evidence suggests that even comatose patients process information. In fact, it may be unethical in many instances for the therapist to be completely candid about his or her thoughts in front of the client. For example, Greenwood and King (1995) asked the nurses in their study to selectively filter out any distressing information when providing think-aloud reports at the patient's bedside. Because of the difficulties associated with thinking aloud in front of the client, this approach to data collection is more common when simulated clients, or written case studies, are used (Elstein, Shulman & Sprafka, 1978; Fonteyn & Fisher, 1995). For example, Lamond and colleagues (1996) used written case vignettes with the think-aloud method to establish the sources of information that acute care nurses used when making assessment judgments about their patients. Sources of patient-related information such as verbal interaction and file notes, were included in the vignettes to enhance ecological validity.

Ericsson and Simon (1993) developed Verbal Protocol Analysis (VPA) to analyze think-aloud data, and this approach is described in the last section of the chapter. In brief, when using VPA, it is the job of the researcher to identify the participant's reasoning processes and related stimuli and responses, rather than the participant's. Hence, the researcher theorizes about the causes and consequences of the therapist's knowledge state (Carroll & Johnson, 1990; Ericsson & Simon, 1993; Newell & Simon, 1972). The analysis involves coding and mapping the subject's verbalizations. However, in the health sciences literature, researchers often analyze concurrent or retrospective think-aloud data within one of the qualitative frameworks such as phenomenology or grounded theory (sometimes including the participants in the analysis) rather than using VPA. For example, in my own clinical reasoning research, I have used the retrospective think-aloud technique to gather data, but then analyzed the data within an ethnographic framework using thematic analysis techniques (Unsworth 2001b; Unsworth 2004; Unsworth 2005). Mattingly and Fleming used the retrospective think-aloud technique, but as part of an action research approach from a phenomenological perspective. In addition, many clinical researchers, including myself, choose to include Level 2 or 3 verbalizations in the data collection whereas a true think-aloud technique with VPA relies solely on the collection of Level 1 verbalizations.

Limitations Associated with Concurrent Reports

When considering written notes using vignettes, the validity of data collected using **concurrent reports** relies on the therapist's ability to write about his or her thought processes. As noted by Roberts (1996), writing one's thoughts can be more difficult than verbalizing them, given the natural tendency to censor what is documented in writing and the more laborious nature of writing down rapid thought processes, which may lead to hasty abbreviations. It can also be argued that clinical reasoning inspired by written cases lacks ecological validity, since vignettes cannot present all the information the therapist has in the real environment, nor reproduce the complex and dynamic environment in which real clinical reasoning occurs (Unsworth, 2001c).

As noted earlier, another limitation of the concurrent think-aloud technique in the clinic is the small number of clients with whom therapists can speak freely. However, the major limitation of this approach is that simply "speaking while thinking" can actually change the subject's underlying thought processes. This may be due to the added insights that talking through a problem may afford, or the intrusive and disruptive nature of having to speak out loud when the therapist is normally silent (Ericsson & Simon, 1993). Hence, the act of speaking may interfere with or even change the course of the therapy session. We may be conscious of this or completely unaware that we are changing what we are actually thinking. Therefore, retrospective reports, in which participants are required to recount their reasoning after the therapy session, are far more common.

Retrospective Reports

In ideal situations, the **retrospective report** of a therapy session occurs directly after the session concludes. This is done to ensure that as much information from the session as possible is retained in the participant's short-term memory. Ericsson and Simon (1993) report that retrospective reports on any immediately preceding cognitive activity can be accessed and described without the experimenter needing to instruct the participant on what information to retrieve. The general instruction of "report everything you can remember about your thoughts during the last therapy session" can be given. If the participant is asked to recall his/her thinking without any other prompting than verbal encouragement from the researcher, then the method is described as free recall. If the therapist is prompted to recall while listening to an audio recording of the session, then the method is described as audio-assisted recall; if the therapist watches a video recording of a session, then this is referred to as video-assisted recall. In all cases, the researcher either transcribes or makes notes directly, or an audiotape or videotape (explained later) is made of the clinician's thoughts. These three techniques are sometimes referred to as retrospective think-aloud procedures (Embrey, Guthrie, White & Dietz 1996). In a true retrospective think-aloud approach, the subject is required to provide current sphere thinking (i.e., the subject's thoughts during the therapy session) and does not provide information concerning his or her reasoning (Unsworth, 2001c). However, as illustrated in the research examples below, free, audio- and video-assisted recall methods used in clinical research generally require the subject to talk about what happened, as well as the reasoning related to the session (i.e., provide Level 2 and/or Level 3 verbalizations).

Free Recall

When the researcher is gathering data using free recall, the therapist is asked to recount the events of therapy (and in some cases their reasoning) after the session ends (Carroll & Johnson, 1990). When eliciting a free-recall report, the researcher may give a prompt such as ". . . tell me what you were thinking at each moment during the therapy session you have just completed." The main advantage of this approach to data collection is that no equipment is introduced into the treatment setting; however, the major disadvantage is that the therapist must rely solely on memory to tell the therapy story (and recount his or her reasoning).

For example, in a study that described the reasoning and decision-making processes of experienced occupational therapists when deciding on intervention for a familiar type of case, Hagedorn (1996) used the free-recall technique. Hagedorn asked therapists to tape record an account of their decision-making processes and conclusions reached as ". . . near in time to the point of decision making as possible" (p. 217). The tapes were then transcribed and subjected to qualitative analysis using immersion and crystallization. Member-checking was also undertaken using follow-up interviews to ensure the accuracy of the emerging interpretation. The free-recall technique was also used by Barnitt and Partridge (1997) when investigating the ethical reasoning of a sample of physical and occupational therapists. These researchers interviewed therapists and asked, "Can you tell me the story of an ethical dilemma you have experienced at work during the past six months" (1997, p.182). Each interview was tape recorded, and the 16 participants in this study were also involved in the data analysis, which drew on the multiple readings methods from hermeneutic phenomenology. Because the researchers interviewed therapists quite some time after the incident and asked for their ethical reasoning specifically related to the incident, the data collected may be described as Level 3 verbalizations (Ericsson & Simon, 1993). In other words, the therapist's recollections included not only information about the incident, but also his/her reasoning, and reflections about their reasoning and their satisfaction with this. Although Hagedorn (1996) and Barnitt and Partridge (1997) asked participants to free-recall events, they also used an interview technique to obtain information about clinical reasoning, and this approach is described later in the chapter.

Audio-Assisted Recall

When using the audio-assisted recall method, researchers audiotape the therapy session and play this back to prompt the therapist's recall of conversations and events (and associated reasoning) immediately after the session ends (Carroll & Johnson, 1990; Meichenbaum & Butler, 1979). A new audiotape or written notes are then made by the researcher regarding the participant's recollections of events and supporting reasoning. This new audiotape is then transcribed, and this transcript (or the written notes) forms the data for analysis. Although an audiotape recorder is usually unobtrusive in the therapy setting, a limitation of this approach is that most individuals are used to information being presented in visual formats. Hence, it is believed that observations of the participant's performance triggers the best recall of reasoning, and therefore videotapes are more commonly used to prompt therapist recall of thinking and reasoning.

Video-Assisted Recall

The use of a videotape of a clinical session to prompt recall of mental events was first described by Kagan (1976) as a means of assisting counselors to improve their interpersonal skills. This method comprises three steps: (1) the therapist/ client interaction is captured using a video camera, (2) the video is shown to the therapist to aid recall, and (3) the resulting thinking and reasoning of the therapist are recorded and the resulting transcript forms the data for analysis. These processes are described in detail below.

Capturing Therapy Sessions Using Video

Therapist and client interactions can be captured by video to prompt therapist reasoning, using a stand-alone video camera (Embrey et al., 1996; Mattingly & Fleming, 1994) or head-mounted video camera (Unsworth, 2001c). When using a stand-alone video camera (in which the video camera is mounted on a tripod), video footage is captured of both therapist and client during a clinical session. For example, Mattingly and Fleming (1994) conducted an in-depth study of 14 occupational therapists from a physical rehabilitation setting in Boston using a standard stand-alone video camera. They used a variety of research methods to study clinical reasoning including participant observation, in-depth interviews, and videotaping clinical sessions with therapists and clients using a stand-alone video camera. A total of 30 videotapes of clinical interactions were shot and transcriptions made from the resulting therapist debriefing sessions. However, the use of a video camera on a tripod to capture data has several limitations, including the following:

1. Difficulty recording the detail of an activity (for example on a table top), since the camera is usually placed some distance away from the action.
2. If the therapist and client move around during the session, a researcher or camera operator needs to be present to ensure that the subjects are in center view; having this other person present may be intrusive or disruptive.
3. Data are captured from the camera's perspective, which is different from that of the therapist, which is believed to impair the therapist's capacity to recall his or her reasoning when viewing the videotape (Omodei & McLennan, 1994).

When using a head-mounted video camera to capture a therapy session, the video camera is attached to a headband worn by the clinician, and a cord running at the back of the headband connects the camera to the video unit (handycam), which is worn in a waist pouch. With this approach to videotaping the session, the clinician can move around freely, the researcher does not need to be present, and the camera is close to the action and captures footage from the viewpoint of the therapist (Unsworth, 2001c). Hence, the use of a head-mounted video camera overcomes all the limitations of a stand-alone video camera, as listed above. When viewing footage from a head-mounted video camera, the therapist "sees" exactly what he or she saw as therapy unfolded (i.e., has the same visual and cognitive perspective); this is believed to significantly enhance reasoning recall (Omodei & McLennan, 1994). Omodei and McLennan argue that having the camera focus on the environment rather than the subject (therapist) minimizes self-awareness and enhances psychological immersion in the original events. Kipper (1986) also demonstrated that video footage from a camera that moves through the environment as if it were a human visual system is much more informative for the viewer than traditional video footage.

The camera used in this method can be any kind of small security or computer-type of camera available through electronics stores. The headband is the type worn by hikers and caving enthusiasts who need to wear a lamp on their head to have both hands free. The video recorder contained in the waist pouch may be any of the small "handycam" units available today. No external microphone is required because the microphone built into the video recorder is powerful enough to record sound. Researchers and technical officers at La Trobe University and Swinburne University of Technology in Melbourne, Australia, have been developing this equipment for use in sporting and health research since 1995. The apparatus used in my own research, as shown in *Figure 15-1*, was built at La Trobe University.

One disadvantage of using video cameras to capture therapy sessions to aid recall is that the presence of a camera on a tripod or on the therapist's head may be distracting to the client and therapist. However, in my experience in using

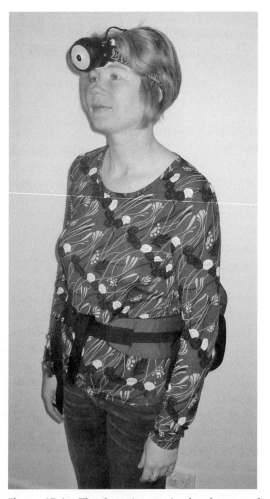

Figure 15-1 The therapist wearing head-mounted camera and video (handycam located in waist bag).

both techniques, both therapists and clients quickly forget about the camera and carry on with the session as usual. In addition, emerging technology options are likely to permit the use of less distracting video capture options.

DEBRIEFING USING VIDEO-ASSISTED RECALL

Having captured the therapy session on video using either a standard stand-alone or head-mounted camera system, the therapist is then required to watch the footage as soon as possible and recount his or her thinking and reasoning. The researcher may assist the therapist using nondirective prompts such as "Say some more about what you are considering doing now" or "What else is going on in your mind here?" (Kagan, 1976). The kinds of prompts depend on the kind of framework the researcher is working in and the level of verbalizations required. Three main approaches to prompting are generally reported in the clinical reasoning literature.

In the most common approach to prompting, the researcher attempts to capture the therapist's reasoning without any evaluation of that reasoning. The therapist is instructed to "recall" rather than "evaluate" the session. For example, the therapist may comment ". . . just now, the client seems to look a bit tired and . . . well . . . fed up, so I thought it would be a good moment to take a break and I'm just explaining to the client how well she is doing, to reinforce her attempts, and then I'll continue on in a moment." However, many therapists find it difficult to refrain from critically analyzing their performance, and therapists are discouraged from making the following kinds of evaluative comments ". . . I probably should have changed activities about five minutes ago, as it seems she just got too disheartened working on this activity." A therapist may become less self-conscious and critical if the researcher reassures the therapists that s/he is not critical of the therapist's performance. This kind of critical reflection on reasoning might form part of a future evaluation of the data or may be used in the second kind of approach to prompting, where the therapist is required to review their performance. Ericsson and Simon (1993) refer to this second approach as requiring Level 3 verbalization. For example, in an 8-year study of the clinical reasoning of 130 nurses working in critical care, Benner, Hooper-Kyriakidis and Standard (1999) prompted retrospective reports with questions such as, "What are you thinking about in this situation?" "What are you watching out for in this situation?" "What are you feeling about this situation?" "Is the situation going as expected?" (1999, p. 559).

A third approach to prompt therapist reasoning was described by Yinger (1986). Yinger suggested that subjects should focus on their immediate thoughts when providing an account of a session rather than trying to remember their thoughts at the time of the actual event. Yinger argued that individuals gain new cues from viewing a video that were not used during the event. If using this kind of approach, the research might instruct the therapist to "verbalize what you are thinking at this point in time, not what you may have been thinking during the treatment session" (Embrey et al., 1996, p. 24). For additional descriptions of the prompts that can be used to elicit thinking and reasoning, the reader is also referred to Ericsson and Simon (1993).

As the therapist watches the video recording of his/her session, the researcher must select a method for recording the therapist's verbalizations, because these utterances form the data for analysis. Most researchers capture the therapist's reasoning by taking notes and/or audio recording his or her commentary; this was the approach used by Mattingly and Fleming (1994). Similarly, Alnervik and Sviden (1996) asked five therapists to watch a videotape of one of their treatment sessions on two occasions. On the first viewing, the therapists were asked to narrate what they saw happening. On the second viewing, the therapists were asked to describe the thoughts and considerations on which their clinical decisions were based (in other words, to provide Level 3 verbalizations). In both instances, audiotapes were made of the resulting descriptions and reasoning and these were transcribed for analysis.

Instead of making an audio recording of therapist verbalizations of their thinking and reasoning, a new video recording can be made. This new video contains the video footage of the therapy session as captured using a head-mounted camera or standard video camera, together with a new soundtrack of the therapist's reasoning. In other words, the therapist's verbal debriefing of the therapy session is superimposed onto the video of the unfolding therapy session. When undertaking the debriefing, the original audio soundtrack of the video is turned down very low so that the therapist can still hear what is said (as a prompt for their reasoning), but his/her description of, and reasoning supporting the session, can be clearly heard on the new videotape. The therapist is given the remote control for the video player during the debriefing session and is asked to pause the video at any point where the description and reasoning may take longer than the running of the film. The advantage of this approach to data capture is that the researcher has the added visual perspective of what was happening as the clinician describes the session and his/her reasoning, when analyzing the data. The circuitry required to capture data in this form is illustrated in *Figure 15-2*.

In my own research, I use a head-mounted video camera to record therapy sessions, and a video-prompted debrief added to a new video-tape to form the data for analysis. For example, differences in the clinical reasoning of experts and novices (Unsworth 2001b) and current conceptualizations of clinical reasoning

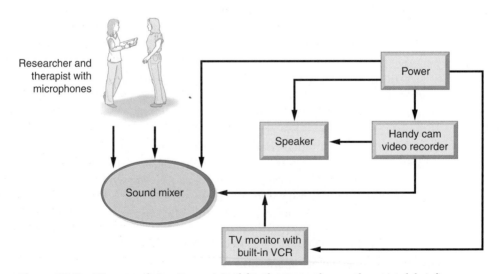

Figure 15-2 Diagram of circuitry required for the researcher or therapist debriefing.

(Unsworth 2004; Unsworth, 2005) have been studied using a sample of 15 therapists from several different physical rehabilitation settings. The data were collected and analyzed within a focused ethnographic framework (as described in the final section of the chapter). In addition, a colleague and I have used this method to study the clinical reasoning of five expert and five novice community health occupational therapists (CHOT) during home visits (Mitchell & Unsworth, 2005). A head-mounted video camera was used to record the visits, followed by subjects verbally reporting their clinical reasoning using a video-assisted debrief method. The transcripts from these verbal reports were analyzed quantitatively and qualitatively.

As described earlier, one of the main advantages of a head-mounted video camera to capture footage and video-assisted recall to prompt thinking and clinical reasoning is that the therapist has a clear picture of the session from his or her own point of view. Omodei and McLennan (1994) reported that subjects involved in competitive orienteering (a sport in which participants find their way in unfamiliar countryside using a map and compass) recollected and described between two and four times the amount of detail when using own-point-of-view video-assisted recall compared with free recall. However, a limitation of this approach is that some therapists find the speed and movement of the videotape difficult to watch. In fact, some therapists who have made small rapid head movements during the filming report feeling nauseous (similar to motion sickness) when watching the resulting videotape. Therefore, although Omodei and McLennan (1994) document that most people report rapid perceptual adaptation to on-screen movement, this method of data filming may be unsuitable for use with some therapists. Finally, when using a head-mounted video camera, the therapist's facial expressions are not captured. Two therapists involved in my own research have reported that they find viewing their own expressions useful to prompt recall of thinking and reasoning.

Limitations Associated with Retrospective Reports

As Newell and Simon (1972) point out, retrospective accounts allow therapists to mix current knowledge with past knowledge, thereby providing opportunity for therapists to be involved in evaluating their thinking in addition to presenting their thinking. Researchers who are true to the retrospective think-aloud method do not want therapists to evaluate their reasoning. Hence, it is very important for researchers who wish to adhere to this method to guide the therapist to recount what she or he was thinking at the time the event was happening rather than evaluating what should have happened using hindsight.

Another criticism of the retrospective reporting method is the reliance on subjects' memories of their thoughts. The length and complexity of any task mean that large gaps and distortions of events are often noted when a memory-dependent approach is used to elicit subjects' reasoning (Martin, 1992). Researchers may attempt to minimize these difficulties by conducting debriefing sessions immediately after the therapy session and reassuring therapists that there are no right or wrong answers. Other limitations of this method include participants reconstructing their reasoning based on what they think they were supposed to do or what the researcher might like to hear, or on rationalizing their thoughts to create a logical story rather than what they were actually thinking. Finally, the processes underlying the therapist's actions may be unconscious and thus not accessible for verbal reporting. For example, when reporting the clinical reasoning and decision-making processes of occupational therapists choosing the first intervention in a familiar type of case, Hagedorn's (1996) participants stated that they were unaware of any models or frames of reference to guide their decisions. However, Hagedorn suggested that ". . . it was quite plain that a variety of biomechanical, cognitive-perceptual, and neurodevelopmental approaches were being utilized" (1996, p. 221). The fact that the participants in this research were not able to articulate theories used or make the connection between theory and practice supports the idea that not all thoughts are brought to a level at which they are available for verbal reporting.

The reader should note that think-aloud retrospective reporting as described by Ericsson and Simon (1993) was borne from a quasi-quantitative research tradition in which the accuracy of the subject's recollections is of paramount importance. In the spirit of the qualitative frame of reference in which most occupational therapy clinical reasoning studies are conducted, researchers should consider that the reasoning provided by the therapist is an accurate representation of their thoughts at the time of the debrief or interview and that reliance on memory is not a significant limitation of the method. Therefore, although these issues are listed as limitations, the degree to which they are truly a problem in data analysis is debatable.

Interviews

The retrospective debrief method described above asks clinicians to provide their thinking and reasoning about a client immediately after the session ends. Although rather one-sided, this approach to data collection may be loosely described as an interview. More directly, the therapist may participate in an in-depth interview in which he or she is asked to describe his/her clinical reasoning in general, or reasoning concerning specific events. When using a semistructured or structured interview format to study clinical reasoning, the researcher should consider the interview as a conversation in which she/he actively listens to what the subject is saying (Rice & Ezzy, 1999). The researcher may compose a theme or topic list to guide the interview or may develop a set of specific questions to ask participants. Excellent references for conducting structured and unstructured interviews include De Vaus (2004), Minichiello et al. (1995), Morse and Field (1995), and Rice and Ezzy (1999). These resources contain valuable suggestions for managing difficult participants and disasters and overcoming pitfalls and strategies the interviewer can use to assist participants to reveal sensitive or personal information. This may be important when interviewing therapists about sensitive or personal issues such as their beliefs and values and how these impact clinical reasoning. For example, Hooper interviewed an occupational therapist on three occasions using a semistructured format concerning "what constitutes her reality" (1997, p. 330), which included questions relating to practice assumptions and beliefs about human nature, occupation, and health and illness. There are other examples of occupational therapy researchers attempting to understand clinical reasoning through the use of in-depth interviews alone or the use of a combination of techniques (triangulation) such as retrospective think aloud during debriefing sessions and general interviews to understand clinical reasoning. For example, Gibson et al. (2000) used semistructured interviews to prompt two therapists to describe their reasoning about a written case vignette. Similarly, Fondiller, Rosage, and Neuhaus (1990) provided nine occupational therapists with a written case vignette and interviewed them using a range of questions such as: "How would you treat this patient?" "What strengths do you have that would enhance your ability to carry out occupational therapy with this patient?" (1990, p. 46).

Using a more unstructured approach, Ward (2003) interviewed her subject over a 3-hour period about her experiences of being an occupational therapist in community mental health, and the nature of clinical reasoning when working with groups of clients. Interviewing clinicians about their reasoning has the advantage of being flexible in the time and place and can access a great deal of reflective information from the therapist. However, although global information about how the therapist "reasons in general" may be captured in an in-depth interview, reasoning related to the specific conduct of therapy is better captured using concurrent or retrospective reporting with a debriefing interview. Both in-depth and debriefing interviews are required to be transcribed for later analysis, and information on transcription is detailed in the next section.

DATA TRANSCRIPTION

Participant's verbal accounts of thinking and reasoning are typed (verbatim, including laughter, pauses, sighs, and so on) so they can be analyzed more easily; this process is referred to as *transcription*. The transcriptions of the therapist's clinical reasoning form the data for analysis. Audiotapes are easily transcribed by the researcher using an audio transcription machine. These machines enable the researcher to pause the tape with a foot pedal while typing. Audiotapes may also be sent to professional transcribers, who are generally faster and more accurate (on the first run) than those of us who are not trained typists. In my own research, I use medical transcription services for transcribing audiotapes and judicial system transcription services for transcribing therapist reasoning from videotapes, since specialist equipment is required to transcribe from videotapes. It takes a professional transcriber approximately five times longer to transcribe the tape compared with the running time, and a novice transcriber may take considerably longer than that. Once the transcription is checked against the original tape to ensure accuracy, it is ready for analysis (Morse & Field, 1995). If the transcription is made from an audiotape, then the typed document is all the researcher requires to undertake this analysis. However, if the transcription was made from a videotape, the researcher has the advantage of reading the transcription while watching the video of the unfolding therapy session. This may enhance analysis of the material, since the reasoning soundtrack is supported by rich visual images and the context for the clinician's comments is preserved.

QUALITATIVE FRAMEWORKS FOR CONDUCTING CLINICAL REASONING RESEARCH AND ANALYZING DATA

The final section of this chapter is concerned with the qualitative frameworks that guide clinical reasoning research and approaches to analyzing and interpreting clinical reasoning data. Although some clinical reasoning researchers simply claim to be using a qualitative framework to guide the study and analyze data (e.g., see

Alnervik & Sviden, 1996; Embrey et al., 1996; Creighton, Dijkers, Bennett & Brown, 1995), we need to understand what these qualitative approaches are, differences between them, and possible advantages or limitations. Researchers have the choice of several qualitative frameworks when conducting clinical reasoning research and analyzing the resulting data. Although the methods for capturing clinical reasoning data as previously described are unique to this field of study, these qualitative frameworks are generic and therefore used across many disciplines and research topics. The most common qualitative frameworks for conducting clinical reasoning research and analyzing data are grounded theory, phenomenology, focused or broad-based ethnography, and action research. A brief overview of these approaches is provided here, and the reader is referred to more extensive descriptions and reviews. Occupational therapy researchers are also beginning to use discourse analysis to analyze verbal reports, and although this form of analysis has not yet been applied to occupational therapy clinical reasoning data, a brief review of the technique is provided.

Finally, although verbal protocol analysis (VPA) is reviewed, this is a very structured (semiqualitative) approach to data analysis that has rarely been adopted in occupational therapy clinical reasoning research. When reading this section of the chapter, the reader should note two points: Clinical reasoning data can be collected and analyzed by the researcher as an outsider or as a participant in the study (and this distinguishes many of the approaches); and since several of the approaches (i.e., grounded theory, ethnography and action research) use similar techniques for data analysis, a summary of these techniques is provided once rather than repeated in each section.

Grounded Theory

In **grounded theory** (Strauss & Corbin, 1990), the researcher has no preconceived ideas or theories prior to the research, and the primary goal of a grounded analysis is to generate explanatory theories of human behavior (Morse & Field, 1995). Whereas **ethnography** focuses on macro aspects of action and interaction as occurs between institutional structures and people, grounded theory focuses on micro actions and interactions occurring between people. In research using grounded theory, data collection and analysis occur together, and further data collection and analysis is based on the emerging theory (Morse & Field, 1995). The phenomenon is studied in its real-world context (Grbich, 2004). Theoretical sampling is used in this method, and therefore participants are selected on the basis of their knowledge of the topic. Data collection techniques include interviews and observation. When analyzing clinical reasoning data in such a framework, the researcher may work alone or as part of a team. Analysis involves systematically examining, arranging and interpreting the data so it can be understood and presented in a meaningful way to others. Analysis of the data requires lateral thinking, reflection, and dialogue with self and others about emerging ideas (Browne, 2004). A summary of analysis techniques is provided in the section that follows. Examples of occupational therapy clinical reasoning research using a grounded theory approach include the work of Fondiller, Rosage, and Neuhaus (1990) (described earlier), which contains an excellent description of the method, and Hooper (1996), when examining the internal beliefs of an occupational therapist and the influence of these on service delivery. For further descriptions of grounded theory, the reader is referred to Creswell (1998), Denzin and Lincoln (2000), Browne (2004), and Miles and Huberman (1994).

Phenomenology

As described earlier, research questions that ask about the structure and essence of occupational therapists' experience of the phenomenon of clinical reasoning are best answered using a phenomenological approach. Unlike grounded theory, in which the goal is to develop theory, the aim of **phenomenology** is to provide a full description of the phenomenon of clinical reasoning. A phenomenological study attempts to understand reality from the perspective of the participant(s) in their natural environment (Morse & Field, 1995). In this approach, the researcher may be a detached observer (as in the clinical reasoning research of Crabtree and Lyons, 1997) or an involved participant (as in the clinical reasoning research of Mattingly and Fleming, 1994). Data collection may consist of debriefing interviews following therapy sessions, semistructured interviews, and observation. The aim of a semistructured interview is to gather rich descriptions of the therapist's experiences to gain a deep understanding of what these experiences mean (Morse & Field, 1995). Again, analysis techniques are summarized below, but these may include coding, thematic analysis, and for the researcher to reflexively analyze his/her own beliefs and feelings prompted by the data.

Other occupational therapy research on clinical reasoning from a phenomenological perspective includes the work of Hallin and Sviden (1995), who described the clinical reasoning of six expert therapists working in neurology. They asked the therapists to view a videotape of a client performing self-care tasks and kitchen tasks and then to "try and think-aloud and tell me: what are your impressions of the patient" (p. 70). Ward (2003) and Barnitt and Partridge (1997) have also conducted research investigating clinical reasoning using hermeneutic phenomenology. Hermeneutic enquiry focuses more on the language and environmental aspects of everyday experiences, and the researcher deliberately detaches him- or herself from the task. For further descriptions of these approaches, the reader is referred to Creswell (1998), Morse and Field (1995), Denzin and Lincoln (2000), and Kelly (1999).

Ethnography and Situated Cognition

Ethnography is the study of groups of people whose beliefs, actions, and artifacts are constructed by the multitude of influences that have shaped their culture (Grbich, 2004). As an interpretive method, ethnography is interested in considering the social construction of shared meaning. Rather than investigating the topic as an outsider, the researcher is part of the community and therefore a participant. In a focused ethnography, the researcher focuses on the subject's perspectives and interpretations of an aspect of their world (Muecke, 1994; Spencer, Krefting & Mattingly, 1993; Fetterman, 1989), such as clinical reasoning. For example, in my own research using focused ethnography (Unsworth 2004; Unsworth 2005), the aim was to describe the clinical reasoning of 13 experienced occupational therapists, explore the meaning of clinical reasoning, and examine the interrelationships of the components of clinical reasoning. This was achieved through analysis of a longitudinal series of three debriefing interviews following real therapy encounters recorded on head-mounted video camera. After a priori category coding of the data, analysis included the multiple reading method to look for patterns, themes, and relationships between the reasoning modes (Miles & Huberman, 1994) and for modes of reasoning that did not fit within the categories already established.

Researchers are now increasingly aware of the contextual aspects of cognition and thinking, as discussed in some depth in previous chapters. What is happening around the clinician has a direct impact on thinking and reasoning. If the researcher is interested in considering the impact of context on clinical reasoning, then rich ethnographic descriptions are made of the clinician interacting with the client and others who are present as well as their environment. An approach that involves consideration of the environment in understanding the participants thinking is termed *situated cognition* (Greeno, 1989). In this case, the term is used to reflect a data collection approach that is sensitive to the context as well as to the persons acting in that context. Similar to an ethnographic approach, the researcher uses "thick description" to record verbal data. However, additional detailed descriptions are made of the actions and tasks of the participant and the people the participant interacts with (Patel & Arocha, 2000). The situated cognition approach relies on analyzing data captured on videotape (as opposed to audiotape) to ensure that the whole situation in which the reasoning occurs is captured. This includes capturing nonverbal information such as gestures, movements, and expressions. In this approach, the analysis may include classification of streams of behavior into a coding scheme developed a priori and based on a theoretical understanding of the topic under study (Patel & Arocha, 2000).

Action Research

A variety of terms and strategies may be broadly classified as **action research,** and these include action science, action inquiry, action learning, participatory action research, cooperative inquiry, and community development research (Street, 2004). Researchers using action research often combine this with one of the main qualitative approaches such as grounded theory, ethnography, or phenomenology (Rice & Ezzy, 1999). In action research, the everyday actions of the participants are the basis for learning, knowing, and changing what is done (Rice and Ezzy, 1999). Hence, action research is often chosen when there is a desire for change in the way things are done.

In action research, the boundaries that usually exist between the researcher as an outsider and the participant as an insider under study do not exist because the design and implementation, and data analysis and interpretation, are undertaken by all persons in the study. For example, Mattingly and Fleming (1994) described how they formed a partnership with their participants and noted that their research interests married well with the practical self-examination and staff development goals of the therapists. In this study, participants were asked to view videotapes of therapy sessions, responding to the prompt to "tell the story" (1994, p. 7) of the video. It is interesting to note that in Mattingly and Fleming's study, the participants were asked to analyze the videos of other therapists to (a) title the unfolding story from the perspective of the therapist and client; (b) "pick out what strategies or decisions the therapist appeared to be making"; or (c) "identify where they saw the therapist getting stuck" (1994, p. 8). This is somewhat different from the majority of clinical reasoning research in occupational therapy in which therapists view only their own videotapes. However, this was undertaken in the spirit of action research in which the group works together to examine practice and gain new insights to therapy and the supporting reasoning. Combining action research with a phenomenological approach helped Mattingly and Fleming to "excavate the tacit dimension" (1994, p. 13) of therapy and to create a new language to illuminate aspects of practice concerned with meaning-making.

There is some disagreement in the literature over the terminology used in action research, and the reader's attention is also drawn to the term Participatory Action Research (PAR) (Rice & Ezzy, 1999). This is also a form of collaborative study between researchers and participants, but seems to have a particular focus on power inequities, for example, with marginalized groups or communities. Rice and Ezzy draw on the work of Ritchie (1996) and note that while "action research has been undertaken by and with people who have considerable power . . . participatory [action] research has been developed with disempowered people" (Rice & Ezzy, 1999, p. 175).

For further information and a clinical example of PAR, the reader is referred to Cockburn & Trentharn (2002) and to the foundation text in the area by de Koning and Martin (1996). However, since in an occupational therapy clinical reasoning study, the partnerships formed by researchers and clinicians are on an equal and professional level, the term action research (rather than PAR) is used. Readers are referred to Barnitt and Partridge for another example of an action research approach (from a hermeneutic phenomenological perspective) to studying clinical reasoning (1997) and to Roth & Esdaile (1999) and Spaulding (2004) for general discussions on the technique.

Analysis Techniques Commonly Used in Grounded Theory, Phenomenology, Ethnography, and Action Research

When using a qualitative approach, principles of data analysis include:

1. To analyze is to interpret.
2. The focus of analysis is to study, explain, or synthesize how individuals construct meaning.
3. Ethical principles are maintained during data analysis as well as data collection.
4. Theoretical sensitivity (having insight, being able to extract meaning from the data and to determine what is and is not important to the analysis) ensures a comprehensive analysis.
5. The outcomes of the analysis range from description to generation of theory (Browne, 2004).

Data analysis generally involves the researcher(s) (and participants in action research) to read and become very familiar with the data transcripts. The researcher(s) then think, reflect, question, discuss, and compare (between participants or situations) the data. The researchers may also consult the literature on topics related to emerging themes. Some form of coding or categorization of the data is also undertaken in which similar concepts are labeled and grouped (Browne, 2004). The researcher(s) may use the assistance of data management software such as Nvivo (Bazeley & Richards, 2000) or The Ethnograph to assist the researcher to organize, code, and retrieve data. Some programs even assist the researcher with theory building. A review of these computer programs may be found in Miles and Huberman (1994). Analysis techniques commonly adopted include constant comparison (in which all pieces of data are compared to produce new understandings of the phenomenona under study), thematic analysis (which requires the researcher to identify themes running through the data), content analysis (topics are chosen and interviews are segmented into these topics), and matrices (from which relationships between data categories can be examined). Full descriptions of these techniques may be found in Creswell (1998), Morse and Field (1995), Miles and Huberman (1994), and Denzin and Lincoln (2000). One of the last steps in the analysis process is to verify the conclusions drawn. Techniques that researchers may use include conducting member checks in which findings and data interpretations are sent to participants for confirmation and comment, triangulating results (providing comparison and convergence of perspectives from sources), looking for negative evidence, following up surprises, and checking out rival explanations. The reader is referred to Morse and Field (1995) for further details on analyzing data, issues of rigor, and writing up qualitative research.

Discourse Analysis

Although the use of discourse analysis to examine clinical reasoning data is rare, its potential use is included here for completeness. Discourse analysis is a method of analyzing the content of text. Lupton (1994) states that the term "discourse" is used to describe patterns in the ways in which phenomena are presented in talk or text. In many cases, the text of newspapers and other published works are analyzed. Data are gathered in unobtrusive ways, in which the researcher does not interact with the participants unless it is to interview the participant to further understand the text that forms the primary source of analysis. Hence, it is an approach to examining the ways humans impart meaning to the physical and social world and interact with each other without directly asking them about these issues (Lupton, 2004). When analyzing the discourse, a linguistic approach (focusing on the structure and content of the language used) may be used, or a more sociological approach may be taken when the focus is on the cultural and social context in which the discourse is produced and understood. Using discourse analysis in a clinical setting, Lupton (2004) describes the interactions between neonatal nursery nurses and the mothers of ill babies. This is done using transcripts of crib-side conversations as well as transcripts of interviews with the nurses and with the mothers. In this example, the analysis focused on the ways the nurses talked about the infants and their mothers and the mothers' stories of their experiences in the nursery unit, specifically looking at how both nurses and mothers described a "good mother" and the language subjects used to describe what behavior was considered appropriate for mothers in the nursery. In the future, transcripts of occupational therapists and clients working together in a clinical settings could be analyzed using discourse analysis to shed new insights on clinical reasoning. This kind of approach could be particularly useful in examining interactive reasoning. For more details on this method of study, the reader is referred to the work of occupational therapy researcher Claire Ballinger (Ballinger, 2000; Ballinger & Payne, 2000), who has used the technique to examine accounts about falling in older people.

Verbal Protocol Analysis

VPA is described last since this approach to data analysis is quite different from the others described above. This quasi-quantitative approach was developed specifically to analyze think-aloud data, based on information processing theory. VPA is described in detail by Ericsson and Simon (1993, pp. 261–373) and requires repetitive analysis of verbal data and labeling the cognitive processes evident in the transcript. Initially, the transcripts are segmented by phrases (following the natural contours of speech). Next, a coding system is set up using vocabulary from the subject and that of the particular problem. Any assumptions made are defined, and the extent to which the context will be considered in the analysis is decided. The reliability of data coding may also be examined. For example, Fowler (1997) examined the inter-rater reliability of coding undertaken by the researchers in her study of the clinical reasoning of five nurses planning care for a newly admitted, chronically ill client. Segments of data are then analyzed for both basic, subordinate, and superordinate concepts and cognitive strategies used. Greenwood and King (1995) used this segmenting process in their research examining the clinical reasoning of nine pairs of expert and novice orthopedic nurses using both concurrently and retrospectively reported data. Greenwood and King (1995) describe basic concepts as including the optimal amount of information required for efficient everyday functioning. Subordinate concepts flow on from basic ones and include more specific information. Finally, superordinate concepts, which are inferred from the logic of basic and subordinate concepts, are examined. When using VPA, problem behavior graphs or decision trees may then be generated to map and illustrate the subject's steps in reasoning or making a decision. Note that occupational therapy researchers have not adopted a VPA approach, probably because when this approach is used, clinical reasoning is dissected into components and examined with great precision. Occupational therapy researchers to date have preferred to take a more phenomenological approach to studying clinical reasoning, in which the whole of a situation is considered from the perspective of the subject. However, the reader is referred to an excellent clinical description of the technique by Greenwood and King (1995) and generalist texts such as Ericsson and Simon (1993) and Carroll and Johnson (1990) for further information.

SUMMARY

This chapter has provided an overview of all the methods available for researchers wishing to explore the phenomenon of clinical reasoning. After some brief comments on posing research questions before contrasting the more quantitative approaches to studying medical decision making with the more qualitative approaches used in occupational therapy research on clinical reasoning, details are provided about techniques to capture and transcribe clinical reasoning data. Finally, theoretical frameworks for conducting qualitative research and analyzing data are presented. The text is illustrated with examples of clinical reasoning research from the health sciences literature. These examples show that researchers in the field adopt a variety of combinations of methods when studying clinical reasoning. This methodological pluralism has the advantage of contributing different pieces of information to our growing knowledge of clinical reasoning. However, further research is urgently required to: expand and refine the language established to assist clinicians to articulate their thinking; increase our understanding of the complex reasoning processes used by therapists in their remarkably varied work; and explore how clinical reasoning changes over the continuum of novice to expert so we can support students and beginner therapists on their journeys to expertise. It is hoped that the presentation of research methods outlined in this chapter will inspire therapists to undertake such research.

LEARNING ACTIVITY 15-1

How Can the Researcher Access What a Therapist is Thinking?

Purpose

To examine ways that a therapist's thinking and reasoning can be accessed

Connections to Major Clinical Reasoning Constructs

Information processing theory

Directions for Learners

1 Describe four techniques a researcher can use to access what a therapist is thinking when working with a client (i.e., his or her clinical reasoning) either during or immediately after a therapy session.
2 What are some of the advantages and limitations of each of these approaches?

LEARNING ACTIVITY 15-2

Studying Clinical Reasoning as an Insider

Purpose

During fieldwork, students become part of the OT department and its culture. The aim of this activity is to develop a methodology suitable to study the clinical reasoning of the therapists in the department.

Connections to Major Clinical Reasoning Constructs

Types of research methods suitable to use as a participant in the research

Directions for Learners

Consider that you are about to embark on your final Level II fieldwork. First, you should decide what sort of facility it is (there are at least five therapists in the department). You will be part of the therapy department for 12 weeks. Before the placement, you have been asked to conduct a small pilot study on the conduct of initial interviews by the occupational therapists. You decide to specifically examine the clinical reasoning that supports the conduct of initial interviews, and decide to conduct some interviews with a couple of therapists and also conduct some debriefing interviews using the retrospective think-aloud approach. You need to plan this pilot research.

1 What is your research question?
2 What will be your theoretical framework?
3 How many interviews and debriefings do you think it is possible to conduct?
4 What sorts of questions might you ask therapists in the interviews?
5 How will you analyze the data (keep in mind the theoretical framework chosen so the approach to analysis is compatible)?
6 How would you write up the results of this pilot study? What would the headings of your report be?

LEARNING ACTIVITY 15-3

Coding Clinical Reasoning Transcripts

Purpose

To examine what a transcript looks like and explore ways transcripts can be coded

Connections to Major Clinical Reasoning Constructs

Techniques for analyzing clinical reasoning data
Using the construct of the "therapist with the three-track mind" when coding transcripts.

Directions for Learners

1 Read the clinical reasoning transcript below. This is the first portion of a transcript from an assessment session between a therapist and her client (with his family). The client sustained an acquired brain injury several weeks before the session.
2 Think about the kinds of issues that have been raised in the transcript about the clinical reasoning that supports therapy for clients who have cognitive and perceptual problems. These might form themes in an analysis. What might these themes be? Highlight the relevant sections in the transcript and give names to these themes.
3 Often researchers code the whole of a transcript for different kinds of reasoning. Using the information from this text, and that provided in Mattingly and Fleming (1994), try highlighting the clinician's comments using three colors to represent the three tracks of procedural, interactive, and conditional reasoning.

Transcript

Interviewer: OK, we'll now watch the assessment session of the video we've just made and I'd like you to tell me about what you're doing with the client and why you're doing it and if it helps. You could imagine that

I'm a fourth-year student and how you would explain it to them. If your comments run for longer than the tape, we can pause the tape so you can explain what is happening, okay? And also if you want more sound from the session, I can turn that up.

Clinician: Yes, we'll probably want a bit of sound, that will prompt me.

(Client is seated at table, mother and sister on other side.)

Interviewer: Okay. So can you tell me what is happening here?

Clinician: So this is a young gentleman who has been involved in a motor vehicle accident. We're about to do an upper limb functional assessment type session here. We're always assessing as we're treating at the same time with someone like this. At the start here, just before we started these activities I gave J., the young man, the choice of what he wanted to do. I always give him lots of choices, as well as a variety of activities with basically the same aim or a few different aims. But I give him the choice of what he wants to do when, because there might be something he doesn't want to do and we always need to make sure that he is empowered in the sessions as well.

(Client has right hand on mat on table.)

Clinician: At the moment we're doing some simple basic exercises that are like a warm-up so we need to warm him up so we can complete the functional activities later down the track.

Interviewer: I notice that your hand is on his shoulder.

Clinician: Yes, I'm supporting his torso there so that he doesn't substitute movement patterns there. So, what we are encouraging J. to do there is forward shoulder flexion and elbow extension, and he likes to move his trunk forward at the same time. He's got some associated tonal patterns there. My prompt on the shoulder is just controlling that trunk involvement so we get the right movement coming back, yes. He's got limited use of his upper limb, so that's what our session involves— facilitating return of the movement that he's got, building strength and endurance there. You can't see much there, can you?

Interviewer: We can also notice the other two ladies there. Can you just explain their role?

Clinician: That's J.'s mother and younger sister; they are very, very involved in his rehab and very committed to J.'s rehab program as well. They're invited to come to every therapy session whenever they want as are all of our family members. J. responds really well to them, and they like to be involved in the process. They're here every day, so we encourage them to be involved in sessions whenever possible. Also, it helps out therapy, because they understand the rationale and reasons why we're doing what we're doing and the goals we want to achieve. They can facilitate those out of therapy sessions and they're actually doing that, they're an excellent family. They have a good understanding of J.'s injury and the things he needs to work on. And if I ask them to do something at home, they do; that's really nice to see. They are a good motivating factor for J., too. He always wants to perform well in front of his family as well.

Interviewer: So what is happening now?

Clinician: Now, I'm getting J. to do some hand activities there on the table. . . . He's still doing some finger movements, yes.

Interviewer: Yes.

(Client is extending his wrist.)

Clinician: He's still on the warm-ups. He's doing a bit of wrist extension stuff here. . . . What I'm doing, I'm actually modeling and showing to J., so demonstrating to J. what is going on there and then he's copying my actions.

Interviewer: So why do you do that?

Clinician: So that J. can see the right movement patterns. Verbally, yes, he understands, but if I just said J. can you bend your wrist up, he could bend it in the wrong pattern or the wrong way. So always a verbal is followed up with a demonstration as well to facilitate your client's understanding of what you're doing.

Interviewer: Okay.

Clinician: So you saw before I was watching up his arm to make sure he didn't have any associated reactions, what's happening here is I just want to see movements from his wrist here.

Interviewer: Okay.

Clinician: And using lots of layman's terms, because if I said we were going to do ulnar and radial activities now (we have lots of nicknames, [like] do some of that side-to-side wrist stuff), [since] J. likes to know all the clinical terms for everything as well, so I explain it to him and he then forgets it because he does have problems with his memory but he thinks it's funny all the terms and so…again he had some substitution patterns at his elbow while he was trying to use it, turning his shoulder; he was externally rotating his shoulder and bring his elbow in whilst he was trying to move his trunk there. So I stabilized his forearm and shoulder and brought his attention to it, so we were just concentrating on the isolated movement patterns we wanted to see there.

Interviewer: So you were using other prompts besides the visual and the auditory?

Clinician: Yes, tactile and touching . . . at the same time. He's a young man who a couple of months ago, whenever you touched his hand, he would get a bit excited and be a bit inappropriate and say "[the therapist's] holding my hand," so you had to be careful about how you touched J. or used touch in a clinical manner and stuff. He's settled down into that now and that doesn't bother him; he understands that we need to touch him and hold his hand to do certain things that he . . .

Interviewer: Right.

Clinician: . . . got a bit excited inappropriately. We used to do things like that. Now when I say "push" I'm just encouraging him to get the greatest range of motion with his forearm there. He's always quite motivated and he's really keen to do it, to try his hardest, so he's a lovely patient to work with because he is well motivated and you don't often get that in the ABI field.

REFERENCES

Alnervik, A. & Sviden, G. (1996). On clinical reasoning: Patterns of reflection on practice. *Occupational Therapy Journal of Research*, 16, 98–110.

Ballinger, C. & Payne, S. (2000). Discourse analysis: Principles, applications and critique. *British Journal of Occupational Therapy*, 63(11), 566–572.

Barnitt, R. & Partridge, C. (1997). Ethical reasoning in physical therapy and occupational therapy. *Physiotherapy Research International*, 2, 178–194.

Bazeley, P. & Richards, L. (2000). *The Nvivo qualitative project book*. London: Sage.

Benner, P, Hooper-Kyriakidis, P. & Stanard, D. (1999). *Clinical wisdom and interventions in critical care: A thinking-in-action approach*. Philadelphia: WB Saunders.

Benner, P. E, Tanner, C. A. & Chesla, C. A. (1996). *Expertise in nursing practice: Caring, clinical judgement and ethics*. New York: Springer.

Benner, P. E. (1984). *From novice to expert: Excellence and power in clinical nursing practice*. Menlo Park, CA: Addison-Wesley.

Browne, J. (2004). Grounded theory analysis: Coming to data with questioning minds. In V. Minichiello, G. Sullivan, K. Greenwood & R. Axford (Eds.), *Research methods for nursing and health science* (2nd ed., pp. 624–669). Frenchs Forest NSW: Pearson Education Australia.

Carroll, J. S. & Johnson, E. (1990). *Decision research: A field guide*. Newbury Park, CA: Sage.

Cockburn, L. & Trentharn, B. (2002). Participatory action research: Integrating community occupational therapy practice and research. *Canadian Journal of Occupational Therapy*, 69(1), 20–30.

Crabtree, M. & Lyons, M. (1997). Focal points and relationships: A study of clinical reasoning. *British Journal of Occupational Therapy*, 60, 57–63.

Creighton, C., Dijkers, M., Bennett, N. & Brown, K. (1995). Reasoning and the art of therapy for spinal cord injury. *American Journal of Occupational Therapy*, 49, 311–317.

Creswell, J. W. (1998). *Qualitative enquiry and research design: Choosing among five traditions*. Thousand Oaks, CA: Sage.

De Vaus, D, (2004). Structured questionnaires and interviews. In V. Minichiello, G. Sullivan, K. Greenwood & R. Axford (Eds.), *Research methods for nursing and health science* (2nd ed., pp. 347–392). Frenchs Forest NSW: Pearson Education Australia.

De Koning, K. & Martin, M. (1996). *Participatory research in health: Issues and experiences*. London: Zed Books.

Denzin, N. K. & Lincoln, Y. S. (2000). *Handbook of qualitative research* (2nd ed.). Thousand Oaks, CA: Sage.

Elstein, A. S., Shulman, L. S. & Sprafka, S. A. (1978). *Medical problem-solving*. Cambridge, MA: Harvard Press.

Embrey, D. G., Guthrie, M. R., White, O. R. & Dietz, J. (1996). Clinical decision making by experienced and inexperienced pediatric physical therapists for children with diplegic cerebral palsy. *Physical Therapy*, 76, 20–33.

Ericsson, K. A. & Simon, H. A. (1993). *Protocol analysis: verbal reports as data* (Rev. ed.). Cambridge, MA: MIT Press.

Fetterman, D. M. (1989) *Ethnography step by step*. Newbury Park, CA: Sage.

Fleming, M. H. (1994). The therapist with the three track mind. In C. Mattingly & M. H. Fleming (Eds.), *Clinical reasoning: Forms of inquiry in a therapeutic practice* (pp. 119–136). Philadelphia: F. A. Davis.

Fondiller, E. D., Rosage, L. J. & Neuhaus, B. E. (1990). Values influencing clinical reasoning in occupational therapy: An exploratory study. *Occupational Therapy of Research*, 10, 41–55.

Fonteyn, M. & Fisher, A. (1995). Use of think aloud method to study nurses' reasoning and decision making in clinical practice settings. *Journal of Neuroscience Nursing*, 27, 124–128.

Fowler, L. P. (1997). Clinical reasoning strategies used during care planning. *Clinical Nursing Research*, 6, 349–361.

Gibson, D., Velde, B., Hoff, T., Kvashay, D., Manross, P. L., Moreau, V. (2000). Clinical reasoning of a novice versus an experienced occupational therapist: A qualitative study. *Occupational Therapy in Health Care*, 12, 15–31.

Grbich, C. (2004). Qualitative research design. In V. Minichiello, G. Sullivan, K. Greenwood & R. Axford (Eds.), Research methods for nursing and health science (2nd ed., pp.151–175). Frenchs Forest NSW: Pearson Education Australia.

Greeno, D. M. (1989). The situativity of knowing, learning and research. *American Psychologist*, 53, 5–26.

Greenwood, J. & King, M. (1995). Some surprising similarities in the clinical reasoning of 'expert' and 'novice' orthopaedic nurses: Report of a study using verbal protocols and protocol analysis. *Journal of Advanced Nursing*, 22, 907–913.

Hagedorn, R. (1996). Clinical decision making in familiar cases: A model of the process and implications for practice. *British Journal of Occupational Therapy*, 59, 217–222.

Hallin, M. & Sviden, G. (1995). On expert occupational therapists' reflection-on practice. *Scandinavian Journal of Occupational Therapy*, 2, 69–75.

Harries, P. A. & Harries, C (2001). Studying clinical reasoning: Part 2 Applying Social Judgment Theory. *British Journal of Occupational Therapy*, 64(6), 285–292.

Harries, P. A. & Gilhooly, K. (2003a). Generic and specialist occupational therapy casework in community mental health. *British Journal of Occupational Therapy*, 66, 101–109.

Harries, P. A. & Gilhooley, K. (2003b). Identifying occupational therapists' referral priorities in community health. *Occupational Therapy International*, 10(2), 150–164.

Hooper, B. (1997). The relationship between pretheoretical assumptions and clinical reasoning. *American Journal of Occupational Therapy*, 51(5), 328–338.

Kagan, N. (1976). *Interpersonal process recall: A method of influencing human action*. East Lansing, MI: University of Michigan.

Kelly, G. (1996). Understanding occupational therapy: A hermeneutic approach. *British Journal of Occupational Therapy*, 59(5), 237–242.

Kipper, P. (1986). Television camera movement as a source of perceptual movement. *Journal of Broadcasting and Electronic Media*, 30, 295–307.

Klein, G. A., Orasanu, J., Claderwood, R. & Zsambok, C. E. (1993). *Decision making in action: Models and methods*. Norwood, NJ: Ablex.

Lamond, D., Crow, R., Chase, J., Doggen, K. & Swinkels, M. (1996). Information sources used in decision making: Considerations for simulation development. *International Journal of Nursing Studies*, 33, 47–57.

Lupton, D. (2004). Discourse analysis. In V. Minichiello, G. Sullivan, K. Greenwood & R. Axford (Eds.), *Research methods for nursing and health science* (2nd ed., pp. 483–496). Frenchs Forest NSW: Pearson Education Australia.

Martin, J. (1992). Intentions, responses, and private reactions: Methodological, ontological and epistemological reflections on process research. *Journal of Counseling and Development*, 70, 742–743.

Mattingly, C. & Fleming, M. H. (1994). *Clinical reasoning: Forms of inquiry in a therapeutic practice*. Philadelphia: F. A. Davis.

Miles, M. B. & Huberman, A. M. (1994). *Qualitative data analysis* (2nd ed.). Thousand Oaks, CA: Sage.

Minichiello, V., Aroni, R., Timewell, E. & Alexander, L. (1995). *In-depth interviewing: Principles, techniques and analyses*. Melbourne: Longman.

Mitchell, R. & Unsworth, C. A. (2005). Clinical reasoning during community health home visits: Expert and novice differences. *British Journal of Occupational Therapy*, 68(5), 215–223.

Morse, J. M. & Field, P. A. (1995). *Qualitative research methods for health professionals* (2nd ed.). Thousand Oaks, CA: Sage.

Newell, A. & Simon, H. A. (1972). *Human problem solving*. Englewood Cliffs, NJ: Prentice-Hall.

Omodei, M. M. & McLennan, J. (1994). Studying complex decision making in natural settings: Using a head-mounted video camera to study competitive orienteering. *Perceptual and Motor Skills*, 79, 1411–1425.

Patel, V. & Arocha, J. F. (2000). Methods in the study of clinical reasoning. In J. Higgs & M. Jones (Eds), *Clinical reasoning in the health professions* (2nd ed., pp. 78–91). Melbourne: Butterworth Heineman.

Rice, P. L. & Ezzy, D. (1999). *Qualitative research methods*. Oxford: Oxford University Press.

Ritchie, J. E. (1996). Using participatory research to enhance health in the work setting: An Australian experience. In K. De Koning & M. Martin (Eds.), *Participatory research in health: Issues and experiences* (pp. 200–220). London: Zed Books.

Roberts, A. E. (1996). Clinical reasoning in occupational therapy: Idiosyncrasies in content and process. *British Journal of Occupational Therapy*, 59, 372–376.

Roth, L. M. & Esdaile, S. A. (1999). Action research: A dynamic discipline for advancing professional goals. *British Journal of Occupational Therapy*, 62(11), 498–506.

Spaulding, N. J. (2004). Using vignettes to assist reflection within an action research study on a preoperative education program. *British Journal of Occupational Therapy*, 67(9), 388–398.

Spencer, J., Krefting, L., Mattingly, C. (1993). Incorporation of ethnographic methods in occupational therapy assessment. *American Journal of Occupational Therapy*, 47, 303–309.

Street, A. (2004). Action research. In V. Minichiello, G. Sullivan, K. Greenwood & R. Axford (Eds.), *Research methods for nursing and health science* (2nd ed., pp. 278–292). Frenchs Forest NSW: Pearson Education Australia.

Strong, J., Gilbert, J., Cassidy, S. & Bennett, S. (1995). Expert clinicians' and students' views on clinical reasoning in occupational therapy. *British Journal of Occupational Therapy, 58,* 119–123.

Tesch, R. (1990). *Qualitative research analysis: Types of software.* New York: Falmer Press.

Thomas, S. A., Wearing, A. J. & Bennett, M. (1991). *Clinical decision making for nurses and health care professionals.* Sydney: Harcourt Brace Jovanovich.

Unsworth, C. A. (2001a). Selection for rehabilitation: Acute care discharge patterns of stroke and orthopaedic patients. *International Journal of Rehabilitation Research, 24,* 103–114.

Unsworth, C. A. (2001b). Clinical reasoning of novice and expert occupational therapists. *Scandinavian Journal of Occupational Therapy, 8,* 163–173.

Unsworth, C. A. (2001c). Using a head-mounted video camera to study clinical reasoning. *American Journal of Occupational Therapy, 55,* 582–588.

Unsworth, C. A. (2004). Clinical reasoning: How do worldview, pragmatic reasoning and client-centredness fit? *British Journal of Occupational Therapy, 67,* 10–19.

Unsworth, C. A. (2005). Using head-mounted video camera to confirm and expand knowledge of clinical reasoning in occupational therapy. *American Journal of Occupational Therapy, 59,* 31–40.

Unsworth, C. A. & Thomas, S. A. (1993). Information use in discharge accommodation recommendations for stroke patients. *Clinical Rehabilitation, 7,* 181–188.

Unsworth, C. A., Thomas, S. A. & Greenwood, K. M. (1997). Decision polarization among rehabilitation team recommendations concerning discharge housing for stroke patients. *International Journal of Rehabilitation Research, 20,* 51–68.

Unsworth, C. A., Thomas, S. A. & Greenwood, K. M. (1995). Rehabilitation team decisions concerning discharge housing for stroke patients. *Archives of Physical Medicine and Rehabilitation, 76,* 331–340.

Ward, J. D. (2003). The nature of clinical reasoning with groups: A phenomenological study of an occupational therapist in community mental health. *American Journal of Occupational Therapy, 57*(6), 625–634.

Yinger, R. L. (1986). Examining thought in action: A theoretical and methodological critique of research on interactive teaching. *Teaching and Teacher Education, 2,* 263–282.

Theory and Practice: New Directions for Research in Professional Reasoning

Barbara A. Boyt Schell, Carolyn A. Unsworth, and John W. Schell

CHAPTER OUTLINE

OBJECTIVES

After reading this chapter, the learner will be able to:

1 Discuss the current state of theory development in clinical and professional reasoning in occupational therapy.
2 Articulate several models for guiding research on clinical and professional reasoning.
3 Articulate a model for guiding research on teaching and learning professional reasoning.
4 Identify gaps in the current knowledge about professional reasoning in occupational therapy.
5 Critically consider appropriate methodologies for researching professional reasoning.

KEY TERMS

Fidelity	Principle
Concepts	Proposition

This chapter has the feel of a comprehensive exam question of the sort given to doctoral students. We are writing, hopefully insightfully, about what it is we know, what we do not know, and how we should go about developing new knowledge related to clinical and professional reasoning. As Kielhofner (2005) noted, the accumulation of knowledge rarely proceeds in an orderly fashion. Therefore, it is essential to punctuate the growing body of literature in the fields of clinical and professional reasoning by a cogent assimilation and synthesis of the current knowledge. For ease of expression we are going to use the term *professional reasoning* to include the reasoning that occurs in service to clients (typically referred to as clinical reasoning) as well as reasoning about supervisory, management, and educational activities in support of service provision. Our reflections here are based on an analysis of all the chapters in this book, as well as our scrutiny of published research, literature reviews, and other pertinent articles. A complete bibliography is included in the Appendix.

To begin, we fit clinical and professional reasoning into the broader concerns of OT practice as a way of situating our current knowledge. We then speak to our emergent understanding of clinical and professional reasoning. In that section, we have identified gaps in the literature and attendant needs for research that could address these unmet needs. In the last part of this chapter, we discuss the status of research about teaching students to adopt professional reasoning as a part of their everyday practice. Additionally, we discuss educational strategies that continue the development of expertise in clinical and professional reasoning. Arrayed throughout this chapter are text boxes containing research questions that could guide future investigations into professional reasoning.

Thinking About Thinking 16-1

The great winds of change are blowing, and that either gives you imagination or a headache.
—Catherine the Great

WHY STUDY PROFESSIONAL REASONING?

Perhaps the most basic question to ask is, "Why do we study professional reasoning?" Our answer is to improve practice. Early studies and much of the present literature are focused on uncovering how therapists think. This was because we needed better ways to explain to students the thinking that is deemed necessary for good practice. The assumption of early studies was that students would become better therapists if they were taught to think like practitioners (Mattingly & Fleming, 1994). Other studies examined how well therapists' actions matched

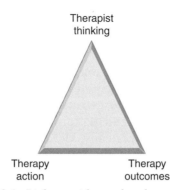

Figure 16-1 Links must be explored among professional reasoning, professional action, and the outcomes of those actions.

their espoused beliefs about practice (Rogers & Masagatani, 1982). Still other studies explored how theoretical perspectives influenced patterns of practice (Burke, 1997, 2001). Although much remains to understand, we propose that it is time for professional reasoning to be more explicitly reconnected to practice. By that we mean the questions should no longer be just "what is the therapist thinking?" and "how well does what the therapist is thinking match what we think the therapist should be thinking?" The time has come to explore the links between what the therapist is thinking and what the therapist is doing, and then to examine what the outcomes are from these therapy actions (*Figure 16-1*). Although admittedly an ambitious agenda, there is scholarship occurring in the field, such as fidelity studies described in the next section, and outcome measures that could be linked to the professional reasoning research.

Professional Reasoning and Therapy Fidelity

Relating therapy thoughts to therapy action provides a clearer picture of how therapist reasoning impacts actual practice patterns. Burke's (1997, 2001) description of pediatric therapists' evaluation practices provides one model of such a study. Such an approach might be further enhanced by examining the degree to which therapy actions are faithful to espoused theoretical explanations, or practice fidelity.

Fidelity is a concept used to describe how accurately the therapy provided matches the principles or theories that are the rationale for the therapy. For instance, fidelity studies emerged in clinical psychology literature when researchers were attempting to discern the relative effectiveness of one psychotherapy approach over another (Moncher & Prinz, 1991). These authors noted that there are two aspects to fidelity: *treatment integrity* (the degree to which treatment is implemented as intended) and *treatment differentiation* (how different treatments actually are when implemented) (p. 248). Occupational therapy is in need of fidelity studies, because it is difficult to demonstrate that outcomes are connected to a particular therapy approach, if there are no well-tested measures of whether that particular approach was used. Responding to this concern, Parham and her colleagues (Parham et al., 2007) are reporting on fidelity in sensory integration therapy. Similarly, Schell has presented preliminary research on the development of a fidelity measure related to occupation-based practice (Schell, 2002).

The emergence of practice descriptions in the form of fidelity measures provides a rich opportunity to connect professional reasoning research with professional action. These could be further connected to research that examines therapist interventions and patterns of treatment found in surveys of treatment media use (i.e., McEneany, McKenna & Summerville, 2002) or therapy implementation (Cleland, Onksen, Swanson & McRae, 2004). Over time, research on reasoning and related therapy action could perhaps be connected with research on the outcomes of therapy. In this way, we could get a clearer understanding of how professional reasoning promotes and supports evidence-based practice.

BOX 16-1

Research Questions About Reasoning and Therapy Action

- What are the connections and disconnections between therapists' reasoning and the actual observed therapy?
- How does therapist reasoning relate to treatment fidelity?
- How does therapist reasoning relate to treatment differentiation?
- What patterns of therapist reasoning promote optimum therapy outcomes?
- What is the connection between therapist reasoning, therapy action and therapy outcomes?
- How does the practice context support or inhibit effective therapy reasoning and related action?

Professional Reasoning and Evidence-Based Practice

Evidence-based practice (EBP) is ". . . the conscientious, explicit and judicious use of current best evidence in making decisions about the care of individuals" (Sackett et al., 2000, p. 71). In considering this definition, two important points concerning professional reasoning are discussed. The first is concerned with the fact that all therapists need to "consume" research and use evidence to reason about daily practice, and the second is concerned with the reasoning processes used in the pursuit of evidence-based practice. Sackett's definition of evidence-based practice assumes that evidence is available to support clinician reasoning and decision making. In many areas of occupational therapy, mounting evidence supports or refutes different therapy approaches, whereas in others there is a great deal less information. Although only some research therapists conduct studies to contribute to the knowledge base, all therapists can be involved in evaluating the outcomes of therapy and contributing to discussions on the effectiveness of therapy.

Thinking About Thinking 16-2

Evidence-based practice is like a toolbox of methods available to the occupational therapy practitioner to aid clinical reasoning.

—Tickle-Degnen, 2000, p.102)

The nexus between evidence-based practice and professional reasoning has been raised in several of the chapters in this text, and in summarizing directions for future research it seems important to make this link more explicit. Both components of the definition of evidence-based practice provided by Sackett involve reasoning and decision making. After locating and reading the evidence, clinicians must reason concerning the quality of the evidence and its contribution to knowledge in the field. Hence, clinicians must be judicious in selecting the best evidence. The second part of the definition of EBP states that therapists use this evidence to reason and make decisions about the care of individuals. *Figure 16-2* provides an illustration of the flow of information as a therapist's reasoning supports and promotes EBP in everyday occupational therapy practice.

Since there are two distinct opportunities for reasoning and decision making when conducting the EBP of occupational therapy, there are two areas when professional reasoning research is required to support therapists. Research is required to examine the types and nature of the reasoning that supports selection of the best quality evidence and the reasoning concerning application of best evidence into daily practice. Craik and Rappolt (2006) suggest that therapists' abilities to integrate research into clinical practice are shaped in part by their engagement in roles and activities such as mentoring students, participating in research, active engagement in continuing education and professional development planning, as well as direct

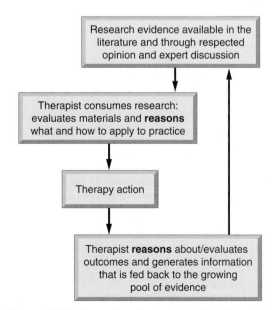

Figure 16-2 Examples of areas in which therapist reasoning intersects with evidence-based practice.

BOX 16-2

Research Questions About Reasoning and EBP

- What are the reasoning processes used by therapists as they search and select best evidence? What factors affect this reasoning (e.g., access to and ability to use library resources, skills to understand statistical material presented in articles)?
- Ideally what reasoning best supports the search for and selection of best evidence?
- How can we facilitate students and professionals to acquire the reasoning they need to search for and select best evidence?
- What are the reasoning processes used by therapists as they determine how to apply best evidence into daily practice?
- What factors affect this reasoning (e.g., therapist's own skill level, motivation, physical resources and other pragmatic factors, practice culture)?
- Ideally, what reasoning best supports therapists to apply best evidence into daily practice?
- How can we help students and professionals to acquire the reasoning they need to apply best evidence into daily practice?

---

service experience. Their discussion provides a useful framework for examining how these activities affect reasoning that incorporates evidence for best practice.

Research examining these questions may be best conducted over three phases involving description, evaluation, and prescription. Initially, research must be directed to uncover and describe how therapists reason as they select evidence and apply this in practice. Once this information is documented and available for scrutiny, the profession can debate the merits of such reasoning and examine how expert reasoning proceeds. Finally, research can then be undertaken to investigate the success of programs to prescribe reasoning strategies that best promote the selection and application of best evidence in daily practice for novice and advanced beginner therapists.

Research on the reasoning supporting EBP must consider both the types and nature of reasoning used. This section of the chapter has focused predominantly on the nature of the reasoning used. However, further research is also required to examine the types of reasoning used. There is no doubt that therapists use all the different types of reasoning we have identified throughout this text when selecting the best-quality evidence and applying findings into daily practice (including interactive, procedural, conditional, ethical, pragmatic, personal, etc.). However, the kinds of evaluative reasoning used as the therapist considers the impact factor of the research and the quality and accuracy of the methods and the statistics used, or calculates confidence intervals to establish the degree of uncertainly associated with the effect on an intervention, must also be researched.

To summarize this section, we will reframe the questions posed by Holm (2000) as she challenged therapists to consider, "Am I an evidence-based practitioner?" New challenges face us as we examine the reasoning that supports us as evidence-based practitioners. Therefore, the questions posed by Holm have been expanded (see italicized questions in Box 16-3) to reflect our interest in the professional reasoning that supports EBP.

BOX 16-3

Am I an Evidence-Based Practitioner?

What reasoning supports me as I conduct evidence-based practice?

- Do I examine what I do by asking clinical questions?
  What and how do I reason about what do and what questions to ask?
- Do I take the time to find the best evidence to guide what I do?
  What and how do I reason as I take the time to find and consider what is the best evidence to guide what I do?
- Do I appraise the evidence I find (or take it at face value)?
  What and how do I reason as I appraise the evidence I find (or take it at face value)?
- Do I use the evidence to do the "right thing right?" (Right person doing the right thing, the right way, in the right place at the right time with the right result?)
  What and how do I reason as I determine how to apply the evidence and do the "right thing right?" (Right person doing the right thing, the right way, in the right place at the right time with the right result?)
- Do I evaluate the impact of evidence-based practice?
  What and how do I reason as I evaluate the impact of evidence-based practice?

NATURE OF PROFESSIONAL REASONING

As research accumulates on reasoning across professions and within occupational therapy specifically, one thing is clear, and that is how complex it is. To understand professional reasoning, we can look at it through neurological, psychological, sociological, and anthropological lenses, to name but a few. Like peeling an onion, there are many layers to be appreciated. In some ways, these perspectives echo the ecological model of occupational performance used by Dunn and her colleagues (Dunn, Brown & Youngstrom, 2003). Although the Ecology of Human Performance was intended as a model to guide occupational therapy, it can be applied to describing why therapists think and act as they do. Viewing clinical reasoning as part of a human ecological system allows us to think about different aspects of the process in a systematic way.

Personal Factors and Professional Reasoning

Each therapist is first a person, with a unique configuration of body, mind, and experiences. Professional reasoning is a human process, and as such it is shaped by the therapist's personal life experiences and demands as well as personal beliefs about meaning of life, spiritual beliefs, the nature of truth, and the like. These personal foundations influence therapists as they engage in the kinds of reasoning overtly related to the client such as procedural, interactive, and conditional reasoning. There are commonalities in the ways in which our biological selves shape the reasoning possibilities. Research from neurology and psychology helps us understand that mechanisms of sensation, perception, memory, and bodily experience all shape our minds and how our minds work. These issues were discussed in Chapters 3 and 4. These mind-body experiences are grounded in the cultures in which we live. Chapters 2, 7, and 8 all make reference to the concepts of worldview, a therapist's personal context, ethical reasoning, and the ways these shape professional reasoning. Schell and Cevero (1993), Hooper (1997), and Unsworth (2004) have all attempted to explore what personal internal philosophies, beliefs, ethics, and spiritual dimensions are part of our professional reasoning or influence our professional reasoning; yet there is still much to explore. We are just at the beginning of understanding what types or modes of personal reasoning exist, the extent to which we can actively reason with our personal beliefs and worldview and the degree to which our personal reasoning is part of, or influences our daily practice. A deeper understanding of how our personal predispositions and life experiences shape the reasoning process would help explain the individual differences in professional reasoning and related therapy actions. This in turn would provide a deeper understanding of how we can strengthen practice.

Although there is limited occupational therapy research on personal factors, research in several comparable fields suggests that many personal factors do influence our reasoning. For example, research with a variety of health professionals suggests that client personality and physical appearance all influence therapist reasoning despite clinician assurances of objectivity (Drucker, 1974; Eisenberg, 1979). Other research has showed that some health professionals may devalue the skills of people with disabilities, misinterpret their behavior, underestimate their capabilities (DeLoach & Greer,1981; Gething, 1992; Williams, 1998), or be influenced in their decisions by the client's socio-economic status (van-Ryn & Burke, 2000). We would be naive to believe that such effects did not exist in our profession and this requires further examination. Since many of these have negative consequences for clients, it is vital that we conduct further research into the personal aspects of professional reasoning.

It is also hardly surprising that there is relatively little research on the personal aspect of professional reasoning. Many researchers may avoid such study, given its personal nature and therefore be reluctant to journey into the unknown depths of such intimate and intangible concepts. In addition, it is possible that researchers shy away from studies that may have negative or damaging consequences for the profession. Finally, current research methods may be inadequate for attempting to accurately access and describe the personal or worldview factors are a part of, or influence on professional reasoning. Although observing therapists' behavior as they work provides us with very little or only "inferred" information about a therapist's personal thoughts, interviewing therapists about these issues has its own set of limitations. Some of the problems that arise when interviewing therapists about personal reasoning/worldview include whether the participant:

- tells the researcher only what s/he thinks the researcher wants to hear, or what the participant thinks is the correct response
- has ever thought about such issues and is therefore able to discuss them
- is able to articulate his/her thoughts
- changes his/her thoughts/reasoning/simply because of being studied (also referred to as the Hawthorne effect).

Researchers from different philosophical approaches in the qualitative research tradition do not always see these issues as problems. Nonetheless, the fact remains that accurately accessing what therapists think is not straightforward, since there are multiple layers of responses for the researcher to access and then tease out. In a novel approach, Chapparo (1997) used the "Theory of Planned Behavior" (Ajzen, 1991) as a framework for examining the impact of a range of factors including personal context influences on professional reasoning. Although the theory of planned behavior was developed as a means of studying the effect of personal beliefs on social behavior, it offers an interesting approach to studying the effects of personal beliefs on professional behavior. Examples of research questions related to the person are found in Box 16-4.

B O X   1 6 - 4

Personal Variance in Professional Reasoning

- How might theories of adult development assist us in understanding variances in therapist's reasoning?
- Is there a relationship between therapists' unique personal make-up and the overarching processes they use to guide the various modes of reasoning?
- Which perspectives of adult development and learning are most useful for improving professional reasoning that leads to improved client care?
- What technological resources are useful in assisting therapists in organizing and retrieving knowledge for decision making? How practical are these resources to use in the daily rounds of therapy?
- What research strategies are most effective for accessing the effects of personal factors on professional reasoning?

Contextual Factors and Professional Reasoning

In addition to the individual who is engaging in professional reasoning, there is mounting evidence that the context in which this reasoning occurs plays an important role. Taking Lave's position that cognition represents "a complex social phenomenon [which] is a nexus of relations between the mind at work and the world in which it works" (1988, p. 1), it becomes important to examine the various contextual factors that shape both the conceptualization of possibilities and the actual implementation of what the therapist envisions. For instance, from a social learning perspective, the communities in which we practice influence the actual activities that make up practice in that setting as well as how therapists identify and draw meaning from their practices. All these in turn shape and reshape the practice community. To further complicate matters, there are overlapping communities of practice. For example, a therapist who works primarily with individuals who are recovering from acute hand injuries is likely to identify with both occupational therapy professionals and an interdisciplinary group of hand therapists. Furthermore, the nature of practice tends to focus on impairment reduction with the assumption that occupational performance will return when impairments are reduced. Alternatively, someone working with individuals with chronic pain in a program designed to return clients to work or productive activity is likely to focus on occupational performance, with minimal attention to the original impairment. Both of these practitioners may interface with governmental agencies dealing with worker compensation and vocational rehabilitation, as well as employers and attorneys. Going even further, some researchers such as Sladyck and Sheckly ask what "parallel non-clinical processes, such as learning to manage the political nature of the workplace, have on the development of clinical reasoning skills?" (1999, p. 168). Looking at professional reasoning as a social process allows us to ask how professional reasoning is shaped by forces of power, and social constructs such as gender, ethnicity, and social class (Box 16-5).

BOX 16-5

Research Questions Related to Professional Reasoning and Context

- How do physical contextual factors, such as equipment, space, and availability of resources contribute to or limit professional reasoning?
- How do supervisory and managerial practices affect therapist reasoning?
- What are the differences among therapists as they reason about both physical and social resources, and how do these differences affect resulting care?
- What is the impact of class, gender, and ethnicity of the therapist on his or her professional reasoning?
- What impact do class, gender, ethnicity, and other social factors of the client have on therapists' professional reasoning?
- How does the community of practice shape therapists' professional reasoning and therapy actions?
- How do therapists choose among the influences of multiple communities of practice in deciding how to shape their own therapy actions?

Missing Pieces

In addition to the particular questions about both personal and contextual aspects of professional reasoning, there are several obvious gaps in empirical evidence that became evident in the completion of this book. These represent more discrete topical areas, but ones of such importance that they bear highlighting. Included are information processing, personal variances in reasoning, ethical reasoning, supervisory/management reasoning, fieldwork supervision, and reasoning of therapy assistants.

Information Processing

Although a significant amount of research has been done in other professions, notably medicine, about the information processing that occurs during practice, little research has been done with occupational therapists (Roberston, 1996). Since there are plenty of models to choose from (see Patel & Arocha, 2000, for a good review and related citations), this sort of research could be easily implemented and serve to help the occupational therapy community understand the applicability and limitation of information-processing models that are borrowed from research in other professions.

Individual Variances in Reasoning

More research is required to explore individual differences associated with professional reasoning. As discussed earlier in this chapter, there is a great deal to learn about the influence of personal factors on professional reasoning and therapy actions. This is particularly critical, because occupational therapy is a highly constructed form of therapy. By this, we mean that therapists construct the problems to address based on their perceptions of client concerns and their assessment of the intrinsic and extrinsic factors affecting client performance. The influence of therapists' individual differences is also a difficult area to access, owing to their highly tacit nature. However, some factors, such as sensory processing preferences, personality style, and personal values can be accessed and require further explication.

Ethical Reasoning

An important aspect of a therapist's personal reasoning or worldview is his/her ethical reasoning. As described in Chapter 8, there have been several studies related to ethics education and many articles describing methods for teaching ethics and ethical decision making in issues in the practice of occupational therapy. However, there is virtually no research that examines the reasoning used by occupational therapists faced with ethical dilemmas in practice. Likewise, there has been no debate on the relative merits of what could and should happen, or to paraphrase Rogers (1983), of all the things we could do, what ought we to do? This is of particular concern in practice situations with a lack of consistent clinical supervision or with staffing that consists of part-time and per-diem therapists. Such situations lack a cohesive group or environment conducive to discussions of ethical concerns (Horowitz, 2002).

Supervisory and Managerial Reasoning

Although there is a growing literature on occupational therapy management, there is a paucity of research in the occupational therapy literature that examines supervisory and managerial reasoning as it relates to occupational therapy practice. It is reasonable to presume that the way in which managers and supervisors think about the therapy process has an impact on their decision making, which in turn becomes an important aspect of the practice context. Clinic design, documentation and reporting forms, public education materials, and performance expectations are but a few of the ways in which managers influence the actual practice of occupational therapy (Schell & Braveman, 2006). Recent efforts to address this issue in educational texts (Braveman, 2006) may open the door to studies examining the interface among managerial, supervisory, and therapist reasoning.

Fieldwork Supervision

Although there is a large body of scholarship on fieldwork education, the work by Farber and Koenig (1999) raises the question of how the reasoning processes of both fieldwork supervisors and students interact. In addition, research is needed on how those intertwined processes ultimately affect development of both partners as well as the therapy practices that result.

Learning, Teaching, and Professional Reasoning

Despite a growing research tradition of relating educational practices to the development of professional reasoning skills, there is still much to learn. As pointed out earlier, the relationship of individual differences to the nature and quality of professional reasoning has barely been explored. Similarly, these personal differences are not adequately addressed in reports of educational research. Such an approach goes well beyond a simple recital of demographic characteristics if we are to match our nuanced understandings of professional reasoning with equally nuanced educational approaches to support it. Daloz's (1986) work on transformational learning with adults provides a nice model for similar studies with occupational therapy students. On a smaller scope, Neistadt and colleagues provided several excellent models for capturing information about the effectiveness of our methods of teaching clinical reasoning and student approaches to learning this material (Neistadt, 1996, 1997; Neistadt & Atkins, 1996; Neistadt & Smith, 1997; Neistadt & Cohn, 1990; Neistadt, Wight & Mulligan, 1998).

The Development of Expertise in Practice

Once therapists enter practice, the next level of concern is the development of expertise. Our understanding of levels of expertise was founded on the work of Dreyfus and Dreyfus (1986) and expanded for application in health professionals by Benner (1984); Benner, Hooper-Kyriakidis and Stanard (1999); and Benner, Tanner, and Chesla (1996). We have a very good understanding of the characteristics of "experts" and the characteristics of "novices." There has been considerable research on the acquisition of expertise and research on the attainment of expertise focused on novice–expert differences (see OT research such as Unsworth [2001]; Mitchell & Unsworth [2005]; Strong, Gilbert, Cassidy & Bennett [1995]; and Gibson et al. [2000]). In addition, Carr and Shotwell (see Chapter 3) provide a very nice discussion on the differences between experts and novices in their chapter on information processing in clinical reasoning. What we do not know much about are the characteristics of the levels in between such as advanced beginner, competent, and proficient (Box 16-6). Furthermore, we do not have a good understanding of what moves therapists up (or down) the continuum of expertise. The next section proposes a model of learning for the development of professional expertise, which serves as a useful unifying guide for research related to teaching and learning as it relates to professional reasoning.

BOX 16-6

Research Questions About the Development of Professional Reasoning

- What are the characteristics of occupational therapists that denote they have achieved the level of "advanced beginner," "competent," or "proficient" practitioner?
- Are there different patterns of development related to different kinds of reasoning?
- Do information processing patterns change with experience? Do these changes parallel findings in other health professions?
- What facilitates a therapist moving from one level of expertise to the next?
- Why do some therapists never attain expertise?
- What factors support development vs. degradation of expertise?

Reasoning at Differing Professional Levels

As may be obvious by now, the majority of research on reasoning in occupational therapy has been done with professional-level occupational therapists, primarily individuals educated in programs culminating in a bachelor's degree. With the move to entry level master's programs in the United States, Canada, and Australia, along with some programs even progressing to entry with a professional doctorate, it will be interesting to see whether any differences in the patterns of reasoning can be observed as well as the development of expertise. In addition, there is very little research examining how occupational therapy assistants reason in practice (Lyons & Crepeau, 1991).

These "missing pieces" highlight a need for theories or models to further guide and systematize the next generation of research on professional reasoning within occupational therapy. In the next section, several different models are described after brief review of considerations for theory development.

Thinking About Thinking 16-3

Theory helps us to explain ourselves to ourselves and to others. We are not talking about self-justification but about the narrative unity of human agency: how we make sense of our own and others' actions. This aspect of theory is deeply communicative in its insistence on the possibility of transparency.

—Nixon and Creek, 2006

THE EVOLVING THEORY OF PROFESSIONAL REASONING

Professional Reasoning: More Than the Link Between Theory and Practice

In his text, *Conceptual Foundations in Occupational Therapy*, Kielhofner (2005) supports the growing realization in the scientific community that there must be discourse among theory, research, and practice. Traditionally, theory is generated separately from its application and practice and is viewed as a hierarchy. In this approach, theorists and researchers generate new knowledge and professionals must translate this into what should be done in practice. The view that practice is simply the application of theory is now widely debated in the scientific community, and Kielhofner (2005), among others, argues that it is illogical because it results in theory of questionable practical value. Supporters of a new approach to understanding the relationship between theory and practice suggest that theory can arise from practice (Creek & Ormston, 1996). Argyris and Schön (1974) refer to these as "theories-in-use" (p. 6). Although the core paradigm of occupational therapy may be referred to as an "espoused theory" and defines the nature and purpose of occupational therapy, theories-in-use involve the application of practical knowledge. Over the past 15 years, the writings of Kielhofner (2005) and Schön (1983), among others, have enabled these ideas to be translated from other disciplines and understood and accepted in the occupational therapy community (Unsworth & Schell, 2006).

The central goal of the AOTF-funded study on clinical reasoning (Mattingly & Fleming, 1994) was to discover the practical theories-in-use of the profession and develop a language to describe these. As Mattingly and Fleming describe, they did more than this; they also explored "the culture of occupational therapy practice, complete with language, values, and even, in some sense, ceremony" (1994, p. 24). But Mattingly and Fleming's work was not in isolation and they had a strong multidisciplinary base on which to build the construct of clinical reasoning in occupational therapy. Mattingly and Fleming (1994) drew on the work of many others such as Rogers and Masagatani (1992) from occupational therapy and of scholars from many other fields such as Pierce (1931-1935), Dewey (1929), Polanyi (1966), and Schön (1983, 1987). As a result of their work, Mattingly and Fleming did for occupational therapy what Benner (1984) and Benner and Tanner (1987) had done in nursing before them; they opened up for the profession a new way of viewing the generation of knowledge and use of theory. By adopting an ethnographic research method, Mattingly and Fleming worked together with practitioners to examine clinical reasoning in what Kielhofner (2005) refers to as a "scholarship of practice." Hence, what needs explaining in the profession and how it gets explained arises out of practice.

The profession now feels very comfortable in viewing professional reasoning and reflection as a means of excavating, examining, and passing on theories in use. It also accepts the link between espoused theory and practice (e.g., Mitcham, 2003; Kielhofner, 2005; Hagedorn, 1997). Furthermore, over the past 10 years, the terminology and concepts of clinical and professional reasoning have become incorporated into occupational therapy theory. For example, the notion of narrative reasoning is now becoming embedded in conceptual practice models such as the Model of Human Occupation (Kielhofner, 2005). However, although professional reasoning is an essential link between theory and practice, we also propose that it is much more than this. Professional reasoning is itself developing into a theory in its own right (Unsworth & Schell, 2006).

Terms Used to Define Theory

Theory may be broadly defined as an attempt to explain and predict phenomena (Walker & Ludwig, 2004). Theory helps us to recognize what we know and to organize what we do know (Mitcham, 2003). Texts describing theories related to occupational therapy such as Hagedorn's (1997) or Walker and Ludwig's (2004) provide useful tables that summarize the different terms used to describe theory by their developers. Hence, like all academics and practitioners working on theory building or trying to teach theory to students, the initial struggle that we face in proposing the developing theory of clinical reasoning is what terminology to use. In the interests of simplicity and flexibility for the field to develop a theory of professional reasoning, we will talk about theory building in general. This is followed by different models of clinical and professional reasoning that are being put forth that contribute to developing theory.

Definitions of Theory

Reed (1984) draws on the work of Kerlinger (1973) in stating that theories are made up of a set of interrelated **concepts** (constructs if these are not tangible or observable) and principles or propositions. A concept may be defined as words that express mental images of a phenomenon, whereas a **principle** is a rule or law concerning the phenomenon or truths, laws, or assumptions about the phenomenon (Walker & Ludwig, 2004). **Propositions** describe the nature of the relationship between the concepts or constructs. Theories vary enormously in complexity and scope. Hence, at one end of the continuum lie theories that are very broad and complex; at the other extreme are those that are narrow in focus and deal with a specific phenomenon. Reed (1984) and Walker and Ludwig (2004) use the general divisions proposed in the nursing literature to describe meta- and grand theories (the most abstract and over-arching of all theories), middle-range theories, and practical theories (those that provide goals and actions for the practitioner).

Theory Construction

To map the progress of professional reasoning on the continuum of theory development, the stages of theory development must be described. Mitcham (2003) describes the process of theory generation as involving six sequential steps (as shown in Box 16-7), starting with observation and ending with tested theory.

BOX 16-7
Steps of Theory Development

1. Observation of the phenomena over time
2. Recognition that phenomena present themselves in certain ways
3. Organization of the phenomena into a conceptual framework
4. Empirical testing of the propositions and concepts that hold the conceptual framework together
5. Refinement and re-testing propositions and concepts
6. Acceptance of the new theory (Adapted from Mitcham, 2003)

This description of theory development implies a coordinated, concerted approach to theory generation. Although Mitcham's model is very prescriptive, the three-stage model of theory development proposed by Lewin (1947) (as described in Walker and Ludwig, 2004) is probably more useful for us as we wallow in the early stages of the development of a theory of professional reasoning:

Speculative period—the field puts forth theoretical models to attempt to explain phenomena.
Descriptive period— the field gathers facts through research to describe what really is happening and to test the theoretical models.
Constructive period—The field revises old theories and develops new ones that are grounded in facts rather than based on speculation (Walker & Ludwig, 2004).

In summary, we construct theory by "developing collaborative models of thoughtful practice that challenge assumptions and suggest new lines of inquiry" (Nixon & Creek, 2006).

Current Progress Toward a Theory of Professional Reasoning

Lewin's (1947) writings provide a useful framework for understanding theory development in relation to professional reasoning. Using his description of the three stages, it appears that we have made some progress toward the first two steps—in a somewhat blurred fashion. Lewin's descriptions rely on an understanding of the term *model* (Unsworth & Schell, 2006). Models may be described as a way of describing the phenomenon in a familiar way so as to increase our understanding (Young & Quinn, 1992). Furthermore, Young and Quinn (1992, p. 14) define the chief functions of a model to "provide a framework for complex data, facilitate visualization of phenomena, facilitate communication of ideas, and suggest predictions about the real world and stimulate the development of theories." Three models have been described in the literature to explain the phenomenon of clinical/professional reasoning. These models were developed using what was described earlier as a "scholarship of practice" approach (Kielfofner, 2005). In other words, some of this information was generated from pure speculation, whereas other aspects were derived from study in environments where professional reasoning occurs such as the clinic. A fourth model is being added in this chapter, reflecting views of professional reasoning that have emerged in editing this book. The four models are the linear model as outlined by Dewey (1930s) and described by Ryan (1998); Higgs and Jones' spiral model (1995), Unsworth's (2004) conceptualization of a three-tier hierarchy of clinical reasoning, which draws heavily on the work of Mattingly and Fleming (1994), and Schell's ecological model of professional reasoning. Although Ryan (1998) also describes a narrative model of clinical reasoning, there is insufficient information on the components and definitions of this model to describe it in any detail. The other three models are briefly described, and their contributions to the evolving theory of clinical reasoning are outlined in the next section.

Dewey's Linear Model of Clinical Reasoning

John Dewey (1929, 1934) developed the classic description of general reasoning (Ryan, 1998). This model has many similarities to the hypothetico-deductive model of reasoning used in early medical studies and reported in Mattingly and Fleming (1994) and Rogers and Holms' work on diagnostic reasoning (1991). Basically, this model is linear and consists of five stages: reflecting on ideas, formulating hypotheses, evaluating hypotheses for truths, determining a course of action, and formulating a verbal statement to represent the hypothesis (Ryan, 1998). This model works well in problem-solving situations such as when a diagnosis is required; however, this model is less well suited to explaining reasoning in the health sciences.

Higgs and Jones' Spiral Model of Clinical Reasoning

Higgs and Jones (2000) describe an integrated, patient-centered model of clinical reasoning. They depict an expanding spiral that reflects the clinician's growing understanding of the client and the clinical problem (*Figure 16-3*).

At the beginning of the spiral is the clinician's encounter with the client; at the end is the final outcome. The tubing of the spiral represents the interaction of the six elements that make up the model. These are:

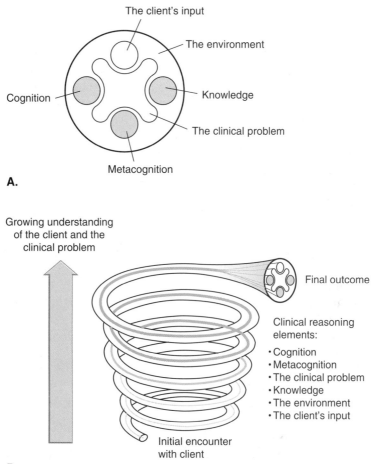

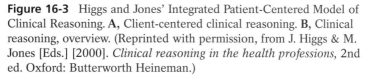

Figure 16-3   Higgs and Jones' Integrated Patient-Centered Model of Clinical Reasoning. **A,** Client-centered clinical reasoning. **B,** Clinical reasoning, overview. (Reprinted with permission, from J. Higgs & M. Jones [Eds.] [2000]. *Clinical reasoning in the health professions,* 2nd ed. Oxford: Butterworth Heineman.)

Cognition (reflective inquiry)
Metacognition (the integrative element between cognition and knowledge)
The clinical problem (the influence of the nature of the clinical problem or task on reasoning)
Knowledge (a discipline-specific knowledge base)
The environment (interaction between the decision makers and the environment or situation)
The client's input (the role of the client in the decision making process).

Unsworth's Hierarchical Model of Clinical Reasoning

Unsworth (2004, 2005) proposed a three-tier hierarchy to depict the relationship between the different types of clinical reasoning found through her own research and as articulated by Mattingly and Fleming (1994); Schön (1983, 1987); Barris (1987); Hooper (1997); and Schell and Cervero (1993) (*Figure 16-4*).

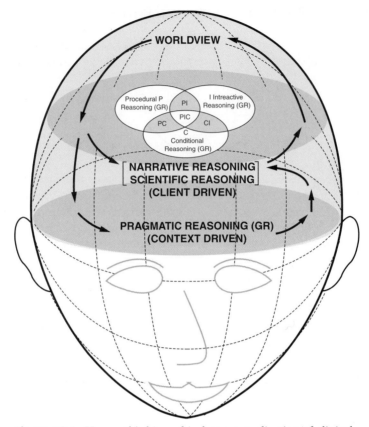

Figure 16-4 Unsworth's hierarchical conceptualization of clinical reasoning in the client-centered practice of occupational therapy (Unsworth, 2004). (Reprinted with permission of the *British Journal of Occupational Therapy.*)

Hence, this model is based on practice, research, and existing theoretical concepts. At the top of Unsworth's model is worldview, which influences and modifies all the other modes of reasoning. The concept of worldview represents sophisticated thinking, which includes one's moral beliefs and sociocultural perspective (Wolters 1989). The middle level of the diagram contains the three main forms of reasoning: procedural, interactive, and conditional. The fact that therapists also seemed to use two or three forms of procedural/interactive/conditional reasoning simultaneously is presented by the use of a Venn diagram (Unsworth, 2005). These modes of reasoning are either more scientific (procedural reasoning) or more narrative/phenomenological in nature (interactive and conditional). Finally, the last level of the diagram contains pragmatic reasoning. Pragmatic reasoning deals with what can be achieved given the practical constraints or benefits of the environment (financial, clinic, client home, etc.). In contrast to scientific and narrative modes of reasoning, which are client driven, pragmatic reasoning is context driven. The arrows that flow around this model indicate that to a greater or lesser extent these modes of reasoning or influences on reasoning all have an impact on each other. This model of clinical reasoning operates in the client-centered practice of occupational therapy (Unsworth, 2004).

Ecological Model of Professional Reasoning

The Ecological Model of Professional Reasoning was introduced at the World Federation Occupational Therapy Conference (Unsworth & Schell, 2006) and represents Barbara Schell's synthesis of research and scholarship in clinical and professional reasoning. This model describes professional reasoning as a process directly linked to therapy action, and it is shaped by factors intrinsic to the therapist and client, as well as extrinsic factors in the practice context. Professional action is the result of the interplay among therapist, the client, and the setting (*Figure 16-5*). Like the previous two models, it draws on the work of many. Its general form and key components were prompted in part by a brief article by Törnebohm (1991), in which he described the interface between the therapist paradigm and the patient's paradigm. The ecological perspective echoes the occupational therapy theory entitled the Ecology of Human Performance (Dunn, Brown & Youngstrom, 2003), as well as the literature on situated cognition and communities of practice (Wenger, 1998; Lave & Wenger, 1991). The major kinds of reasoning are drawn from Mattingly and Fleming (1994), Schell and Cervero (1993), and the many subsequent studies of clinical reasoning as a multi-track process (e.g., Crepeau, 1991; Creighton, Dijkers, Bennett & Brown, 1995; Unsworth, 2004, 2005).

The Ecological Model of Professional Reasoning describes professional reasoning and resulting therapy action as the interface of the therapist, the client and the practice content (see *Figure 16-5*). The model postulates that each practitioner brings to the therapy situation knowledge and skills that are grounded in

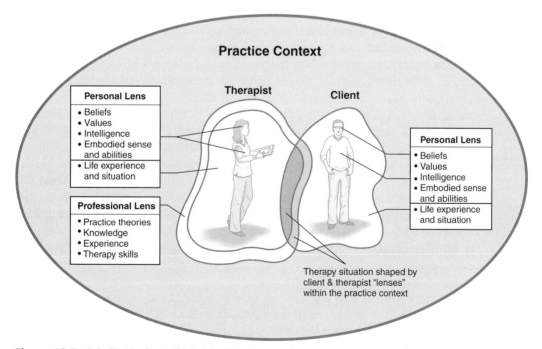

Figure 16-5 Schell's Ecological Model of Professional Reasoning. The therapist views the client through personal and professional lenses, just as the client views the therapist through the lens of his or her life experiences. Much of the task of professional reasoning in occupational therapy is to develop effective collaboration necessary for therapy to occur.

life experiences including personal characteristics such as physical capacities, sensory profile (see Chapter 4; Harris, 2005), personality, and intelligence profile (Gardner, 2004), as well as enculturated factors such as values, beliefs, and preferences (Fondiller, Rosage & Neuhaus, 1990; Hooper 1997; Unsworth, 2004; Chapter 2). These form a *personal self,* which is an inescapable lens through which the therapist frames the therapy encounter. Layered over or entwined with this personal self is the *professional self,* which includes the therapist's professional knowledge from education, experiences from prior clients, and therapy beliefs, along with knowledge of specific technical skills and therapy routines available for use in the practice context (Burke, 1997; Fondiller & Rosage, 1990; Mattingly & Fleming, 1994; Törnebohm, 1991). The personal and professional selves act in concert to respond to various problems of practice. Some problems are primarily related to the *client* (Rogers & Holm, 1991; Mattingly & Fleming, 1994), and some are related more to the *practice context* (Schell & Cervero, 1993; Unsworth, 2004). Similarly, the client comes to therapy with his or her own life experiences and personal characteristics, life situation, as well as the performance problems that prompted the need for therapy. A significant portion of professional reasoning is directed toward developing a shared understanding of problems as well as eliciting collaboration required to develop and implement therapy action (Crepeau, 1991; Mattingly & Fleming, 1994).

The therapist and the client function within a community of practice that shapes the nature, scope, and trajectory of the therapy process (Lave & Wenger, 1991; Wenger, 1998; Schell, 1994; Barris, 1987; Rogers & Masagatani, 1982). Different forms of reasoning occur in response to problems raised from the client or the therapy context or the therapist's personal characteristics as they interface with the client and therapy context. These include scientific, procedural, narrative, interactive, and pragmatic reasoning. Less commonly documented in the research are ethical and conditional reasoning.

Scientific reasoning involves the use of applied logical and scientific methods, such as hypothesis testing, explicit pattern recognition, theory-based decision making, and statistical evidence. One form of scientific reasoning is diagnostic reasoning, which is used to understand the client's occupational problems (Rogers & Holms, 1991). Scientific reasoning is generally directed toward the client, or in the case of managerial or educational activities, toward the development of therapy programs that are supported by evidence and critical thinking.

Procedural reasoning is used when therapists are thinking about what typically works with a client in a given situation or what treatment protocols are used in that setting for a given diagnosis (Barris, 1987; Rogers & Masagatani, 1982; Fleming, 1991). It represents an interaction among the therapist, the client and the practice context. Managers are postulated to engage in procedural reasoning when developing orientation programs and support documents for therapist reference as well as records of service.

Narrative reasoning is a process in which therapists attempt to understand the meaning of the condition to the client, as well as to figure out a common trajectory on which to base intervention planning (Mattingly, 1991). Although narrative reasoning primarily involves obtaining information from the client's perspective, there are also times when the therapist attempts to match a "story" from his or her own life with a client for whom one is having difficulty eliciting a personal perspective. An example is when a student therapist decides to play checkers with an older man, because she could not get him to tell her what he would like to do and because her grandfather always liked to play checkers. *Interactive reasoning* guides the communicative acts that the therapist undertakes with the client, generally to elicit cooperation or facilitate collaboration (Crepeau, 1991; Fleming, 1991). Both narrative reasoning and interactive reasoning primarily address the interactions among the client, the client life situation, and the therapist's personal and professional selves.

Pragmatic reasoning is a form of reasoning used to fit therapy possibilities into the current realities of service delivery. Some of these realities include scheduling options, payment for services, equipment availability, management directives, and the like (Schell, 1994; Mitchell & Unsworth, 2005; Unsworth, 2004). There is some evidence that the practice context can support or hinder the range of possible therapy actions, based on therapist beliefs and experiences about what is practical in the particular setting. There are also factors that therapists consider as being related more to their own situations. Some of these are related to the professional self, such as the therapist's repertoire of therapy skills. Others are related to the personal self, such as outside obligations and activity preferences. From these perspectives, pragmatic reasoning is focused more on the practice context or on the therapist's personal situation than it is on the client per se.

Ethical reasoning is introduced as needed to solve perceived conflicts about the just or right course of action (Rogers, 1983). *Conditional reasoning* is a form of futuristic thinking that occurs as therapists consider possibilities over time for the client, given the client's particular situation and the therapist's experiences with other clients (Fleming, 1991). Conditional reasoning can involve all the other forms of reasoning and is a synthesis used to guide current intervention based on imagined possibilities.

Because professional reasoning is a dynamic process directed toward action, the development of expertise is likewise affected by the interface among the therapist, the clients seen, and the practice context, which includes both physical and sociological factors. In this way, professional reasoning is a form of situated cognition that is shaped by the various communities in which one practices. As stated initially, this model has not been researched directly, but represents a meta-synthesis of the research that has been done in the field.

CONTEXTUAL TEACHING FOR PROFESSIONAL REASONING

Because we are concerned about promoting clinical and professional reasoning, it is important to provide a model for contextual teaching that promotes such higher-order thinking. Earlier in this book, we wrote about the how experiences and reflection can be thought of as twin instructional dynamics (Schell, 2001). John Schell has developed a circular model that illustrates the intersection of learning and teaching. This model is, in part, based on John Dewey's point of "emancipation and enlargement of experience" (Jeffs & Smith, 2005, pp. 2–3). For Dewey and others, authentic experiences provide an excellent setting for interaction between student and teacher as a way (a) to provide instruction and co-construction of knowledge, (b) for learners to articulate their constructed knowledge, and then (c) to reflect on that constructed knowledge as a way to make meaning. The circle is then completed as the learner reinterprets the

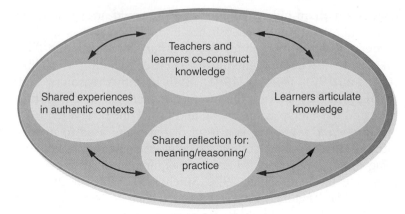

Figure 16-6 John Schell's Model for Contextual Teaching for Professional Reasoning.

environment in light of his or her more advanced perspective(s). This continuous cycle means additional opportunities to reengage in the learning cycle when the learner has obtained higher and higher levels of expertise. This brings about even greater levels of sophistication and insight as learners and teachers continue the learning-teaching cycle. The model is illustrated in *Figure 16-6*.

Shared Experiences in Authentic Contexts

This model of instruction begins with the same assumption made by John Dewey in the late 19th Century: Experience, learning, and reflection are all connected. Learners begin to learn professional reasoning as they engage in OT experiences purposely set in authentic learning environments. As we have stated in many places in this book, learning and teaching are most effective when experience-based and should occur in genuine contexts when practical. Given financial, institutional, ethical, and practical reasons, it is not always possible to provide instruction in the context of actual occupational therapy. However, our belief is to promote the idea that contexts should be authentic. Or, as we stated earlier—the "realer the better." It is important for the instructor to also be engaged with the students as they encounter an experience. In this way, the teacher has a common repertoire upon which to draw later during instructional phases. Teachers can arrange for learners to have specific experiences that will cause them to engage in specific behaviors that are germane to the purpose of the lesson. Our basic assumption for this overarching part of the model is consistent with Wenger's model for *Communities of Practice* (1998). We believe that learning is essentially social in nature. It is the complex patterns of interplay between the student and significant actors (teachers, practicing OTs, patients, and their families) that are crucial to the authenticity of the learning environment. In fact, these rich social dynamics are very difficult to replicate in a simulation but are critical to making learning seem more real, important, and even urgent. An example of an authentic context is when a novice OT (preservice) is required to conduct parent interviews of two different families, one of which has a typically developing child and the other a child with a developmental delay. It should be obvious that this experience varies greatly from these students just interviewing each other for practice in class or lab.

Teachers and Learners Co-Construct Knowledge

After—or sometimes during—a contextualized learning experience, the instructor is engaged in assisting the learner to construct new knowledge. This is a form of constructivism. A variety of types of constructivism ranging from internal to external cognitive processes was discussed in Chapter 11. This model is based on a combination of those perspectives known as *blended* or *dialectical constructivism* in which the source of cognition begins with either the teacher or the learner. We assume that at times the source of instruction resides with the teacher, who has an obligation to meet instructional objectives and/or professional standards. At other times, it is appropriate for learners to advocate for themselves and become emancipated from the tyranny of linear teaching to determine their own path for learning.

Teaching methods that promote co-construction of knowledge can be drawn from the model of cognitive apprenticeship teaching (Brown, Collins & Duguid, 1989). Such teaching initiated by the teacher might draw on "modeling" methods in which a demonstration of the desired technique is provided. Working toward independence or pushing what Vygotsky (1978) called the Zone of Proximal Development (ZPD), teachers can call on "coaching" methods followed as needed by "scaffolding and fading." For example, as an OT student learns to safely transfer a client from wheelchair to bed, the teacher might demonstrate or model appropriate techniques. Having seen a transfer, it is reasonable to have the student try one with another student, who plays the patient while the instructor watches and give suggestions. As the student attempts their first transfer of an actual patient, the instructor is on the sideline coaching or giving instruction as needed. At all times, client safety is the highest priority. When the teacher believes that the student cannot safely accomplish the transfer, he or she can scaffold by performing a small part of the procedure that ensures safety. As the learner becomes more competent, however, the teacher can fade out and allow much greater independence for the student. We see this as a co-construction of knowledge, since the teacher's role is to facilitate and guide while the learner is seeking to interpret the material in light of their prior knowledge and its fit with their previously established mental frameworks.

Learners Articulate Knowledge

After students have accomplished some level of expertise, the teacher might ask students to articulate their newly acquired knowledge or skill. Usually when we hear the term articulate, it can be assumed that we are asking the learner to tell you what they have learned. This is a very important step and certainly can and should be accomplished orally. Yet, left at this level, the probability for recall and application in actual practice remains small. It is important to use a range of instructional strategies that promote a variety of ways for students to articulate their knowledge in many ways. Very few complex tasks are learned in a single attempt, so teachers should arrange for students to articulate their knowledge many times using a variety of media. For example, students can be asked to write the traditional paper with regard to what they have learned. Obviously, this is a tried and true approach. However, students who are additionally asked to present their work in the form of an audio or video Podcast demonstrating their skills are more likely to have engaged with the topic in a deeper and more meaningful way.

Shared Reflection for Meaning/Reasoning/Practice

Articulation and reflection on meaning are closely associated instructional techniques. As stated earlier in this book, many teachers ask students to reflect on their knowledge. We suspect that few teachers find ways to "connect" the construction of knowledge with its articulation and then find a systematic way to facilitate deep reflection as an exercise in meaning-making. We strongly suggest that when the teacher is able to make these connections transparent, students are more likely to assign a value to the knowledge they have acquired. This is because the question of When will I ever use this stuff? has been answered as a matter of instructional practice. We also contend that meaning-making is only part of the possible outcomes from systematic reflection. After teaching, reflection gives opportunities to build on reflective judgment and to have good discussions with regard to the "truth of the matter" and the level and quality of evidence that the learner uses to support their position. This is a natural instructional practice for those who want to promote evidence-based practice. Of course, the Holy Grail of reflection is to facilitate ways in which teachers and learners co-construct connections with everyday OT practice. Reflection should ask the student to engage in questions such as: How does this knowledge impact my practice? How can I use supporting evidence for this knowledge so that I can make choices among practice alternatives that make sense for the needs and contexts of the client? How do I know to do this?

A Learning Cycle That Never Ends

There are very few things that can be said with certainty about learning and teaching, but one that can probably stand is: Once is never enough. Benner's work on expertise (Benner, 1984; Benner, Tanner & Chesla, 1996) suggests that advanced competency comes after many years of repetition and practice. So it is with teaching and learning. In the case of teaching for professional practice, students and teachers must continue the cycle on many occasions seeking nuance and changing conditions. Eventually, learners must complete these revolutions on their own.

METHODOLOGIES TO SUPPORT FUTURE RESEARCH

The discussions in this chapter focus on the kinds of research into professional reasoning that we envision are required to further support occupational therapy practice. The kinds of quantitative and qualitative research methods that can be used to explore professional reasoning were reviewed in Chapter 15. Our aim here is to examine what methods can best help us further develop and validate models of professional reasoning, as well to explore the links among reasoning, action, and outcome. Furthermore, we propose some conventions that we feel might be useful in strengthening the quality of the research conducted.

Methods and Rigor

Professional reasoning research in occupational therapy needs to move beyond uncritical examination of reasoning to a more nuanced examination of the differential effects of different reasoning approaches to the development and implementation of therapy actions that result in desired outcomes of meaning to the client. This is because an important commitment that professions make to society is to use specialized knowledge in a manner most likely to benefit the client. This requires a shift in design of professional reasoning studies. For instance, self-report paper or web-based surveys are likely to provide only superficial and incomplete information. This is for a number of reasons:

1. There are obviously social factors that limit what a therapist is likely to reveal.
2. Much therapist knowledge is tacit, requiring skilled "excavation" practices to stimulate therapist memory. Even observation and interview based in actual practice settings are subject to these limitations.
3. As convincingly argued by Benner and colleagues (Benner, 1984; Benner, Hooper-Kyriakidis & Stanard, 1999; Benner, Tanner & Chesla, 1996), professional reasoning is deeply embedded in the actual practice situation, as is the relative level of expertise. Therefore, designs need to incorporate the natural context as much as possible to obtain more credible information.

Therefore, research designs that use broader methods of triangulating of data are required. Equally important is the need to find and use sensitive techniques designed to minimize degradations in memory, socially based editing, and the generation of espoused (rather than practiced) theories. The use of technology that is minimally disturbing to the therapy setting and that can also be used to monitor physiological functions of the therapist while reasoning in actual practice situations is one hopeful avenue. Careful use of participant observation, peer informants, and document review can also help to put the pieces together for a more valid picture of what the therapist is thinking.

Studying Reasoning Over Time

Another consideration in methodology is the need to study therapists over time, particularly if we are to understand what moves therapists from one level of expertise to another. Although cross-sectional studies of therapists as they reason in everyday practice can provide some clues as to differences, longitudinal studies are required to fully explore this phenomenon. Given the cost and complexity of longitudinal studies, careful selection of quantitative measures as well as qualitative methods are required. In addition, the scope of these studies may need to address both individual factors and the systems in which the practitioner is functioning.

Connecting Thought, Action, and Outcome

Related to the careful exploration of what the therapist is thinking is careful data collection about what the therapist is actually doing. "Doing" in this sense needs to encompass a wide range of therapist and client interactions, both verbal and nonverbal. These "doings" can then be related to the thinking, to begin to form an understanding of how and why therapists think about what they are doing. Much has been made of the landmark study by Mattingly and Fleming (1994), in part because the findings seem to strike a chord of recognition in the occupational therapy community. One of the strengths of this study was its in-depth and prolonged use of ethnographic and action research methods. Videotapes captured what was actually going on, and interviews and group discussions used these to surface what the therapist thought about. Similarly, we need to conduct studies in a whole range of practice settings to surface what therapists are thinking and connect that with what they are doing. Because the work of Mattingly and Fleming was restricted to medically based practice by one group (or community) of practitioners, it is possible that different understandings of the process and practice would emerge from different practice contexts. When doing these studies, we need to also characterize the therapy practice using creditable approaches, such as the use of fidelity instruments or peer review, along with observations. Finally, we need to link all these to observable outcomes to complete the cycle.

THE FUTURE OF THEORY DEVELOPMENT ON PROFESSIONAL REASONING

There is an old pop tune that croons something like "the future's so bright I gotta wear shades," and so it is in the field of theory development in professional reasoning. The research and study required in the future is exciting and dazzling. As described above, it seems that we are still working on the first and second phases of Lewin's approach for developing the theory of professional reasoning. We are still speculating on the nature of professional reasoning and developing models to describe what we are finding in our research. Likewise, we are exploring models to support the education of new practitioners as well as the development of expertise. The challenge for us now is to test out these emerging models. From there, we must enter the constructive phase of theory development and merge or further develop these models into a comprehensive theory of professional reasoning. This emerging theory will be grounded in studies of professional reasoning from both the qualitative and quantitative research traditions. When entering this constructive period, the work of Reed (1984) will be useful.

Reed (1984, based on the work of Thomas [1979] and Overton and Reese [1973]) proposed that in order to be useful to health professionals, models should attempt to accomplish nine things: (1) It is important that a theory accurately reflects what people actually do in their everyday lives and (2) it should provide an explanation of the phenomena being studied. A theory should also be (3) understandable and (4) should explain the occurrence of past events and predict future events. A theory should (5) assist an individual to solve everyday problems by giving practical guidelines; should (6) stimulate new knowledge, techniques, or understanding; and should (7) be economical when in use. A theory should be (8) internally consistent, meaning that aspects of the theory work in harmony rather than contradicting each other; and finally, a theory should (9) be intuitively satisfying because it explains human performance using common sense (Reed, 1984).

It is exciting to be part of the generation that develops a theory of professional reasoning and to watch the form that it takes. We urge you to be part of this exciting development as well.

SUMMARY

This chapter draws together key elements and issues concerning professional reasoning from across the text and extends these by identifying where further research and development in the field are required. The chapter has provided an overview of the nature of clinical and professional reasoning, and the purpose of that reasoning. Overt links have been made between relating therapy thoughts to actions (described as practice fidelity) and professional reasoning as the vehicle that enables evidence-based practice. Descriptions of different types of reasoning and personal variance in clinical reasoning have been provided. The idea has been presented that professional reasoning is evolving into a theory, and models that contribute to this goal, including a model for guiding research on teaching and learning professional reasoning, have been described. Finally, some strategies to connect thought, action, and outcome through research are described. Although outlining what we need to accomplish to explicate professional reasoning forms the concluding chapter for this text, we hope readers will rise to the challenges and opportunities this provides for new beginnings in professional reasoning research.

LEARNING ACTIVITY 16-1

Developing the Field of Professional Reasoning Through Research

Carolyn A. Unsworth

Purpose

To develop a plan for conducting research in an area of professional reasoning that requires further development of knowledge

Connections to Major Clinical Reasoning Constructs

Information processing theory, models of clinical reasoning as described in the chapter

Directions for Learners

This chapter describes our current research progress in the area of professional reasoning and charts these developments against the criteria for building a theory of clinical reasoning. We also described many of the areas that required further research exploration.

1 Choose an area that excites your interest for further professional reasoning research.
2 What are the main research questions in this area that require answering?
3 What sorts of methods might be most suitable to explore this kind of reasoning?
4 Using the theory development information provided, describe how your research would contribute to theory development.

LEARNING ACTIVITY 16-2

Examining Teaching Practices
Carolyn A. Unsworth

Purpose

To develop a plan for conducting research about teaching, learning, and the development of expertise

Connections to Major Clinical Reasoning Constructs

Provides an opportunity to think about how to test educational models, such as the Model of Contextual Teaching for Professional Reasoning.

Directions for Learners

This chapter describes models of professional reasoning as well as a model for contextual teaching and learning. Considering this information:

1 Identify a current teaching practice in your setting.
2 Develop a plan for evaluating the current teaching practice in terms of:
   a Demonstration of learning gains
   b Fit with proposed model of contextual teaching
3 Evaluate your plan and reflect on what you might find through its implementation.
4 Discuss how findings from your proposed research might contribute to our understanding of how to teach professional reasoning.

REFERENCES

Ajzen, I. (1991). The theory of planned behaviour. *Organisational Behavior and Human Decision Processes, 50,* 179–211.

Argyris, C. & Schön, D. A. (1973). *Theory in practice: Increasing professional effectiveness.* San Francisco: Jossey-Bass.

Benner, P. E. (1984). *From novice to expert: Excellence and power in clinical nursing practice.* Menlo Park, CA: Addison-Wesley.

Benner, P., Hooper-Kyriakidis, P. & Stanard, D. (1999). *Clinical wisdom and interventions in critical care: A thinking-in-action approach.* Philadelphia: W. B. Saunders.

Benner, P E., Tanner, C. A & Chesla, C. A. (1996). *Expertise in nursing practice: Caring, clinical judgement and ethics.* New York: Springer.

Braveman, B. (Ed.) (2006). *Leading and managing occupational therapy services: An evidence-based approach.* Philadelphia: F. A. Davis.

Barris, R. (1987). Clinical reasoning in psychosocial occupational therapy: The evaluation process. *Occupational Therapy Journal of Research, 7,* 147–162.

Brown, J. S., Collins, A. & Duguid, P. (1989). Situated cognition and the culture of learning. *Educational Researcher, 18*(1), 32–42.

Burke, J. P. (2001). How therapists' conceptual perspectives influence early intervention evaluations. *Scandinavian Journal of Occupational Therapy, 8,* 49–61.

Burke, J. P. (1997). Frames of meaning: An analysis of occupational therapy evaluations of young children. *Dissertation Abstracts International, 58*(3), 644. (UMI Number: 9727199).

Chapparo, C (1997). Influences on clinical reasoning in occupational therapy. PhD thesis. Macquarie University, Australia.

Cleland, J. A., Onksen, P., Swanson, B. & McRae, M. (2004). Attributes of expert and novice clinicians: A brief review and investigation of the differences in peripheral sympathetic nervous system activity elicited during thoracic mobilization. *Physical Therapy Review*, 9, 31–38.

Craik, J. & Rappolt, S. (2006). Enhancing research utilization capacity through multifaceted professional development. *American Journal of Occupational Therapy*, 60, 155–164.

Creighton, C., Dijkers, M., Bennett, N. & Brown, K. (1995). Reasoning and the art of therapy for spinal cord injury. *American Journal of Occupational Therapy*, 49, 311–317.

Crepeau, E. B. (1991). Achieving intersubjective understanding: Examples form an occupational therapy treatment session. *American Journal of Occupational Therapy*, 44, 1016–1024.

Creek, J. & Ormston, C. (1996). The essential elements of professional motivation. *British Journal of Occupational Therapy*, 59, 7–10.

Daloz, L. A. (1986). *Effective teaching and mentoring: Realizing the transformation power of adult learning experiences.* San Francisco: Jossey-Bass.

DeLoach, C. P. & Greer, B. G. (1981). *Adjustment to severe physical disability. A metamorphosis.* New York: McGraw-Hill.

Dewey, J. (1929). *Experience and nature.* New York: W. W. Norton.

Dewey, J. (1934). *Art as experience.* New York: Minton, Balch & Co.

Dreyfus, H. L. & Dreyfus, S. E. (1986). *Mind over machine: The power of human intuition and expertise in the era of the computer.* New York: Free Press.

Dunn, W., Brown, C. & Youngstrom, M. J. (2003). Ecological model of occupation. In P. Kramer, J. Hinojosa & C. B. Royeen (Eds.), *Perspectives in human occupation: Participation in life.* (pp. 222–263). Philadelphia: Lippincott Williams & Wilkins.

Drucker, E. (1974). Hidden values and health care. *Medical Care*, 12, 266–273.

Eisenberg, J. (1979). Sociologic influences on decision making by clinicians. *Annals of Internal Medicine*, 90, 957–964.

Farber, R. S. & Koenig, K. (1999). Examination of fieldwork educators' responses to challenging fieldwork situations. *Innovations in Occupational Therapy Education*, 89–104.

Fleming, M. H. (1991). The therapist with the three-track mind. *American Journal of Occupational Therapy*, 45, 1007–1014.

Fondiller, E. D., Rosage, L. J. & Neuhaus, B. E. (1990). Values influencing clinical reasoning in occupational therapy: An exploratory study. *Occupational Therapy Journal of Research*, 10, 41–55.

Gething, L. (1992). Judgements by health professionals of personal characteristics of people with a visible physical disability. *Social Sciences and Medicine*, 34, 809–815.

Gardner, H. (2004). *Frames of mind: The theory of multiple intelligences* (Twentieth anniversary ed.). New York: Basic Books.

Gibson, D., Velde, B., Hoff, T., Kvashay, D., Manross, P. L., & Moreau, V. (2000). Clinical reasoning of a novice versus an experienced occupational therapist: A qualitative study. *Occupational Therapy in Health Care*, 12, 15–31.

Hagedorn, R. (1997). *Foundations for practice in occupational therapy* (2nd ed.). London: Churchill Livingstone.

Harris, D. L. (2005). *Therapist's sensory processing and its influence upon occupational therapy interventions in children with autism.* Unpublished manuscript, Brenau University at Gainesville, GA.

Higgs, J. & Jones, M. (Eds) (2000). *Clinical Reasoning in the Health Professions* (2nd Ed.). Oxford: Butterworth Heineman.

Holm, M. B. (2000). Our mandate for the new millennium: Evidence-based practice. *American Journal of Occupational Therapy*, 54, 575–585.

Hooper, B. (1997). The relationship between pretheoretical assumptions and clinical reasoning. *American Journal of Occupational Therapy*, 51(5), 328–338.

Jeffs, T. & Smith, M. K. (2005). *Informal education: Conversation, democracy and learning.* Nottingham: Educational Heretics Press.

Kerlinger, F.N. (1973). *Foundations of behavioural research* (2nd ed.). New York: holt, Rinehart & Winston.

Kielhofner, G. (2005). *Conceptual foundations of occupational therapy* (3rd ed.). Philadelphia: F. A. Davis.

Lave, J. &, Wenger, E. (1991). *Situated learning: Legitimate peripheral participation.* Cambridge: Cambridge University Press.

Lave, J. (1988). *Cognition in practice: Mind, mathematics and culture in everyday life,* Cambridge: Cambridge University Press.

Lewin, K. (1947). *Principles of topological psychology.* New York: McGraw-Hill.

Lyons, K. D. & Crepeau, E. B. (2001). Case report. The clinical reasoning of an occupational therapy assistant. *American Journal of Occupational Therapy*, 55(5), 577–581.

Mattingly, C. (1991). The narrative nature of clinical reasoning. *American Journal of Occupational Therapy*, 45, 998–1005.

Mattingly, C. & Fleming, M. H. (1994). *Clinical reasoning—forms of inquiry in a therapeutic practice*. Philadelphia: F. A. Davis.

McEneany, J., McKenna, K. & Summerville, P. (2002). Australian occupational therapists working in adult physical dysfunction settings: What treatment media do they use? *Australian Occupational Therapy Journal*, 49(3), 115–127.

Mitcham, M. D. (2003). Integrating theory and practice: Using theory creatively to enhance professional practice. In G. Brown, S. A. Esdaile & S. E. Ryan (Eds.), *Becoming an advanced healthcare practitioner*. New York: Butterworth Heinemann.

Mitchell, R. & Unsworth, C.A. (2005). Clinical reasoning during community health home visits: Expert and novice differences. *British Journal of Occupational Therapy*, 68(5), 215–223.

Moncher, F. J, & Prinz, R. J. Treatment fidelity in outcomes studies. *Clinical Psychology Review*, 11(3), 247–266.

Neistadt, M. E. (1996). Teaching strategies for the development of clinical reasoning. *American Journal of Occupational Therapy*, 52(3), 221–229.

Neistadt, M. E. (1997). Teaching diagnostic reasoning: Using a classroom-as-clinic methodology with videotapes. *American Journal of Occupational Therapy*, 51, 360–368.

Neistadt, M. E. & Atkins A (1996). Analysis of the orthopedic content in an occupational therapy curriculum from a clinical reasoning perspective. *American Journal of Occupational Therapy*, 50(8), 669–675.

Neistadt, M. E. & Cohn, E. S. (1990). Evaluating a Level I Fieldwork model for independent living skills. *American Journal of Occupational Therapy*, 44, 392–399.

Neistadt, M. E. & Smith, R. E. (1997). Teaching diagnostic reasoning: Using a classroom-as-clinic methodology with videotapes. *American Journal of Occupational Therapy*, 51, 360–368.

Neistadt, M. E., Wight, J. & Mulligan, S. E. (1998). Clinical reasoning case studies as teaching tools. *American Journal of Occupational Therapy*, 52, 125–132.

Nixon, J. & Creek, J. (2006). Towards a theory of practice. *British Journal of Occupational Therapy*, 69, 77–80.

Overton, W. F. & Reese, H. W. (1973). Life span development: Methodological implications. In J. R. Nesselroade & H. W. Reese (Eds.), *Life span developmental psychology—methodological Issues*. New York: Academic Press.

Parham, L. D., Cohn, E. S., Spitzer, S., et al. (2007). Fidelity in sensory integration intervention research. *American Journal of Occupational Therapy*, 61, 216–227.

Patel, V. L., & Arocha, J. F. (2000). Methods in the study of clinical reasoning. In J. Higgs & M. Jones (Eds). *Clinical Reasoning in the Health Professions*, (2nd ed, pp 78–91). Oxford: Butterworth Heineman.

Pierce, C. S. (1931–1935). *Collected papers of Charles Sanders Pierce* (vols. 1–6). In C. Hartshorne & D. Weiss (Eds.). Cambridge, MA: Harvard University Press.

Polyani, M. (1966). The Tacit Dimension. New York: Anchor Books.

Reed, K. L. (1984). *Models of practice in occupational therapy*. Baltimore: Williams & Wilkins.

Robertson, A. E. (1996). Approaches to reasoning in occupational therapy: A critical exploration. *British Journal of Occupational Therapy*, 59, 233–236.

Rogers, J. C. (1983). Clinical reasoning: The ethics, science, and art. *American Journal of Occupational Therapy*, 37, 601–616.

Rogers, J. C. & Holm, M. B. (1991). Occupational therapy diagnostic reasoning: A component of clinical reasoning. *American Journal of Occupational Therapy*, 45, 1045–1053.

Rogers, J. C. & Masagatani, G. (1982). Clinical reasoning of occupational therapists during initial assessment of physically disabled patients. *Occupational Therapy Journal of Research*, 2, 195–219.

Ryan, S. (1998). Influences that shape our reasoning. In J. Creek (Ed.). *Occupational therapy: New perspectives*. London: Whurr.

Sackett D. L., Straus S. E., Richardson W. S., Rosenberg W., & Haynes R. B. (2000). *Evidence-based medicine: How to practice and teach* (2nd ed.). Toronto: Churchill Livingstone.

Schell, B. & Braveman, B. (2006). Turning theory into practice: Managerial strategies. In B. Bravemen (Ed.), *Leading and managing occupational therapy services: An evidence-based approach* (pp. 245–271). Philadelphia: F. A. Davis.

Schell, B. A. & Cervero, R. M. (1993). Clinical reasoning in occupational therapy: An integrative review. *American Journal of Occupational Therapy*, 47, 605–610.

Schell, B. A. B. (1994). *The effect of practice context on occupational therapy practitioner's clinical reasoning*. (Doctoral dissertation, University of Georgia, 1994). *Dissertation Abstracts International*.

Schell, B. A. B.(2002) Occupational Therapy Intervention Scale, panel presentation. B. Hooper, R. Farber & B. Schell: *Emerging concepts in clinical reasoning: Implications for teaching and research,* World Federation of Occupational Therapy, Stockholm, Sweden.

Schell, J. W. (2001*) Contextual teaching and learning.* Retrieved May 15, 2006 from University of Georgia College of Education web site: www.coe.uga.edu/ctl/theory

Schön, D. A. (1983). *The reflective practitioner: How professionals think in action.* New York: Basic Books.

Schön, D. A. (1988). *Educating the reflective practitioner.* San Francisco: Jossey-Bass.

Sladyk, K. & Sheckley, B. (1999). Differences between clinical reasoning gainers and decliners during fieldwork. In P. A. Crist (Ed.), *Innovations in occupational therapy education 1999* (pp. 157–170). Bethesda, MD: American Occupational Therapy Association.

Strong, J., Gilbert, J., Cassidy, S. & Bennett, S. (1995). Expert clinicians' and students' views on clinical reasoning in occupational therapy. *British Journal of Occupational Therapy, 58,* 119–123.

Taylor, C. M. *Evidence-based practice for occupational therapists* 2000. Oxford: Blackwell Science.

Thomas, R. M. (1979). *Comparing theories of child development.* Belmont, CA: Wadsworth.

Tickle-Degnen L. (2000). Gathering current evidence to enhance clinical reasoning. *American Journal of Occupational Therapy, 54*(1), 102–105.

Törnebohm, H. (1991). What is worth knowing in occupational therapy? *American Journal of Occupational Therapy, 45,* 451–454.

Unsworth, C. A. (2001). Clinical reasoning of novice and expert occupational therapists. *Scandinavian Journal of Occupational Therapy, 8,* 163–173.

Unsworth, C. A. (2004). Clinical reasoning: How do worldview, pragmatic reasoning and client-centredness fit? *British Journal of Occupational Therapy, 67,* 10–19.

Unsworth, C. A. (2005). Using head-mounted video camera to confirm and expand knowledge of clinical reasoning in occupational therapy. *American Journal of Occupational Therapy, 59,* 31–40.

Unsworth, C. A. & Schell, B. A. (2006). Clinical reasoning: Development of a theory-in-use. *Proceedings of the 14th International Congress of the World Federation of Occupational Therapists. Sydney, 24-28th July. Sydney Convention Centre.*

van-Ryn, M. & Burke, J. (2000). The effect of patient race and socio-economic status on physician's perceptions of patients. *Social Science and Medicine, 50,* 813–828.

Vygotsky, L. S. (1978). *Mind in society.* Cambridge, MA: Harvard University Press.

Walker, K. F. & Ludwig, F. M. (2004). *Perspectives on theory for the practice of occupational therapy,* (3rd ed.). Austin, Texas: Pro-ed.

Wenger, E. (1998). *Communities of practice.* Cambridge, U.K.: Cambridge University Press.

Williams, M. (1998). Critical thinking as an outcome of nursing education. What is it? Why is it important to nursing practice? *Journal of Advanced Nursing, 28,* 323–331.

Wolters, A. M. (1989). On the idea of worldview and its relationship to philosophy. In P. A. Marshall, S. Griffioen & R. Mouw (Eds.), *Stained glass: Worldviews and social science* (pp. 14–26). New York: University Press of America.

Young, M. E. & Quinn, E. (1992). *Theories and principles of occupational therapy.* London: Churchill Livingstone.

Bibliography of Clinical and Professional Reasoning

Compiled by Barbara A. Boyt Schell and Barbara Hooper

This compilation of research and scholarly work related to clinical and professional reasoning is included as a resource for our readers. This list includes materials from within occupational therapy, as well as references from a number of other disciplines. These research and scholarly works draw upon a wide variety of interdisciplinary sources for their conceptual foundations and frameworks, which constitute another important category of resources for the scholar of clinical and professional reasoning. Readers are encouraged to consult the reference lists within each of the works cited here in order to follow the trail of knowledge development.

This bibliography is divided into several categories:

- Empirical studies focused on occupational therapy clinical and professional reasoning
- Other scholarly literature about reasoning in occupational therapy
- Selected empirical studies about clinical and professional reasoning from other disciplines
- Empirical studies in occupational therapy clinical reasoning education
- Other scholarly literature on occupational therapy education related to clinical and professional reasoning
- Other scholarly literature about clinical and professional reasoning in other disciplines

We attempted to include all research within occupational therapy that focuses directly on clinical and/or professional reasoning and that is published in English. Similarly, we attempted to be comprehensive in our listing of educational research directly focused on clinical and/professional reasoning within the field. Beyond that, we do not claim to be inclusive, but did attempt to reflect major work that we feel contributes to theoretical understanding. Because one can make the case that almost all education is relevant to clinical and professional reasoning, our listings reflect those references that included key words such as clinical reasoning, problem solving and the like in the titles or key words. A silent partner over many years in developing and maintaining this bibliography is Mary Binderman, the inestimable librarian at the American Occupational Therapy Foundation, to whom we are most grateful.

EMPIRICAL STUDIES FOCUSED ON OCCUPATIONAL THERAPY CLINICAL AND PROFESSIONAL REASONING

Alnervik A. & Sviden, G. (1996). On clinical reasoning: Patterns of reflection on practice. *Occupational Therapy Journal of Research*, 16(2), 98–110.

Barrett, L., Beer, D. & Kielhofner, G. (1999). The importance of volitional narrative in treatment: An ethnographic case study in a work program. *Work*, 12, 79–92.

Barris, R. (1987). Clinical reasoning in psychosocial occupational therapy: The evaluation process. *Occupational Therapy Journal of Research*, 7, 147–162.

Burke, J. P. (1997). Frames of meaning: An analysis of occupational therapy evaluations of young children. *Dissertation Abstracts International*, 58(03), 644 (UMI Number: 9727199).

Burke, J. P. (2001). How therapists' conceptual perspectives influence early intervention evaluations. *Scandinavian Journal of Occupational Therapy*, 8, 49–61.

Clark, F. (1993). Occupation embedded in real life: Interweaving occupational science and occupational therapy. *American Journal of Occupational Therapy*, 47, 1067–1078.

Creighton, C., Dijkers, M., Bennett, N. & Brown, K. (1995). Reasoning and the art of therapy for spinal cord injury. *American Journal of Occupational Therapy*, 49, 311–317.

Crepeau, E. B. (1991). Achieving intersubjective understanding: Examples form an occupational therapy treatment session. *American Journal of Occupational Therapy*, 44, 1016–1024.

Crepeau, E. B. (1994). Three images of interdisciplinary team meetings. *American Journal of Occupational Therapy*, 48, 717–722.

Doumanov, P. & Rugg, S. (2003). Clinical reasoning skills of occupational therapists and support staff: A comparison. *International Journal of Therapy and Rehabilitation*, 10(5), 195–203.

Drake, V. & Truital, V. (1997). Clarifying ambiguity in problem fieldwork placements: Picking up and dealing with problem signals. *Australian Occupational Therapy Journal*, 44, 62–70.

Dysart, A. M. & Tomlin, G. S. (2002). Factors related to evidence-based practice among U.S. occupational therapy clinicians. *American Journal of Occupational Therapy*, 56, 275–284.

Fleming, M. H. (1991a). The therapist with the three-track mind. *American Journal of Occupational Therapy*, 45, 1007–1014.

Fleming, M. H. (1991b). Clinical reasoning in medicine compared with clinical reasoning in occupational therapy. *American Journal of Occupational Therapy*, 45, 988–995.

Fondiller, E. D., Rosage, L. J. & Neuhaus, B. E. (1990). Values influencing clinical reasoning in occupational therapy: An exploratory study. *Occupational Therapy Journal of Research*, 10, 41–55.

Gibson, D., Velde, B., Hoff, T., Kvashay, D., Manross, P. L. & Moreau, V. (2000). Clinical reasoning of a novice versus an experienced occupational therapist: A qualitative study. *Occupational Therapy in Health Care*, 12(4), 15–31.

Hansen, R. A. (1984). *Moral reasoning of occupational therapists: Implications for education and practice*. Doctoral dissertation. Detroit: Wayne State University.

Harris, D. L.(1995). *Therapist's sensory processing and its influence upon occupational therapy interventions in children with autism*. Manuscript in preparation.

Hooper, B. (1997). The relationship between pre-theoretical assumptions and clinical reasoning. *American Journal of Occupational Therapy*, 51, 328–338.

Humbert, T. K. (2004). *The use of clinical reasoning skills by experienced occupational therapy assistants*. Unpublished doctoral dissertation, Pennsylvania State University. DAI-A 65/07. AAT 3140036.

Kanny, E. M. (1996). Occupational therapists' ethical reasoning: Assessing student and practitioner responses to ethical dilemmas. (Doctoral dissertation, University of Washington, 1996). University Microfilms, 1490 Eisenhower Place, P.O. Box 975, Ann Arbor, MI 48106.

Katzman, L. N. (1993). Linking patient and family stories to caregivers' use of clinical reasoning. *American Journal of Occupational Therapy*, 47, 169–173.

Kouloumpi, M., Ryan, S. & Savaris, I. (2002). From psychiatric asylum to mental health hospitals: Clinical reasoning in transition. (2002). Paper presented at the meeting of the World Federation of Occupational Therapy Stockholm, Sweden.

Lyons, K. D. & Crepeau, E. B. (2001 Sep-Oct). Case report. The clinical reasoning of an occupational therapy assistant. *American Journal of Occupational Therapy*, 55(5), 577–581.

Mattingly, C. (1998). *Healing dramas and clinical plots: The narrative structure of experience*. New York: Cambridge University Press.

Mattingly, C. (1991a). What is clinical reasoning? *American Journal of Occupational Therapy*, 45, 979–986.

Mattingly, C. (1991b). The narrative nature of clinical reasoning. *American Journal of Occupational Therapy*, 45, 998–1005.

Mattingly, C. & Fleming, M. H. (1994). *Clinical reasoning-forms of inquiry in a therapeutic practice*. Philadelphia: F. A. Davis.

McKay, E. A. & Ryan, S. (1995). Clinical reasoning through story telling: Examining a student's case story on a fieldwork placement. *British Journal of Occupational Therapy*, 58, 234–238.

Mekkes, M. P. (2003). *The influence of occupational therapist's worldview on clinical reasoning: A Qualitative study*. Unpublished thesis, Grand Valley State University, Grand Rapids, MI. AAT 1413315.

Mew, M. M. & Fossey, E. (1996). Client-centred aspects of clinical reasoning during an initial assessment using the Canadian Occupational Performance Measure. *Australian Occupational Therapy Journal*, 43(3/4), 155–166.

Mitchell R. & Unsworth, C. A. (2005). Clinical reasoning during community health home visits: Expert and novice differences. *British Journal of Occupational Therapy*, 68(5), 215–223.

Mitchell, R. & Unsworth, C. A. (2004). Role perceptions and clinical reasoning of community health occupational therapists undertaking home visits. *Australian Occupational Therapy Journal*, 51(1), 13–24.

Munroe, H. (1996). Clinical reasoning in community occupational therapy. *British Journal of Occupational Therapy*, 59(5), 196–202.

Pace, J., Vernon, D. & Yenny, C. (2000). *Understanding clinical reasoning and clinical actions through the exploration of therapists' assumptions*. Unpublished Master's research project, University of North Carolina, Chapel Hill.

Roberts, A. E. (1996). Clinical reasoning in occupational therapy: Idiosyncrasies in content and process. *British Journal of Occupational Therapy*, 59, 372–376.

Robertson, A. E. (1996). Approaches to reasoning in occupational therapy: A critical exploration. *British Journal of Occupational Therapy*, 59, 233–236.

Robertson, L. J. (1996). Clinical reasoning, part 2: Novice/expert differences. *British Journal of Occupational Therapy*, 59, 212–216.

Rogers, J. C. & Holm, M. B. (1991). Occupational therapy diagnostic reasoning: A component of clinical reasoning. *American Journal of Occupational Therapy*, 45 (11), 1045–1053.

Rogers, J. C. & Masagatani, G. (1982). Clinical reasoning of occupational therapists during initial assessment of physically disabled patients. *Occupational Therapy Journal of Research*, 2, 195–219.

Ryan, S. E. (1999). How are narratives being used? In S. E. Ryan & E. A. McKay (Eds.). *Thinking and reasoning in therapy: Narratives from practice* (pp. 1–15). Cheltenham, England: Stanley Thornes (Publishers) Ltd.

Schell, B. A. B. (1994). The effect of practice context on occupational therapy practitioner's clinical reasoning (Doctoral dissertation, University of Georgia, 1994). *Dissertation Abstracts International*.

Scheirton, L., Mu, K. & Lohman, H. (2003). Occupational therapists' responses to practice errors in physical rehabilitation settings. *American Journal of Occupational Therapy*, 57, 307–314.

Slater, D. Y. & Cohn, E. S. (1991). Staff development through analysis of practice. *American Journal of Occupational Therapy*, 45, 1038–1044.

Strong, J., Gilbert, J., Cassidy, S. & Bennett, S. (1995). Expert clinicians and student views on clinical reasoning in occupational therapy. *British Journal of Occupational Therapy*, 58, 119–123.

Svidén, G. & Hallin, M. (1999). Differences in clinical reasoning between occupational therapists working in rheumatology and neurology. *Scandinavian Journal of Occupational Therapy*, 6(2), 63–69.

Svidén, G. & Söljö, R. (1993). Perceiving patients and their nonverbal reactions. *American Journal of Occupational Therapy*, 47, 491–497.

Trigillo, J .T. (2003) *Variations in clinical reasoning among occupational therapy practitioners*. Dissertation Abstracts International-A 64/01, Publication Number AAT 3076538, Obtained from http://proquest.umi.com 1/13/2006.

Unsworth, C. A. (2001). The clinical reasoning of novice and expert occupational therapists. *Scandinavian Journal of Occupational Therapy*, 8, 163–173.

Unsworth, C. A. (2004). How do pragmatic reasoning, worldview and client-centredness fit? *British Journal of Occupational Therapy*, 67(1), 10–19.

Unsworth, C. A. (2005). Using a head-mounted video camera to explore current conceptualizations of clinical reasoning in occupational therapy. *American Journal of Occupational Therapy*, 59, 31–40.

Ward, J. D. (2003). The nature of clinical reasoning with groups: A phenomenological study of an occupational therapist in community mental health. *American Journal of Occupational Therapy*, 57, 625–634.

OTHER SCHOLARLY LITERATURE ABOUT REASONING IN OCCUPATIONAL THERAPY

Chapparo, C. & Ranka, J. (2000). Clinical reasoning in occupational therapy. In J. Higgs & M. Jones (Eds.). *Clinical reasoning in the health professions* (pp. 128–127). Oxford: Butterworth Heineman.

Clark, F., Ennevor, B. L., Richardson, P. L. (1996). A grounded theory of techniques for occupational storytelling and occupational story making. In R. Zemke & F. Clark (Eds.). *Occupational science: The evolving discipline* (pp. 373–392). Philadelphia: F. A. Davis.

Crabtree, M. (1998). Images of reasoning: A literature review. *Australian Occupational Therapy Journal*, 45, 113–123.

Cohn, E. S. (1991). Clinical reasoning: Explicating complexity. *American Journal of Occupational Therapy*, 45(11), 969–971.

Dunn, W. (2000). Clinical reasoning for best practice services for children and families. In W. Dunn (Ed.). *Best practice occupational therapy: In community service with children and families* (pp. 19–25). Thorofare, NJ: SLACK.

Gillette, N. P. & Mattingly, C. (1987). Clinical reasoning in occupational therapy. *American Journal of Occupational Therapy*, 41(6), 399–400.

Hall, L., Robertson, W. & Turner, M. A. (1992). Clinical reasoning process for service provision in the public school. *American Journal of Occupational Therapy*, 46, 927–936.

Harries, P. A. & Harries, C. (2001). Studying clinical reasoning, part 2: Applying social judgement theory. *British Journal of Occupational Therapy*, 64(6), 285–292.

Harries, P. A. & Harries, C. Studying clinical reasoning, part 1: Have we been taking the wrong 'track'? *British Journal of Occupational Therapy*, 64(4), 164–168.

Holm, M. B. & Rogers, J. C. (1989). The therapist's thinking behind functional assessment: Part II. In C. Royeen (Ed.). *Assessment of function: An action guide*. Rockville, MD: American Occupational Therapy Association.

Horowitz, B. P. (2002). Ethical decision-making challenges in clinical practice. *Occupational Therapy in Health Care*, 16 (4), 1–13.

Howard, B. S. (1991). How high do we jump? The effect of reimbursement on occupational therapy. *American Journal of Occupational Therapy*, 45, 875–881.

Kanny, E. M. & Kyler, P. L. (1999). Are faculty prepared to address ethical issues in education? *American Journal of Occupational Therapy*, 53(1), 72–74.

Kyler, P. (1998, April 2). The merger of clinical and ethical competence. *OT Week*, 12, 22–23.

Leicht, S. B. & Dickerson, A. (2001). Clinical reasoning, looking back. *Occupational Therapy in Health Care*, 14(3/4), 105–130.

Mattingly, C. & Gillette, N. (1991). Anthropology, occupational therapy and action research. *American Journal of Occupational Therapy*, 45, 972–978.

Neuhaus, B. E. (1988). Ethical considerations in clinical reasoning: The impact of technology and cost containment. *American Journal of Occupational Therapy*, 42, 288–294.

Opacich, K. J. (1997). Moral tensions and obligations of occupational therapy practitioners providing home care. *American Journal of Occupational Therapy*, 51, 430–435.

Opacich, K. J. (2003). Ethical dimensions of occupational therapy management. In McCormack, Jaffe, Goodman-Lavey (Eds). *The occupational therapy manager*. Rockville, MD: American Occupational Therapy Association.

Parham, D. (1987). Nationally speaking—toward professionalism: The reflective therapist. *American Journal of Occupational Therapy*, 41, 555–561.

Pelland, M. J. (1987). A conceptual model for the instruction and supervision of treatment planning. *American Journal of Occupational Therapy*, 41, 351–359.

Peloquin, S. M. (1993). The depersonalization of patients: A profile gleaned from narratives. *American Journal of Occupational Therapy*, 49, 830–837.

Peloquin, S. (1990). The patient-therapist relationship in occupational therapy: Understanding visions and images. *American Journal of Occupational Therapy*, 44(1), 13–21.

Peloquin, S. (1993). The patient-therapist relationship: Beliefs that shape care. *American Journal of Occupational Therapy*, 47(10), 935–942.

Purtilo, R. B. (1993). *Ethical dimensions in the health professions* (2nd ed). Philadelphia: W. B. Saunders.

Purtilo, R. B., Jensen, G. M. & Brasic Royeen, C. (Eds.) (2005). *Educating for moral action: A sourcebook in health and rehabilitation ethics*. Philadelphia: F. A. Davis.

Rogers, J. C. (1983). Clinical reasoning: The ethics, science, and art. *American Journal of Occupational Therapy*, 37, 601–616.

Rogers, J. C. & Holm, M. B. (1989). The therapist's thinking behind functional assessment: Part I. In C. Royeen (Ed.). *Assessment of function: An action guide*. Rockville, MD: American Occupational Therapy Association.

Rogers, J. C. & Holm, M. B. (1997). Diagnostic reasoning: The process of problem identification. In C. H. Christiansen & C. M. Baum (Eds.). *Occupational therapy: Enabling function and well-being* (2nd ed, pp. 137–156). Thorofare, NJ: Slack.

Rogers, J. C. (1986). Clinical judgement: The bridge between theory and practice. In American Occupational Therapy Association (Ed.), *Target 2000: Occupational therapy education* [Proceedings]. Rockville, MD: Author.

Rosa, S. A. & Hasselkus, B. R. (1996). Connecting with patients: The personal experience of professional helping. *Occupational Therapy Journal of Research, 16*(4), 245–260.

Ryan, S. E. & McKay, E. A (Eds.) (1999). *Thinking and reasoning in practice*. Cheltenham, England: Stanley Thornes (Publishers) Ltd.

Schell, B. (2003). Clinical reasoning and occupation-based practice: Changing habits. *OT Practice, 8*(18), Suppl. CE-1–CE-8.

Schell, B. (2003). *Clinical reasoning: The basis of practice*. In Crepeau, B., Cohn, E. & Schell, B. A. B. *Willard & Spackman's occupational therapy*. Philadelphia: Lippincott Williams & Wilkins.

Schell, B. A. & Cervero, R. M. (1993). Clinical reasoning in occupational therapy: An integrative review. *American Journal of Occupational Therapy, 47*, 605–610.

Schwartz, K. B. (1991). Clinical reasoning and new ideas on intelligence: Implications for teaching and learning. *American Journal of Occupational Therapy, 45*(11), 1033–1037.

Slater, D. Y. (September 6, 2004). Legal and ethical practice: A professional responsibility. *OT Practice*, 1–4.

Sinclair, K. (2004). Focus on research . . . A model for the development of clinical reasoning in occupational therapy. *British Journal of Occupational Therapy, 67*(10), 456.

Sinclair, K. (2003) *A model for the development of clinical reasoning in occupational therapy*. Unpublished doctoral dissertation. Hong Kong Polytechnic (People's Republic of China), DAI-A 64/10. AAT 3107452.

Tickle-Degnen, L. (2000). Evidence-based practice forum—gathering current research evidence to enhance clinical reasoning. *American Journal of Occupational Therapy, 54*, 102–105.

Tickle-Degnen, L. (1998). Using research evidence in planning treatment for the individual client. *Canadian Journal of Occupational Therapy, 65*, 152–159.

Tona, J. T. (2003). *Variations in clinical reasoning among occupational therapy practitioners*. Unpublished doctoral dissertation. State University of New York at Buffalo. DAI-A 64/01. AAT 3076538.

Tornebohm, H. (1991). What is worth knowing in occupational therapy? *American Journal of Occupational Therapy, 45*, 451–454.

Unsworth, C. (1999). *Clinical reasoning in occupational therapy*. In Unsworth, C. (Ed) *Cognitive and perceptual dysfunction: A clinical reasoning approach to evaluation and intervention* (pp. 43–73). Philadelphia: F. A. Davis.

SELECTED EMPIRICAL STUDIES ABOUT CLINICAL AND PROFESSIONAL REASONING FROM OTHER DISCIPLINES

Arling, M. (1998). Supervision in psychotherapy: An educational experiment in integrative metalearning. *Transactional Analysis Journal, 28*(3), 224–233.

Baab, D. A. & Bebeau, M. J. (1990). The effect of instruction on ethical sensitivity. *Journal of Dental Education, 54*(1), 44.

Benner, P. (1984). *From novice to expert: Excellence and power in clinical nursing practice*. Menlo Park, CA: Addison-Wesley Publishing Company.

Benner, P., Hooper-Kyriakidis, P., Stannard, D. (1999). *Clinical wisdom and interventions in critical care: A thinking-in-action approach*. Philadelphia: W. B. Saunders.

Benner, P. & Tanner, C. (1987). Clinical judgement: How expert nurses use intuition. *American Journal of Nursing, 87*(1), 23–31.

Biggs, D. A. & Barnett, R. (1981). *Moral judgment development of college students. Research in Higher Education, 14*(2), 91–102.

Biklen, D. (1988). The myth of clinical judgment. *Journal of Social Issues, 44*, 127–140.

Carr, S. M. (2004). A framework for understanding clinical reasoning in community nursing. *Journal of Clinical Nursing, 13*(7), 850–857.

Claessen, J. (2004). A 2:1 clinical practicum, incorporating reciprocal peer coaching, clinical reasoning, and self-and-peer evaluation. *Journal of Speech Language Pathology & Audiology, 28*(4), 156–165.

Dierf, K. (2004). Ethical decision-making by students in physical and occupational therapy. *Journal of Allied Health, 33*(1), 24–30.

Doody, C. & McAteer, M. (2002). Clinical reasoning of expert and novice physiotherapists in an outpatient orthopaedic setting. *Physiotherapy, 88*(5), 258–268.

Edwards I, Jones M, Carr J, Braunack-Mayer A, Jensen, G. M. (2004). Clinical reasoning strategies in physical therapy. *Physical Therapy, 84*(4), 312–335.

Elio, R. (2002). Issues in commonsense reasoning and rationality. In R. Elio (Ed.). *Common sense, reasoning, and rationality* (pp. 3–36). New York: Oxford University Press.

Elstein, A. S., Shulman, L. S. & Sprafka, S. A. (1978). *Medical problem-solving: An analysis of clinical reasoning.* Cambridge, MA: Harvard University Press.

Embrey, D. G., Guthrie, M. R., White, O. R. & Dietz, J. (1996). Clinical decision making by experienced and inexperienced pediatric physical therapists for children with diplegic cerebral palsy. *Physical Therapy, 76*, 20–33.

Ericcson, K. A. (1998). The scientific study of expert levels of performance: General implications for optimal learning and creativity. *High Ability Studies, 9*, 75–100.

Hutchinson S. L., LeBlanc, A., Booth, R. (2002). "Perpetual problem-solving": An ethnographic study of clinical reasoning in a therapeutic recreation setting. *Therapeutic Recreation Journal, 36*(1), 18–34.

James, G. (2001). Clinical reasoning in novices: Refining a research question. *British Journal of Therapeutic Rehabilitation, 8*(8), 286–293.

Joseph, G. M. & Patel, V. L. (1990). Domain knowledge and hypothesis generation in diagnostic reasoning. *Journal of Medical Decision Making, 10*, 31–46.

Katzman, E. M. (1989). Nurses' and physicians' perceptions of nursing authority. *Journal of Professional Nursing, 5*, 208–214.

Kautz, D. D., Kuiper, R., Pesut, D. J., Knight-Brown, P., Daneker, D (2005). Promoting clinical reasoning in undergraduate nursing students: Application and evaluation of the Outcome Present State Test (OPT) model of clinical reasoning. *International Journal of Nursing Education Scholarship, 2*(1), 21.

Khanyile, T., Mfidi, F. (2005). The effect of curricula approaches to the development of the student's clinical reasoning ability. *Curationis, 28*(2), 70–76.

Ladyshewsky, R. K. (2002). A quasi-experimental study of the differences in performance and clinical reasoning using individual learning versus reciprocal peer coaching. *Physiotherapy Theory and Practice, 18*(1), 17–31.

McCarthy, M. C. (2003a). Detecting acute confusion in older adults: Comparing clinical reasoning of nurses working in acute, long-term, and community health care environments. *Research in Nursing Health, 26*(3), 203–212.

Murphy, J. I. (2004). Using focused reflection and articulation to promote clinical reasoning: An evidence-based teaching strategy. *Nursing Education Perspectives, 25*(5), 226–231.

O'Neill, E. S., Dluhy N. M., Chin, E. (2005). Modelling novice clinical reasoning for a computerized decision support system. *Journal of Advanced Nursing Research, 49*(1), 68–77.

Schmidt, H. G. & Baoshuizen, P. A. (1993). On acquiring expertise in medicine. *Educational Psychology Review, 5*(3), 205–221.

Simmons, B., Lanuza, D., Fonteyn, M., Hicks, F., Holm, K. (2003). Clinical reasoning in experienced nurses. *Western Journal of Nursing Research, 25*(6), 701–724.

Spake, E. F. (2003). *Clinical reasoning and decision making of experienced clinicians and entry-level physical therapist students.* Unpublished doctoral dissertation. University of Kansas. DAI-B 64/09. AAT 3106468.

Wise, D. (2000). How practicing physical therapists identify and resolve ethical dilemmas. Doctoral dissertation, Capella University.

EMPIRICAL STUDIES IN OCCUPATIONAL THERAPY CLINICAL REASONING EDUCATION

Ainsworth, E. (2004). *Occupational therapy clinical educators' perceptions of the development of clinical reasoning of their students: A contextual perspective.* Unpublished doctoral dissertation. Pennsylvania State University, DAI-B 65/09, AAT 3147572.

Christie, B. A., Joyce, P. C. & Moeller, P. L. (1985a). Fieldwork experience, Part I: Impact on practice preference. *American Journal of Occupational Therapy, 39*(10), 671–674.

Christie, B. A., Joyce, P. C. & Moeller, P. L. (1985b). Fieldwork experience, Part II: The supervisor's dilemma. *American Journal of Occupational Therapy, 39*(10), 675–681.

Coates, G. & Crist P. A. (2004). Brief or new: Professional development of fieldwork students: Occupational adaptation, clinical reasoning, and client-centeredness. *Occupational Therapy in Health Care,* 18(1/2), 39–47.

Farber, R. S. & Koenig, K. (1999). Examination of fieldwork educators' responses to challenging fieldwork situations. *Innovations in Occupational Therapy Education,* 89–104.

Hammel, J., Royeen, C. B., Bagatell, N., Chandler, B., Jensen, G., Loveland, J. & Stone, G. (1999). Student perspectives on problem-based learning in an occupational therapy curriculum: A multiyear qualitative evaluation. *American Journal of Occupational Therapy,* 53, 199–206.

Hummel, J. (1997) Effective fieldwork supervision: Occupational therapy student perspective. *Australian Occupational Therapy Journal,* 4, 147–157.

Lysaght, R. & Bent M. (2005). A comparative analysis of case presentation modalities used in clinical reasoning coursework in occupational therapy. *American Journal of Occupational Therapy,* 59(3), 314–324.

McCannon, R., Robertson D., Caldwell, J., Juwah, C., Elfessi, A. (2004). Comparison of clinical reasoning skills in occupational therapy students in the USA and Scotland. *Occupational Therapy International,* 11(3), 160–176.

McCarron, K. A. D'Amico F (2002). The impact of problem-based learning on clinical reasoning in occupational therapy education. *Occupational Therapy in Health Care,* 16(1), 1–13.

Martin, M. (1996). How reflective is student supervision? A study of supervision in action. *British Journal of Occupational Therapy,* 59(5), 229–232.

McKay, E. A. & Ryan, S. (1995). Clinical reasoning through story telling: Examining a student's case story on a fieldwork placement. *British Journal of Occupational Therapy,* 58(6), 324–338.

Neistadt, M. E. (1987). Classroom as clinic: A model for teaching clinical reasoning in occupational therapy education. *American Journal of Occupational Therapy,* 41, 631–637.

Neistadt, M. E. (1998). Teaching clinical reasoning as a thinking frame. *American Journal of Occupational Therapy,* 52(3), 221–229.

Neistadt, M. E. (1992). The classroom as clinic: Applications for a method of teaching clinical reasoning. *American Journal of Occupational Therapy,* 46, 814–819.

Neistadt, M. E. (1996). Teaching strategies for the development of clinical reasoning. *American Journal of Occupational Therapy,* 52(3), 221–229.

Neistadt, M. E. (1997). Teaching diagnostic reasoning: Using a classroom-as-clinic methodology with videotapes. *American Journal of Occupational Therapy,* 51, 360–368.

Neistadt, M. E. & Atkins, A (1996). Analysis of the orthopedic content in an occupational therapy curriculum from a clinical reasoning perspective. *American Journal of Occupational Therapy,* 50(8), 669–675.

Neistadt, M. E. & Cohn, E. S. (1990). Evaluating a Level I Fieldwork model for independent living skills. *American Journal of Occupational Therapy,* 44, 392–399.

Neistadt, M. E. & Smith, R. E. (1997). Teaching diagnostic reasoning: Using a classroom-as-clinic methodology with videotapes. *American Journal of Occupational Therapy,* 51, 360–368.

Neistadt, M. E., Wight, J. & Mulligan, S. E. (1998). Clinical reasoning case studies as teaching tools. *American Journal of Occupational Therapy,* 52, 125–132.

Paterson, M. & Adamson, L. (2001). An international study of educational approaches to clinical reasoning. *British Journal of Occupational Therapy,* 64(8), 403–405.

Scaffa, M. E. & Smith, T. M. (2004). Effects of Level II Fieldwork on clinical reasoning in occupational therapy. *Occupational Therapy in Health Care,* 18(1/2), 31–38.

Scaffa, M. E. & Wooster, D. M. (2004). Brief report. Effects of problem-based learning on clinical reasoning in occupational therapy. *American Journal of Occupational Therapy,* 58(3), 333–336.

Sladyk, K. & Sheckley, B. (2000). Clinical reasoning and reflective practice: Implications of fieldwork activities. *Occupational Therapy in Health Care,* 13(1), 11–22.

Sladyk, K. & Sheckley, B. (1999). Differences between clinical reasoning gainers and decliners during fieldwork. In P. A. Crist (Ed.). *Innovations in occupational therapy education, 1999* (pp. 157–170). Bethesda, MD: American Occupational Therapy Association.

Sweeney, G., Webley, P. & Treacher, A. (2001a). Supervision in occupational therapy, Part 1: The supervisor's anxieties. *British Journal of Occupational Therapy,* 64(7), 337–345.

Sweeney, G., Webley, P. & Treacher, A. (2001b). Supervision in occupational therapy, Part 2: The supervisor's dilemma. *British Journal of Occupational Therapy,* 64(8), 380–386.

Sweeney, G., Webley, P. & Treacher, A. (2001c). Supervision in occupational therapy, Part 3: Accommodating the supervisor and the supervisee. *British Journal of Occupational Therapy,* 64(9), 426–443.

Tomlin, G. (2005). The use of interactive video client simulation scores to predict clinical performance of occupational therapy students. *American Journal of Occupational Therapy, 59,* 50–56.

Wittman, P. P. (1990). Cognitive developmental level and clinical behaviors in occupational therapy students: An exploratory investigation. (Doctoral Dissertation, North Carolina State University, 1990).

OTHER SCHOLARLY LITERATURE ABOUT OCCUPATIONAL THERAPY EDUCATION RELATED TO CLINICAL AND PROFESSIONAL REASONING

Bailey, D. M. & Cohn E. S. (2001) Understanding others: A course to learn interactive clinical reasoning. *Occupational Therapy in Healthcare, 15*(1/2), 31–46.

Bailey, D. M. & Schwartzberg, S. L. (2003). *Ethical and Legal Dilemmas* (2nd ed). Philadelphia: F. A. Davis.

Barnitt, R. E. (1993). Deeply troubling questions: The teaching of ethics in undergraduate courses. *British Journal of Occupational Therapy, 56,* 401–406.

Brown, G., Esdaile, S. A. & Ryan, S. E. (2003). *Becoming an advanced healthcare practitioner.* Edinburgh: Butterworth-Heinemann.

Buchanan, H., Moore, R. & van Niekerk, L. (1998). The fieldwork case study: Writing for clinical reasoning. *American Journal of Occupational Therapy, 52*(4), 291–295.

Cohn, E. S. (1989). Fieldwork education: Shaping a foundation for clinical reasoning. *American Journal of Occupational Therapy, 43,* 240–244.

Cohn, E. S. & Crist, P. (1995). Nationally speaking- Back to the future: New approaches to fieldwork education. *American Journal of Occupational Therapy, 49*(2), 103–106.

Coppard, B. M., Jensen, G. M. & Custard, C. L. (1997). Teaching reflection: Integrating clinical reasoning with narrative cases. *OT Practice, 2*(12), 30–35.

Cortellini Benamy, B. (1996). *Developing clinical reasoning skills: Strategies for the occupational therapist.* Therapy Skill Builders.

Coster, W. & Schwarz, L. (June, 2004). Facilitating transfer of evidence-based practice into practice. *Education Special Interest Section Quarterly, 14*(2), 1–3.

Crist, P., Wilcox, B. L. & McCarron, K. (1998). Transitional portfolios: Orchestrating our professional competence. *American Journal of Occupational Therapy, 52,* 729–736.

Cubie, S. H. & Kaplan, K. (1982). A case analysis method for the model of human occupation. *American Journal of Occupational Therapy, 36,* 645–656.

Day, D. J. (1973). A systems diagram for teaching treatment planning. *American Journal of Occupational Therapy, 27,* 239–243.

Dutton, R. (1995). *Clinical reasoning in physical disabilities.* Baltimore: Williams & Wilkins.

Greene, D. (1997). The use of service learning in client environments to enhance ethical reasoning in students. *American Journal of Occupational Therapy, 51*(10), 844–852.

Haddad, A. M. (1988). Teaching ethical analysis in occupational therapy. *American Journal of Occupational Therapy, 42,* 300–304.

Hall, L. Robertson, W., Turner, M. A. (1992). Clinical reasoning process for service provision in the public school. *American Journal of Occupational Therapy, 46*(10), 927–936.

Hinojosa, J. & Blount, M.-L. (1998). Nationally speaking: Professional competence. *American Journal of Occupational Therapy, 52,* 765–769.

Hooper, B. & Wood, W. (2002). Pragmatism and structuralism in occupational therapy: The long conversation. *Journal of Occupational Therapy, 56,* 40–50.

Lewin, J. E. & Reed, C. A. (1998). *Creative problem solving in occupational therapy: With stories about children.* Philadelphia: Lippincott Williams & Wilkins.

Nolinske, T. (1999). Resource list for teaching and learning. *American Journal of Occupational Therapy, 53,* 75–82.

Pelland, M. J. (1987). A conceptual model for the instruction and supervision of treatment planning. *American Journal of Occupational Therapy, 41,* 351–359.

Royeen, C. (1995). A problem-based curriculum for occupational therapy education. *American Journal of Occupational Therapy, 49,* 338–346.

Schell, B. A. B (Oct. 6, 2003). Clinical reasoning and occupation-based practice: Changing habits. Continuing Education Article for *Occupational Therapy Practice.*

Schwartzberg, S. L. (2002) *Interactive reasoning in the practice of occupational therapy.* Upper Saddle River, NJ: Prentice Hall.

Stern, P. (2005). Holistic approach to teaching evidence-based practice. *American Journal of Occupational Therapy, 59,* 157–165.

Tickle-Degnen, L. (1999). Organizing, evaluating, and using evidence in occupational therapy practice. *American Journal of Occupational Therapy, 53,* 537–539.

Tickle-Degnen, L. (2000). Gathering current research evidence to enhance clinical reasoning. *American Journal of Occupational Therapy*, 54, 102–105.

Unsworth, C. (1999). *Cognitive and perceptual dysfunction: A clinical reasoning approach to evaluation and intervention*. Philadelphia: F. A. Davis.

VanLeit, B. (1995). Using the case method to develop clinical reasoning skills in problem-based learning. *American Journal of Occupational Therapy*, 49(4), 34953.

Wood, W., Nielson, C., Humphry, R., Coppola, S., Baranek, G. & Rourk, J. (2000). A curricular renaissance: Graduate education centered on occupation. *American Journal of Occupational Therapy*, 54, 586–597.

OTHER SCHOLARLY LITERATURE ABOUT CLINICAL AND PROFESSIONAL REASONING IN OTHER DISCIPLINES

Argyris, C. (1993). *Knowledge for action: A guide to overcoming barriers to organizational change*. San Francisco: Jossey-Bass.

Argyris, C. & Schön, D. A. (1974). *Theory in practice: Increasing professional effectiveness*. San Francisco: Jossey-Bass.

Bebeau, M. J. & Brabeck, M. M. (1987). Integrating care and justice issues in professional moral education: A gender perspective. *Journal of Moral Education*, 16 (3), 189–203.

Boud, D. & Walker, D. (1998). Promoting reflection in professional courses: The challenge of context. *Studies in Higher Education*, 23, 191–206.

Brookfield, S. D. (1991). *Developing critical thinkers: Challenging adults to explore alternative ways of thinking and acting*. San Francisco: Jossey-Bass.

Brown, J. S., Collins, A. & Duguid, P. (1989). Situated cognition and the culture of learning. *Educational Researcher*, 18(1), 32–42.

Bleakley, A., Farrow, R., Gould, D. & Marshall, R. (2003). Making sense of clinical reasoning: Judgement and the evidence of the senses. *Medical Education*, 37, 544–552.

Bruner, J. (1990). *Acts of meaning*. Cambridge, MA: Harvard University Press.

Bruning, R. H., Schraw, G. H. & Ronning, R. R. (1999). *Cognitive psychology and instruction* (3rd ed.). Columbus, OH: Merrill.

Cervero, R. M. (1988). *Effective continuing education for professionals*. San Cervero, R. M., Wilson, A. L. & associates (2001). *Power in practice*. San Francisco: Jossey-Bass.

Chi, M. T. H., Glaser, R. & Farr, M. J. (1988). *The nature of expertise*. Hillsdale, NJ: Erlbaum.

Daloz, L. A. (1986). *Effective teaching and mentoring: Realizing the transformation power of adult learning experiences*. San Francisco: Jossey-Bass.

Dowie, J. & Elstein, A. (Eds.) (1988). *Professional judgment: A reader in decision making*. Cambridge: Cambridge University Press.

Dreyfus, H. L. & Dreyfus, S. E. (1986). *Mind over machine: The power of human intuition and expertise in the era of the computer*. New York: Free Press.

Elstein, A. S., Shulman, L. S. & Sprafka, S. A. (1978). *Medical problem-solving: An analysis of clinical reasoning*. Cambridge, MA: Harvard University Press.

Ericsson, K. A. & Smith, J. (Eds.) (1991). *Toward a general theory of expertise: Prospects and limits*. Cambridge, MA: Cambridge University Press.

Ferrario, C. G. (2004). Developing clinical reasoning strategies: Cognitive shortcuts. *Journal for Nurses in Staff Development*, 20(5), 229–235.

Ferry, N. M. & Ross-Gordon, J. M.(1998). An inquiry into Schön's epistemology of practice: Exploring links between experience.

Fish, D. & Coles, C. (1998). *Developing professional judgement in healthcare: Learning through the critical appreciation of practice*. Edinburgh: Butterworth-Heinemann.

Gambrill, E. (2005). *Critical thinking in clinical practice: Improving the quality of judgments and decisions about clients* (2nd ed.). Hoboken, NJ: John Wiley & Sons.

Gardner, H. (2004). *Frames of mind: The theory of multiple intelligences (Twentieth anniversary ed.)*. New York: Basic Books.

Gladwell, M. (2005). *Blink: The power of thinking without thinking*. New York: Little, Brown & Company.

Gilovich, T. (1991). *How we know what isn't so: The fallibility of human reason in everyday life*. New York: The Free Press.

Greenwood, J. (1998).Theoretical approaches to the study of nurses' clinical reasoning: Getting things clear. *Contemporary Nurse*, 7(3), 110–116.

Higgs, J., Burn, A., Jones M. (2001). Integrating clinical reasoning and evidence-based practice. *AACN Clinical Issues in Adv Pract Acute Critical Care*, 12(4), 482–490.

Higgs, J. & Jones, M. (Ed.). (2002) *Clinical reasoning in the health professions* (2nd ed.). Oxford: Butterworth-Heinemann.

Hunt, E. (1989). Cognitive Science: Definition, status, and questions. *Annual Review of Psychology,* 40, 603–629.

Johnson, M. L. (1999). Embodied reason. In G. Weiss & H. F. Haber (Eds.). *Perspectives on embodiment: The intersections of nature and culture* (pp. 81–102). New York: Routledge.

King, P. M. & Kitchener, K. S. (1994). *Developing reflective judgment.* San Francisco: Jossey-Bass.

Lakoff, G. & Johnson, M. (1999). *Philosophy in the flesh: The embodied mind and its challenge to Western thought.* New York: Basic Books.

Lave, J. (1988). *Cognition in practice: Mind, mathematics and culture in everyday life.* Cambridge: Cambridge University Press.

Lave, J. & Wenger, E. (1991). *Situated learning: Legitimate peripheral participation.* Cambridge: Cambridge University Press.

Mainzer, K. (1997). *Thinking in complexity: The complex dynamics of matter, mind, and mankind.* Berlin: Springer.

Miller, G. A. (1956). The magic number seven, plus or minus two: Some limits on our capacity for processing information. *Psychological Review,* 63, 81–97.

Rest, J. R. (1988b). Why does college promote development in moral judgment? *Journal of Moral Education,* 17(3), 183–194.

Rest, J. R. & Narvaez, D. (Eds.) (1994). *Moral development in the professions.* Hillsdale, NJ: Lawrence Erlbaum Associates.

Schell, J. W. &, Black, R. S. (1997). Situated learning: An inductive case study of a collaborative learning experience. *Journal of Industrial Teacher Education,* 34(4), 5–27.

Spoon, J. & Schell, J. W. (1997). Aligning student learning styles with instructor teaching styles. *Journal of Industrial-Technical Teacher Education,* 35(2), 38.

Schneider, W. & D. F. Bjorklund (1992). Expertise, aptitude, and strategic remembering. *Child Development,* 63, 461–473.

Schön, D. A. (1983). *The reflective practitioner: How professionals think in action.* New York: Basic Books.

Schön, D. A. (1987). *Educating the reflective practitioner.* San Francisco: Jossey-Bass.

Sheets-Johnstone, M. (1992). *Giving the body its due.* Albany: State University of New York Press.

Schmidt, H. G., Norman, G. R. & Boshuizen, H. P. A. (1990). A cognitive perspective on medical expertise: Theory and implications. *Academic Medicine,* 65, 611–621.

Stephenson RC. (2004). Using a complexity model of human behaviour to help interprofessional clinical reasoning. *International Journal of Therapy and Rehabilitation,* 11(4), 168–175.

Tversky, A. & Kahneman, D. (1974). Judgment under uncertainty: Heuristics and biases. *Science,* 125, 1124–1131.

Vygotsky, L. S. (1978). *Mind in society.* Edited and Translated by M. Cole, V. John-Steiner, S. Scribner &, E. Souberman. Cambridge, MA: Harvard University Press.

Weiss, G. & Haber, H. F. (1999). *Perspectives on embodiment: The intersections of nature and culture.* New York: Routledge.

Wenger, E. (1998). *Communities of practice.* Cambridge, UK: Cambridge University Press.

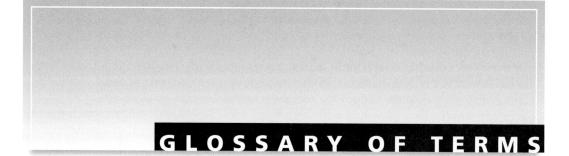

GLOSSARY OF TERMS

John W. Schell and Barbara A. Boyt Schell

The following terms are drawn from the chapters in this book and are intended as a resource to enhance reader understanding. Definitions are based on information provided by chapter authors. Readers should refer to the chapters in which these terms occur to find reference citations and related information. When citing information, readers should cite the chapters in which the terms are used or source material provided in chapter references.

Action research. Research in which the subject is an active participant in the research and therefore may be involved in the research design and data collection, coding and analysis.

Agentic plots. A type of plot classification in which people assume an internalized locus of control and perceive themselves as capable of changing circumstances within their control.

Applied normative ethics. A system of morals with direct applicability to a specified professional area or field. These are the day-to-day deliberations about what is the right thing to do.

Assumption. An understanding or belief that is accepted to be true.

Automaticity. A process of fast and efficient problem solving with little conscious thought.

Autonomy. Ethical principle stating the right to self-determination.

Axiology. The study of values, such as "What is good?" (ethics) and "What is beautiful?" (aesthetics).

Behavioral engineering. An educational philosophy that proposes that (a) people acknowledge supremacy of scientific method; (b) truth is scientifically proved; (c) behaviors are to be controlled; (d) behavior is programmed from birth by culture; (e) learner is conditioned via response to stimuli.

Beneficence. Ethical principle that guides one to act in a way that benefits others, to do good.

Bioethics. A type of normative or applied ethics involving the application of ethical principles to health care delivery.

Chaos narrative. A type of plot classification in which people take a hopeless, despairing stance about the lack of progress and control. Called "anti-narrative" because it lacks plot, narrative sequence, and causal relationships.

Clinical reasoning. The processes used by practitioners to plan, direct, perform, and reflect on client care.

Coda. An optional structural element of a narrative that signals the completion of the narrative by returning the temporal perspective to the present.

Code of Professional Ethics. Formal writings that include rules or principles that apply to a specified group of professionals.

Cognitive apprenticeship. A system of teaching associated with social learning theory and based on four interacting elements: (a) instructional content; (b) instructional methods; (c) instructional sequence; and (d) the sociology of the learning community.

Concurrent report. An approach to eliciting a therapist's clinical reasoning in which the therapist provides his or her reasoning, as it occurs, in relation to a real or simulated client.

Conditional reasoning. A blending of all forms of professional reasoning for the purposes of flexibly responding to changing conditions or predicting possible client futures.

Confidentiality. Ethical principle involving recognition of and respect for the right to privacy.

Constructivism. A view of learning that recognizes the learner's contribution to meaning and learning through individual and/or social activity.

Context (for learning). The social and psychological constructs that the learner brings, including (a) the level of conceptual knowledge; (b) learners' interpretation of instructional goals; and (c) participant roles that the learner brings to bear in the setting.

Cues (in clinical reasoning). Anything in the environment that prompts the therapist to consider a specific diagnosis or client status. A cue can be a smell, information from the client, something the therapist sees or a combination of these.

Deductive reasoning. Using rules of logic with premises to reach irrefutable conclusions.

Diagnostic reasoning. A process of methodical thinking by which problems or needs are detected or inferred.

Dialectical constructivism. A view of knowledge development that proposes that thought and experience are inextricably intertwined with the contexts or settings in which learning occurs.

Disease. An abstract concept of the conditions that cause a pathological state or diagnosis that does not include the person's experience of having the condition.

Embodiment. The appreciation that one's body plays a central role in thinking, and that one's body shapes one's experience of the world.

Empirical. Information or data found in or directly derived from the world of experience.

Endogenous constructivism. Knowledge acquisition that begins with the learner's internal cognition and shapes an understanding of the external environment through that mental lens.

Epistemology. The study of knowledge and the basis for knowing.

Essentialism (realism). An educational philosophy that proposes that (a) people seek essential and universal reality; (b) ultimate good exists—probably unattainable by mortals; (c) truth is absolute even if unknown; (d) education conserves basic principles and values.

Ethical dilemma. A situation in which one moral conviction or action conflicts with another.

Ethical reasoning. Reasoning directed to analyzing an ethical dilemma, generating alternative solutions, and determining actions to be taken. Systematic approach to moral conflict.

Ethnography. The study of groups of people whose beliefs, actions, and artifacts are constructed by the multitude of influences that have shaped their culture.

Evaluation (in narrative). A structural element that gives the narrator's opinion, point of view, or meaning to convey how the narrator wants the listener or reader to interpret the narrative.

Evidence-based practice. Professional actions that reflect the integration of best research evidence with professional expertise and the values of the person/group receiving services.

Existentialism. An educational philosophy which proposes that (a) people must seek their own path; (b) human existence has no universal purpose; (c) humans are free agents to decide for themselves; (d) truth is subjective and open for individual interpretation; (e) education gives courage to seek meaning; (f) there is no promise of external reward.

Exogenous constructivism. A view of knowledge as a true reality that corresponds with the learner's accepted environment. This is consistent with the assumed truth in both essentialist and perennialist philosophic positions—there is little room for truth with shades of gray.

Expertise. The experience and knowledge to work at a high level in a given domain.

Fidelity. An ethical principle guiding one to keep promises and contracts. Also refers to the accurate implementation of assessment and intervention processes in a manner consistent with the guiding theories and procedures.

Generalization. Findings or principles discovered in one setting being applicable to other settings.

Grounded theory. A qualitative research method in which the researcher has no preconceived ideas or theories prior to the study, and the primary goal of analysis is to generate explanatory theories of human behavior.

Habits of expectation. One's assumptions about humans, knowledge, and future, which act to selectively determine the scope of our attention by filtering information and guiding perceptions toward what to notice, what to ignore, what is relevant, and what is irrelevant.

Hypothesis testing. The use of deductive and inductive reasoning to confirm or disconfirm possible explanations of a phenomenon.

Illness. A uniquely personal and subjective perspective of the social, psychological, and occupational experience of having disease or disability.

Illness narrative. A story that shows causal relationships of health, disease, illness, impairment, and disability, and that communicates the experience, alterations, and individual meaning of living life affected by illness or disability.

Inductive reasoning. Use of empirical data and confirming or disconfirming hypotheses to draw conclusions.

Information processing. The organization of our memories and the processes used to learn and use information in those memories.

Interactive reasoning. Thinking directed toward building positive interpersonal relationships with clients, permitting collaborative problem identification and problem solving.

Intrinsicality. The therapist's interior experience that gives meaning to, and guides actions taken within, practice.

Justice. Ethical principle focused on fairness in which actions distribute benefits and harms fairly.

Learning transfer. Use of acquired knowledge across settings. Frequency and reliability of transfer depend on the ability of the individual to interpret the social setting in such a way that enables them to apply and use the knowledge within that setting.

Legitimate peripheral participation. A description of how individuals gain opportunities to use learning as members of a community by having legitimate reasoning for participation and gaining authentic status, thus moving from peripheral to more central roles.

Life story. The uniquely personal account of one's life that interprets and assigns meaning to events, intention, and action in story form, which includes one's perception of self, identity, history, roles, and reality. Serves as a source for making decisions and occupational choices.

Logical or scientific thinking. A mode of thought whose goal is to state consistent truths for defined circumstances by study of empirical, observable facts through procedures and conventions posited by an objective observer. Using carefully defined concepts, scientific thinking starts with generalities and abstractions and narrows and tests to define detailed certainties, which are intended to be generalized within a given set of circumstances.

Logical reasoning. Use of structured rules for drawing inferences that are irrefutable.

Long-term memory. A form of cognition in which memory becomes more compact and streamlined with experience, making retrieval of information into working memory easier and faster.

Metacognition thinking. Processes focused on one's own cognition.

Metaphysics. A branch of philosophy focused on nature of reality and human existence.

Model. A representation of an aspect of reality revealing relationships or processes.

Morals/ethics. The philosophy that deals with systematic approaches to moral conflict. Principles or standards of right and wrong conduct; the ways in which we determine right from wrong so that relations with people can be cooperative and respectful.

Narrative. A cognitive organizational scheme through which the narrator subjectively organizes, shapes, and structures experiences into a coherent whole, which clarifies how each event contributes individually to the whole. Conflict is an inherent factor and narrative's hallmark is a distinct beginning, middle, and end.

Narrative reasoning. The process through which therapists make sense of people's particular circumstances; prospectively imagine the effect of illness, disability, or occupational performance problems on their daily lives; and create a collaborative story that is enacted with clients and families through intervention.

Narrative thinking. A mode of thought dealing in subjective, personalized particulars and specifics of lived experience, human intention, and action that connects events across time and defines possibilities.

Nonmaleficence. An ethical principle that guides one to refrain from inflicting harm, to do no harm.

Novice-to-expert continuum. A stage theory of professional development that describes five stages: (a) novice, (b) advanced beginner, (c) competent, (d) proficient, and (e) expert.

Occupational narrative. A story about occupational experience showing relationships of health and participation, and of illness, disability, or restriction when present; placing occupational performance within specific contexts; and expressing the meaning of specific occupations and the relationships of occupations in one's life.

Occupational storymaking. A collaborative process of prospective narrative reasoning in which people transform their lives by taking occupational narratives in new directions.

Orientation clause. A structural element in narratives that may signal the beginning of a narrative by providing characters, settings, time, and circumstances. May begin the narrative or be interspersed throughout it.

Perceptual filter. A set of assumptions that form the lens or viewpoint through which a therapist interprets practice.

Perennialism (idealism). An educational philosophy that proposes that (a) people seek "ideal" universal order; (b) faith and reason coexist and are mutually supporting; (c) truth is represented by an ideal existence; and (d) past and present exist to achieve divine purpose.

Phenomenology. A qualitative research method in which the focus is on people's lived experience.

Physical resources. The availability or lack of tangible resources such as naturalistic settings, equipment, space, or finances that influence therapist decision making during professional reasoning.

Plot. The pattern of events and circumstances of a narrative or story that links specific events into the whole and suggests relationships, such as cause and effect, between them.

Practice context. The physical and social situation in which therapy occurs.

Practice errors. Empirically discovered mistakes made by professionals in practice.

Pragmatic reasoning. Practical reasoning that is used to attend to the contextual factors that inhibit or facilitate therapy. Attends to fitting therapy possibilities into the current realities of service delivery, such as scheduling options, payment for services, equipment availability, therapists' skills, management directives, and the personal situation of the therapist.

Procedural reasoning. The thinking steps involved in working through the intervention routines for identified conditions.

Professional reasoning. Cognitive processes used to guide professional actions. Includes the actual therapy process, as well as reasoning done by supervisors, fieldwork educators, managers and consultant managers as they conceptualize occupational therapy practice.

Progressive narrative. A type of plot classification in which the person reaches the desired goal characterized by an upward slope of the narrative over time.

Progressivism. An educational philosophy that proposes that (a) people must progress toward better solutions to problems; (b) truth is relative to context; (c) ability to select among options is nurtured; (d) skill in evaluating practical outcomes is critical; (e) democratic society depends on informed participation.

Quest narrative. A type of plot classification in which people accept illness and seek to use it. Characterized by the archetype of the journey, in which illness is viewed as a quest for self-knowledge; often presented in the format of mythological hero's tales.

Reconstructionism. An educational philosophy that proposes (a) that people must participate in achievement of a better society; (b) that truth is relative to context; (c) that education is key to democratic perfection; (d) identification and isolation of those holding power sufficient to deter human progress; (e) that education promotes and protects individual rights and equality; (f) redistribution of power among all social groups.

Regressive narratives. A type of plot classification in which the person is unable to meet goals; characterized by deterioration and a downward slope of the narrative over time.

Restitution narrative. A type of plot classification in which people treat illness as a transitory experience, seek medical cure to curtail the interruption of illness, and seek to regain control of life, body, and occupations.

Retrospective report. An approach to data collection in which the clinician recounts his/her clinical reasoning after it has occurred (preferably immediately).

Scientific inquiry. A disciplined investigation of an empirical question.

Scientific reasoning. A systematic approach that applies logical and scientific method to creating, testing, and using knowledge to make decisions.

Sensibility. The discrimination made about sensory input that informs professional reasoning.

Sensitivity. An awareness or threshold for sensory input that is used for clinical or professional reasoning.

Settings (learning). Physical places or tasks where learning occurs.

Situated cognition. A social view of cognition that describes cognition as a connection between the mind at work and the world in which it is working.

Stable narrative. A type of plot classification in which the person is not progressing toward the goal; characterized by a horizontal slope of the narrative over time.

Statistical reasoning. Using probability and logic under conditions of uncertainty to draw inferences with a quantifiable level of confidence.

Storymaking. A collaborative process through which therapist, client, and family prospectively link the present to the future by imagining the effect of occupational performance problems in scenes of future occupational contexts. The process results in the prospective treatment story through therapeutic emplotment.

Storytelling. An inherently therapeutic process linking past to present that includes the teller's personal interpretation of experience. Throughout the occupational therapy process, storytelling helps reform identity, provides safe re-experiencing of events without consequences, and provides hope.

Syllogism. A scheme of a formal deductive argument with a major and minor premise and a conclusion.

Thick description. A term used to describe data collected in the qualitative research tradition, usually describing the rich and full information provided by the participant or observed by the researcher.

Think aloud. A research technique in which the therapist speaks his/her thoughts as they occur.

Values. Standards or principles that are important/of worth to an individual, society, or profession and that guide actions, e.g., altruism, equality, freedom, human dignity, justice, and truth.

Veracity. Ethical principle focused on being truthful with clients and colleagues.

Victimic plot. A type of plot classification in which people assume an externalized locus of control and perceive themselves as subject to circumstances beyond their control.

Volitional narrative. A type of occupational narrative based on the Model of Human Occupation created by the occupational therapist to express a person's volition (personal causation, interests, and values) and show how volition affects occupational choice and decision making.

Women's ways of knowing. A view of women's knowledge development and use. Progressive divisions included (a) silence; (b) received knowledge; (c) subjective knowledge; (d) procedural knowledge; and (e) constructed knowledge.

Working memory. Also called short-term memory, mediates our perceptions of the world with our memory or knowledge of the world. The primary purpose of working memory is to process, but not store, information.

Zones of proximal development (ZPD). The difference between the level of difficulty that a learner can demonstrate with independence and a level that can be achieved with the help of a facilitating practitioner.

Page numbers in *italics* denote figures; those followed by t denote tables; those followed by b indicate boxed material.